AMTA Monograph Series

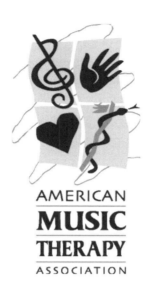

AMERICAN
MUSIC
THERAPY
ASSOCIATION

Effective Clinical Practice in Music Therapy:
Medical Music Therapy for Pediatrics in Hospital Settings

Deanna Hanson-Abromeit, Monograph Editor
Cynthia M. Colwell, Series Editor

The American Music Therapy Association is a non-profit association dedicated to increasing access to quality music therapy services for individuals with disabilities or illnesses or for those who are interested in personal growth and wellness. AMTA provides extensive educational and research information about the music therapy profession. Referrals for qualified music therapists are also provided to consumers and parents. AMTA holds an annual conference every autumn and its seven regions hold conferences every spring.

For up-to-date information, please access the AMTA website at www.musictherapy.org

ISBN: 978-1-884914-22-5

Monograph Editor: **Deanna Hanson-Abromeit**
University of Missouri–Kansas City
Kansas City, Missouri

Series Editor: **Cynthia Colwell**
University of Kansas
Lawrence, Kansas

Copyright Information: **© by American Music Therapy Association, Inc., 2008**
8455 Colesville Road, Suite 1000
Silver Spring, Maryland 20910 USA
www.musictherapy.org
info@musictherapy.org

Technical Assistance: **Wordsetters**
Kalamazoo, Michigan

Cover Design: **Tawna Grasty, Grass T Design**

FSC
Mixed Sources
Product group from well-managed forests, controlled sources and recycled wood or fiber

Cert no. SW-COC-002062
www.fsc.org
© 1996 Forest Stewardship Council

Printed in the United States of America

List of Contributing Authors

Claire M. Ghetti, MME, LCAT, MT-BC, CCLS
    Komansky Center for Children's Health
    New York–Presbyterian Hospital
    Weill Cornell Medical Center

Ann Hannan, MT-BC
    Riley Hospital for Children
    Indianapolis, Indiana

Deanna Hanson-Abromeit, PhD, MT-BC
    Assistant Professor of Music Therapy
    Conservatory of Music and Dance
    University of Missouri–Kansas City

Joanne V. Loewy, DA, MT-BC, LCAT
    Director, The Louis Armstrong Center for Music and Medicine
    Beth Israel Medical Center
    New York, New York

Christine Tuden Neugebauer, MS, MT-BC, LPC
    Child Life Department
    Shriners Hospitals for Children
    Galveston, Texas

Helen Shoemark, PhD, RMT
    Senior Music Therapist for Neonates and Infant Program
    Coordinator, Music Therapy Clinical Research Program
    Royal Children's Hospital
    Melbourne, Australia

Joey Walker, MA, MT-BC
    Iowa City Hospice
    Iowa City, Iowa

Acknowledgments

The editors would like to acknowledge the following individuals with the University of Missouri–Kansas City for their assistance in preparing the manuscript of this monograph.

Jessica Crump
V. Carol Dale
Heather Eakin
Rachel French
Kirsten Meyer

Contents

List of Contributing Authors.. iii

Acknowledgments v

Section I: Music Therapy in Hospital Settings

Chapter 1   Introduction to Pediatric Medical Music Therapy.................................. 3
             Deanna Hanson-Abromeit

Section II: Music Therapy with Pediatric Units

Chapter 2   Newborn Intensive Care Unit (NICU).. 15
             Deanna Hanson-Abromeit
             Helen Shoemark
             Joanne V. Loewy

Chapter 3   Pediatric Intensive Care Unit (PICU) 71
             Claire Ghetti
             Ann Hannan

Chapter 4   General Pediatrics Medical/Surgical... 107
             Ann Hannan

Chapter 5   Hematology, Oncology, and Bone Marrow Transplant....................... 147
             Claire Ghetti
             Joey Walker

Chapter 6   Pediatric Burn Recovery: Acute Care, Rehabilitation.
             and Reconstruction.. 195
             Christine Tuden Neugebauer

Section III: Resources

Glossary of Terms 233
Compiled by Kirsten Meyer

Comprehensive Bibliography 239
Compiled by Kirsten Meyer

Sample Music Therapy Intervention Plans 247

Appendices

    A.   Music Therapy and Medicine 261

    B.   Music Therapy and Pain Management 267

Section I:

Music Therapy in Hospital Settings

CHAPTER 1

Introduction to Pediatric Medical Music Therapy

Deanna Hanson-Abromeit

Music therapy had just finished in the pediatric playroom with the school-age patients. The session had been satisfying for both the patients and the therapist. It had lasted more than an hour. As the patients and their siblings left the playroom, the therapist could hear a child screaming. His voice carried throughout the unit and sounded distressed as he moved from yelling to crying. The therapist continued to clean up and wondered why it seemed like no one was addressing this child's concerns. As she finished, she pushed the equipment cart into the hallway, preparing to move to her next session. The young boy was still screaming and the therapist could hear a woman talking softly to the child, trying to calm him down. The therapist also noticed several staff, including nurses and the child life specialist, watching the room with perplexed looks on their faces. The music therapist approached the staff and inquired as to what was happening with the patient. He had been screaming for quite some time with no apparent pain or medical needs. Several people, including the child's mother who was still in the room, had tried to comfort him. The music therapist asked if she could try. Not knowing what to expect, she approached the child's room with her guitar. At the doorway, the mother looked up and the therapist asked if she could come in. The mother replied, "Please." As the therapist entered the room, the child, about 9 or 10 years of age, looked at her and quieted his screaming. The therapist approached the bedside, looking at the young boy and said, "We just finished a music group in the playroom and I noticed you were not able to join us. Would it be okay if I sat here next to you and sang a song?" The patient nodded. The therapist sang "Puff the Magic Dragon" and proceeded into a song-writing activity using that song to refocus the child to more positive experiences. Within 10 minutes of entering the room, the music therapist, child, and mother were laughing. The therapist stayed several more minutes and then left to see her other patients.

3

This experience illustrates the power of a short musical experience on a pediatric unit and the value of the type of services a pediatric medical music therapist can provide. Music therapists may work within a children's hospital or pediatric unit of a general hospital. The music therapist in the children's hospital will work strictly with pediatrics, whereas the general hospital music therapist may have a patient case load that spans the age range. Regardless of where the pediatric music therapist is working, the structure of the music therapy treatment will differ depending on a variety of factors, such as outpatient or inpatient, length of stay, severity of illness or diagnosis, acute or chronic, short-term or long-term therapy, procedural support or bedside care, inclusion of family members and family dynamics, and patient coping strategies. These factors influence the way the therapist approaches the patient, the type of interventions provided, and the organization of the treatment process.

The pediatric patient may be seen only in the outpatient clinic, or may be hospitalized for overnight or several weeks, months, or years. The patient may be seen once for an injury, illness, or procedure, or he or she may be hospitalized multiple times a year due to a chronic medical condition. The pediatric patient may have a parent or other caregiver attending at all times or may only see his or her parents periodically, or not at all, due to a host of circumstances such as financial and family responsibilities and distance to the hospital. Every patient paints a different picture due to his or her individual experiences and diagnosis. Every family of a patient has its own unique culture that impacts the quality of life and recovery of the pediatric patient. The hospital staff must be able to respond to all of the needs of their patients and families.

The medical music therapist is flexible and adaptable to the changing routines of the hospital day; the variety of diagnoses and levels of care of the patients; the individual needs, cultures, and relationships of the patient and family; and the abundant interactions among hospital personnel. Medical music therapists must be quick thinking, caring, nurturing, and nonjudgmental. They should be aware of boundaries and personal involvement. They are careful listeners and observers, and they must be able to deal with ambiguity and unpredictability. Medical music therapists must know how to put aside their personal beliefs and concerns for the well-being of the patient, and they must be able to recognize the side effects of working in a fast-paced setting that deals with critical illnesses and death. Self-care, such as healthy eating, regular exercise, fun leisure activities, and strong interpersonal relationships outside of the work environment are important to reducing symptoms of stress and burnout.

The chapters in this monograph exemplify pediatric music therapists who illustrate these characteristics. They are dedicated individuals who believe in the efficacious application of music in medical setting. While the chapters are specific to unit and/or diagnosis, the content can be applied to many areas of the hospital setting. Within the broader view of the treatment process in medical music therapy there is recognition of the value of specialization to the hospital setting and the unit or diagnosis.

The pediatric volume of the medical music therapy monograph is a compilation of practice wisdom among clinicians in the pediatric hospital setting. The knowledge in this monograph is based on evidence from the literature; years of clinical experience; and strong relationships between the therapists, their patients and families, and the staff with whom they work. Each chapter relates an understanding of the various patient needs and diagnoses experienced on the unit. The reader is guided through the treatment process with practical knowledge and tips for success. Case studies illustrate the efficacious nature of music therapy in the medical environment. Sample forms are added to provide examples of the written paperwork necessary to the treatment process.

The pediatric volume is divided into five chapters highlighting various units in the pediatric or children's hospital: the Neonatal Intensive Care Unit (NICU); Pediatric Intensive Care Unit (PICU); General Pediatrics Medical/Surgical; **Hematology**, **Oncology**, and Bone Marrow Transplant; and Pediatric Burn Recovery. Each of these chapters has unique contributions relevant to the specific unit; however, much of the information can be transferred to other areas of clinical practice in the hospital. The monograph concludes with a glossary that defines terminology that the reader, unfamiliar with the hospital environment, might find useful. A bibliography provides a quick reference of sources that may or may not be cited in the chapters. Intervention plans by various authors appropriate to many of the units discussed in this monograph are provided as samples. Finally, AMTA Fact Sheets provide additional resources to support the knowledge presented in the monograph. Several concepts help to contextualize music therapy in the hospital setting: a historical perspective of music therapy in pediatrics, a definition of medical music therapy, an understanding of evidence-based practice, and the key concepts of family-centered care.

Historical Perspectives of Music Therapy in Pediatrics

Studies began to emerge in the literature on the effect of music on children in the medical setting in the late 1960s to early 1970s. A meta-analysis of music therapy (Standley & Whipple, 2003) with pediatric patients examined studies that used music, either live or recorded, for noninvasive, minor invasive, and major invasive procedures. Results from the meta-analysis suggest that the use of music in pediatric medical treatment is better than no music, that active engagement with the music is better than passive listening, and that live music is better than recorded. According to the meta-analysis, music therapy functions better for noninvasive and major invasive procedures than for minor invasive procedures. More recently, a systematic review of literature found that music is effective at reducing anxiety and pain in children undergoing clinical procedures and should be considered an **adjunctive** therapy in such situations (Klassen, Liang, Tjosvold, Klassen, & Hartling, 2008). Additional support for pediatric medical music therapy can be found for its use as an adjunctive therapy in improving the immune response and lowering stress levels (Avers, Mathur, & Kamat, 2007).

Little is known about the historical context of clinical practice in pediatric medical music therapy. In 1929, the newly constructed Duke University Hospital installed wall mounted speakers to broadcast radio programming on the infant and children units. In 1938, the *New York Times* published an article describing the use of instrument playing to support rehabilitation on the pediatric and orthopedic units (Taylor, 1981). Early practice primarily addressed the psychological needs in pediatrics (Rudenberg & Royka, 1989; Taylor, 1981). In the 1940s, Pickerell, Metzger, Wilde, Broadbent, and Edwards (1950, as cited in Taylor, 1981) started a project to infuse music in all areas of the hospital. In pediatrics, records were played to provide pleasure and simplify the effort required in cares. This project also involved early procedural support for children going into surgery. The goal of the music was to avoid irreparable psychological and physical damage, and nurses used songs and dolls to explain procedures.

By the 1950s, music therapists were employed in the pediatric setting. For example, the University of Iowa Hospital School, established in 1947, provided educational-based services for children with disabilities. A full-time music therapist was hired in 1955 to provide music experiences for the children. This program eventually grew to include other areas of the hospital, including child psychiatric and pediatric services, and employed multiple therapists (Hanson-Abromeit, in review). Clinical practice emerged in specialty hospitals, such as Shriners Burns Hospital in Galveston, Texas, in the 1970s. This hospital may be one of the first to offer music therapy to children with severe burn injuries, as well as an internship training program established in 1979 that helped to secure a full-time music therapy position in 1992 (C. Neugebauer, personal communication). Based on the work of Mary Rudenberg, the first journal article specific to music therapy in pediatric burn care was published in 1989 (Rudenberg & Royka, 1989). Now many children's hospitals employ music therapists. Other medical music therapy programs grew from beginnings in the pediatric settings, such as the Louis and Lucille Armstrong Music Therapy Program at Beth Israel Hospital in New York. This program, started in 1994 with one music therapist, has grown to serve multiple pediatric settings as well as adult units, employing multiple music therapists (J. Loewy, personal communication). Related publications and clinical work in pediatrics continue to be growing areas for music therapy practice.

Medical Music Therapy

Music therapy is defined by the American Music Therapy Association as

> an established healthcare profession that uses music to address physical, emotional, cognitive, and social needs of individuals of all ages. Music therapy improves the quality of life for persons who are well and meets the needs of children and adults with disabilities or illnesses. Music therapy interventions can be designed to: promote wellness, manage stress, alleviate pain, express feelings, enhance memory, improve communication, promote physical rehabilitation. (American Music Therapy Association, 2004)

This is a broad definition to encompass the various populations, diagnoses, and settings in which music therapists provide services. In the hospital setting, the application of music-based intervention strategies within the context of a therapeutic relationship between the board certified music therapist, the patient, and the patient's family might be referred to as medical music therapy (Dileo, 1999).

The philosophical underpinnings of medical music therapy may differ among clinicians and settings. Due to the variety of clinical problems, individual patient and family needs, medical settings, and treatment strategies presented, the medical music therapist may call upon different theoretical models to support the therapeutic interventions. At times the clinical interventions may have a foundation based on several philosophies, theories, and approaches. Multiple theoretical orientations have been identified in medical music therapy; however, a distinction is difficult to make due to the challenges related to isolating the various components of music therapy and the role of the treatment in the physical, social, psychological, or spiritual needs of the patient and family (Dileo, 1999). The clinician authors in this monograph have demonstrated elements of various theoretical orientations; however, the emphasis is clearly on the patient and the desired outcome. A theoretical orientation, combined with the relevant research, the expertise of the clinician, and the desires of the patient and family form the primary foundation in the application of music therapy treatment in the medical setting.

Evidence-Based Practice

Evidence-based medicine has become the standard in an effort to improve patient outcomes and quality of care, as well as a means to make available the most current treatment. In addition, it is a method to streamline the large amount of research available in the global community (Davidson et al., 2003; Haynes, 2002). The standards for evidence-based medicine were developed by the medical community and primarily address the research methods and epistemology of the physical sciences (Edwards, 2005). However, some of the medical science standards are not applicable to behavioral studies. Efforts are being made to establish consistent evidence-based principles for behavioral medicine (Davidson et al., 2003), of which medical music therapy could be considered a part.

Understanding the concepts of evidence-based research provides a common ground of communication within the medical setting, allowing music therapists to demonstrate the distinct and valuable contributions they make to the hospital environment (Edwards, 2002). An understanding of the music therapy research and how it fits into the evidence-based framework will also allow music therapists to integrate the vast amount of literature into clinical practice (Edwards, 2005).

Clinical practice in an evidence-based manner is the clear, meticulous, and thoughtful use of the research evidence to inform the best intervention strategies for the patient. The clinician studies and interprets the research evidence with regards to the patient's needs, rights, and desires to determine the best course of treatment (Sackett, Rosenberg, Gray, Haynes, & Richardson, 1996). Thus, evidence-based practice involves the clinician's expertise to determine the most efficacious application of the research treatment recommendations in consideration of best interests of the patient. For the music therapist in the hospital setting, evidence-based practice provides clinicians with a system to articulate the value of their work to other professionals (Edwards, 2005). Due to the vast array of diagnoses the medical music therapist encounters and the copious amount of medical literature from music therapy and related fields, evidence-based practice provides a structure in which music therapists can prescribe treatment in the most efficient and beneficial manner to their patients and families.

Web-based Resources about Evidenced-Based Practice

Research Centre for Transcultural Studies in Health, Middlesex University
http://www.mdx.ac.uk/www/rctsh/ebp/main.htm

Social Work Resources, Evidence-Based Practice,
Smith College School for Social Work
http://sophia.smith.edu/~jdrisko/evidence_based_practice.htm#top

Evidence-Based Practice, Tutorial, University of Minnesota
http://www.biomed.lib.umn.edu/learn/ebp/

Evidence-Based Practice, Nursing Library and Information Resources,
Cushing/Whitney Medical Library, Yale University
http://www.med.yale.edu/library/nursing/education/ebhc.html

Family-Centered Care

Practicing in a family-centered manner impacts how music therapy is planned, delivered, and evaluated. The foundation for treatment is found in a mutually beneficial partnership between the patients, their families, and the care providers. Within the hospital, this partnership is exemplified through the relationships that value input from the family members, acknowledge their expertise and strengths, and recognize the significance of their observations and perceptions (Institute for Family-Centered Care, n.d.). According to the Institute for Family-Centered Care (www.familycenteredcare.org), there are four key principles that guide practice in a family-centered care philosophy: dignity and respect, sharing of information, participation, and collaboration. For music therapists, these key principles are exemplified in their interactions and attitudes with patients and staff, the intervention strategies employed, their cultural awareness of different family configurations and experiences, and the types of music utilized.

Listening and honoring the patient and family perspectives and choices advocate dignity and respect. The family's knowledge, beliefs, values, and cultural perspective is integrated into the planning and implementation of services. Information is provided to the patient and family in a manner that communicates and shares complete and unbiased information. Communication is affirming, useful, complete, and timely, and patients and families are encouraged to participate in all aspects and levels of the care and decision making (Institute for Family-Centered Care, n.d.).

Family-centered music therapy addresses issues from the perspective of the patient, parent, sibling, and therapist. The therapist enters into the relationship with an understanding of the disease process and with a nonjudgmental mentality. The music therapist integrates treatment approaches to follow the family throughout hospitalization and to incorporate them into the treatment process. Sometimes this means providing direct service to the parent or sibling rather than the patient. Intervention strategies are employed that support family integration both in and out of the hospital setting (Hanson-Abromeit, Hawkins, Nelson, Oelkers, & Mozena, 2005).

From the parents' perspective, family-centered care can improve perceptions of the quality of care being provided to their child and can help them to better engage in their role as a parent in hospital and in the health of their child. Family-centered music therapy develops a triadic relationship between the patient, family, and the therapist. This relationship may allow the parents to engage at a different level with their child during a music-making experience, receive validation of their efforts toward normalization, and feel comfortable enough to taking a break from attending to their child (Shoemark & Dearn, 2008). Family-centered music therapy can create joyful experiences and positive memories in a sometimes frustrating environment (Hanson-Abromeit et al., 2005; Shoemark & Dearn, 2008). Positive experiences and continuity of care can build a bond of trust that allows for greater support in particularly challenging times during hospitalization (Shoemark & Dearn, 2008).

When treatment becomes completely focused on the patient, the music therapist may not fully engage with the needs of the parent. Obviously, levels of engagement may differ based on parent availability, the parent's desires, and the safety and best interest of the child. However, when music therapy is provided in a truly family-centered manner, treatment considers both the patient and family, with a central focus on the parent. Ultimately, the child benefits from a positive and supportive interaction with the parents. The music therapist with family-centered practice values will possess poise, be approachable and personable, demonstrate consistency of character, and recognize the need to maintain boundaries (Shoemark & Dearn, 2008).

Conclusion

Historical documents demonstrate that music as a therapeutic tool in the hospital has been utilized for decades. Literature outside of the professional music therapy journals demonstrates the current use of music in medical practice by other professions. Much of what is documented historically and in non-music therapy publications advocates the use of pre-recorded music. While recorded music can be used prescriptively, it is music therapy that provides the benefits experienced by the patients, their families, the staff, and the therapist. Medical music therapy considers the relationship that develops between the patient, the family, and the therapist and the therapeutic process they create through the music (Dileo, 1999) in promoting health and well-being. It is the engagement in the musical process within a therapeutic relationship that differentiates music therapy from other professions.

The role of collaboration will be important to the future of medical music therapy. Collaboration with hospital personnel will improve and inform not only music therapy practice, but also other professions and program development in the hospital. Shared clinical services, (e.g., co-treatment and team planning) and the implementation of various types and levels of research will encourage future growth in both clinical practice and evidence-based research. Collaboration with the patients and families will inform new or adapted clinical practice techniques. Expansion of services can be supported through collaboration. The music therapist can triage referrals, providing direct service to the most critical cases and facilitating therapeutic activities that use music to be employed by other staff members.

Through collaboration, the music therapist becomes fully integrated into the family-centered and evidence-based practice approach of the hospital unit. This can create a stronger team approach that facilitates a deeper respect and appreciation for the music therapist and music therapy services. Collaboration will encourage greater knowledge and integration of evidenced-based research and practice relevant to the profession of music therapy.

For many clinicians in the hospital setting, clinical knowledge was built through trial and error. Few clinicians enter their hospital-based internship or employment with the ability to play guitar while wearing protective gloves or to realize the necessity of alternative ways to engage a patient when facial expressions are hidden behind a mask. Understanding the environment and the way music therapy functions in a particular setting is critical to successful programming. This monograph clearly illustrates the value of music therapy in the pediatric hospital environment. Based on years of clinical experience and practice wisdom, the pediatric medical music therapy monograph provides a useful tool to inform the educator teaching medical music therapy; the music therapy student learning about a prospective area of practice or preparing for a hospital-based internship; the experienced clinician looking to expand areas of practice; and the hospital nurse manager, physician, or administrator interested in developing a more comprehensive understanding of the role of music therapy in the pediatric setting.

References

American Music Therapy Association. (2004). *What is music therapy?* Retrieved September 3, 2008, from http://www.musictherapy.org/

Avers, L., Mathur, A., & Kamat, D. (2007). Music therapy in pediatrics. *Clinical Pediatrics, 46*(7), 575–579.

Davidson, K. W., Goldstein, M., Kaplan, R. M., Kauffman, P. G., Knatterud, G. L., Orleans, C. T., Spring, B., Trudeau, K. J., & Whitlock, E, P. (2003). Evidence-based behavioral medicine: What is it and how do we achieve it. *Annals of Behavioral Medicine, 26*(3), 161–171.

Dileo, C. (1999). Introduction to music therapy and medicine: Definitions, theoretical orientations and levels of practice. In C. Dileo (Ed.) *Music therapy and medicine: Theoretical and clinical applications* (pp. 3–10). Silver Spring, MD: American Music Therapy Association.

Edwards, J. (2005). Possibilities and problems for evidence-based practice in music therapy. *The Arts in Psychotherapy, 32*, 293–301.

Edwards, J. (2002). Using the evidence-based medicine framework to support music therapy posts in healthcare settings. *British Journal of Music Therapy, 16*(1), 29–34.

Hanson-Abromeit, D. (in review). Development of the undergraduate music therapy degree program at the University of Iowa. *Journal of Music Therapy.*

Hanson-Abromeit, D., Hawkins, K., Nelson, K., Oelkers, L., & Mozena, E. (2005, November). *Music therapy and family-centered care with hospitalized infants and children.* Paper presented at the annual meeting of the American Music Therapy Association, Orlando, FL.

Haynes, R. B. (2002). What kind of evidence is it that evidence-based medicine advocates want health care providers and consumers to pay attention to? *BMC Health Services Research, 2*(3), 3–15. Retrieved from http://www.biomedcentral.com/1472-6963/2/3

Institute for Family-Centered Care. (n.d.). *Clinicians.* Retrieved September 5, 2008, from http://www.familycenteredcare.org/advance/clinician.html

Institute for Family-Centered Care. (n.d.). *Patient and family centered care core concepts.* Retrieved September 5, 2008, from http://www.familycenteredcare.org/pdf/CoreConcepts.pdf

Klassen, J. A., Liang, Y., Tjosvold, L., Klassen, T. P., & Hartling, L. (2008). Music for pain and anxiety in children undergoing medical procedures: A systematic review of randomized controlled trials. *Ambulatory Pediatrics, 8*(17), 117–128.

Rudenberg, M. T., & Royka, A. M. (1989). Promoting psychosocial adjustment in pediatric burn patients through music therapy and child life therapy. *Music Therapy Perspectives, 7*, 40–43.

Sackett, D. L., Rosenberg, W. M. C., Gray, J. A., Haynes, R. B., & Richardson, W. S. (1996). Evidenced based medicine: What it is and what it isn't: It's about integrating individual clinical expertise and the best external evidence. *British Medical Journal, 312*(7023), 71–72.

Shoemark, H., & Dearn, T. (2008). Keeping parents at the centre of family centred music therapy with hospitalised infants. *Australian Journal of Music Therapy, 19*, 3–24.

Standley, J. M., & Whipple, J. (2003). Music therapy with pediatric patients: A meta analysis. In S. L. Robb (Ed.), *Music therapy in pediatric healthcare: Research and evidence-based practice* (pp. 1–18). Silver Spring, MD: American Music Therapy Association.

Taylor, D. B. (1981). Music in general hospital treatment from 1900 to 1950. *Journal of Music Therapy, 18*(2), 62–73.

Section II:

Music Therapy with Pediatric Units

CHAPTER 2

Newborn Intensive Care Unit (NICU)

Deanna Hanson-Abromeit
Helen Shoemark
Joanne V. Loewy

The Neonatal Intensive Care Unit is an environment of great need. Neonatal music therapists are clinicians who specialize in the application of music-based interventions to support the developmental processes of the young hospitalized infant. Infants may be challenged due to prematurity, critical illnesses, medical complications that require surgery, or other risk factors for developmental delays (e.g., failure to thrive, addiction and/or withdrawal from narcotics due to maternal use). Neonatal music therapists understand the expected developmental processes of infancy, concerns for developmental trajectories due to hospitalization (e.g., attachment, meeting developmental expectations across domains), issues related to specific medical conditions, and the therapeutic function of music as it relates to the fragile states of the hospitalized infant.

The vast level of knowledge required and the challenges to clinical work with such fragile humans make this a highly specialized area of practice that demands the music therapist to stay abreast of the most recent research and medical practice techniques. Clinical practice techniques continue to be refined as they relate to research protocols. The neonatal music therapist must be self-aware and connected to the therapeutic process within each individual session. This allows the music therapist to continually monitor, evaluate, and adapt the appropriate music therapy interventions for an individual infant and his or her family. An interdisciplinary collaborative approach is critical to the success of a music therapy program in the NICU.

Due to the wide body of knowledge required for clinical practice with premature and critically ill infants and the limitations of space, the scope of this chapter will focus on presenting the treatment process of music therapy in the context of the NICU for families and their premature and ill full-term infants. The terminology of the *Newborn Intensive Care Unit* (NICU) will be used in this chapter with the understanding that this nursery in the hospital can provide services to neonates with a variety of medical complications.

General Characteristics of Infants in the NICU

General and specialty hospitals provide services specifically targeting medically fragile infants and their families. The units of care may be referred to as Intensive Care Nurseries, Newborn Intensive Care Nurseries, or Special Care Nurseries. They may be designated at different levels indicating an increasing sophistication and breadth of care. They serve premature and critically ill newborn infants in various levels of medical severity.

The rate of premature birth continues to increase. In 2005, 12.7% of live infants were born premature in the United States (Martin et al., 2007) and 8.1% in Australia (Laws, Abeywardana, Walker, & Sullivan, 2007). Premature birth is defined as a live birth that happens before the end of the 37th week of pregnancy (counting from the first day of the last menstrual period). Infants born before 32 weeks gestation are considered very preterm and those born between 34 weeks to 36 weeks are considered late preterm (American Academy of Pediatrics, American College of Obstetricians and Gynecologists, 2005). These are important distinctions as outcomes for infants are directly related to gestational age and weight at birth (March of Dimes, n.d.).

Full-term newborn surgical patients also cared for in tertiary level NICUs include those with congenital anomalies such as anencephaly, meningomyelocele/spina bifida, cleft lip/palate, syndromes, and other conditions causing cardiac, facial and esophageal abnormalities, **omphalocele/gastroschisis**, and other bowel obstructions. The clinical pathway for these patients may include surgery on the first day of life and further surgeries in the first weeks and months of life.

The newborn infants are cared for in an **extrauterine** environment, which offers stark contrast to the womb. While standards for the NICU are regularly updated (Philbin & Evans, 2006), hospitals vary greatly on the sensory environment provided. While some have continuous or frequent noise and light, leaving little differentiation between day and night, others achieve a predominantly peaceful and muted sensory experience. Causes of excessive noise and its constraints on the developing premature infant have been reviewed (Schwartz, 2004), investigated, and addressed through Environmental Music Therapy (Shoemark, 2007; Stewart & Schneider, 2000). Noise hindrances may include the conversations of staff and family members, equipment alarms, monitors, motors, and the closing of isolettes.

Further, the premature infant will experience multiple caregivers and will receive unnatural stimulation that may be painful, random, and lacking contingent interaction. These experiences may cause the infant's premature neurobehavioral subsystems to become defensive, leading to maladaptive and life-threatening behaviors. Complications of prematurity are vast and individualized to the infant. Prematurity puts an infant at risk for later developmental disabilities (e.g., intellectual impairment, cerebral palsy), medical complications (e.g., lung and gastrointestinal issues), sensory system complications (e.g., vision and hearing), and even death (March of Dimes, 2007). Specific complications related to prematurity include cardiorespiratory problems like apnea (cessation of breathing) and bradycardia (heart rate that is too low),as well as stress behaviors (e.g., state lability, sleep deprivation, and avoidance behaviors) (Gardner & Lubchenco, 1998). Long-term effects could include psychological concerns, attentional and school difficulties, and lower IQ (Wolke, 1998). Follow-up studies investigating experiences of the full-term NICU patient are limited in the literature.

Models of premature infant development and care may guide the modulation and organization of the premature infant's behavior by providing useful indictors of appropriate caregiving and therapeutic interventions (Als, 1982, 1986). Such indicators include autonomic stability, sensitivity to infant orientation, responses to environmental and social stimuli, and motor disorganization. Caregivers, with guidance and an understanding of these indicators, can provide more supportive and less stressful interactions and interventions for the infant (Mouradian, Als, & Coster, 2000).

Medical advances, focusing on the stability of the autonomic system, are able to keep premature infants alive at earlier and earlier gestational ages. The motor, state-organizational, and sensory systems are highly dependent on an adaptive and reciprocal environment in which to develop and function. While best practice offers clear information about patterning care, promotion of sleep, positioning, and swaddling, these systems are still often left unaddressed. Understanding the development and differentiation of each of these systems provides the caregiver, therapist, and medical staff with the theoretical basis to form appropriate and supportive interventions for the whole infant (Als, 1982).

As the rate of premature births increases, the need for medical and developmental services is critical. Understanding the premature infant is complicated, as infants complete their early development in a non-womb-like environment. For the full-term ill infant, we are yet to clearly understand the impact of recurrent pain, disrupted sleep, invasive monitoring, or ongoing treatment. For both the premature and medically compromised infant, medical technology provides the support necessary for physical survival. However, care and interventions that support their psychological development are less understood and more often controversial than development of healthy full-term born infants. The premature and medically compromised infants themselves are informing the direction of care.

Until there is a clearer knowledge-base of the unique development of the premature and medically compromised infant, clinicians, medical personnel, researchers, and families must make their decisions for care based on the cumulative knowledge available and closely guarded consideration for the negative effects and potential benefits of interventions. At this time, interventions that are directed to premature infants are based on the cumulative knowledge about fetal and newborn infant development, and the emerging awareness of premature infant development. For full-term infants, the focus is on successfully retaining opportunities for windows of development to occur despite the compromise of significant medical conditions, and current thinking recommends this be best achieved within a model of family-centered care.

Neonatal music therapy is one intervention that is emerging as a clinical practice in the NICU following more than 20 years of research and protocol development. Music therapy protocols with premature infants are research-based and carefully implemented to provide "best practice" techniques for clinical interventions (Standley, 2003). This work has also provided a transferable interim model for work with full-term medically fragile infants.

While music therapists working within the NICU environment recognize the benefits of music therapy as a therapeutic intervention, they also recognize the criticisms related to the broad, uninformed use of recorded music in the NICU as a form of "music therapy" (Graven, 2000; Philbin, 2000). Board certified (or equivalent) music therapists with specialty education, training, and mentorship in neonatal music therapy recognize and demonstrate the value of music therapy for the family relationships, developmental milestones, and infant mental health of these medically challenged neonates through appropriate clinical applications.

Premature infants are obliged to complete their early development in an environment that is markedly different than that of the womb. In order to support their emerging development, the type and level of care provided to these infants are critical and sometimes controversial. Understanding premature infants involves a dynamic process of learning from the infants themselves within the unique context of their environment and experiences. Professional caregivers must also extrapolate information gleaned from the developmental experiences of the fetus and the neonate, as well as the unique intentions of their caregivers. The latter will allow for creative interventions that can be catered to fostering the parent–child bonding, which is critically important to growth and sustenance (Bowlby, 1988; Stern, 1995). The cumulative knowledge about the fetus, neonate, and premature infant informs medical and developmental interventions. Music therapy can ease caregivers' understanding of premature and medically compromised infants and assist in their capacity to organize the knowledge necessary to provide a framework for care that will best serve the infant's development into a healthy and developmentally competent individual well connected to the world.

Music therapy with hospitalized newborn infants is a relatively new area of clinical practice, with only a few music therapists providing services in the Neonatal Intensive Care Unit (NICU). Research examining music use in the NICU demonstrates positive benefits for the premature infant. The majority of this research has involved the use of recorded music. Clinical evidence indicates that the application of recorded music can support the infant's transition between behavior states, e.g., moving from an agitated to a quieter, drowsy, or sleep state (Shoemark, 1999). Music therapists are developing protocols and standards of practice (Standley, 2003), training programs (Standley et al., 2005; Standley, Whipple, & Abromeit, 2003) and multi-site clinical trials and trainings (Loewy & Stewart, 2008) and are instituting clinical competencies for music therapists serving premature infants (*Clinical Core Competency Training Manual,* 2005; Department of Rehabilitation Therapies, 2003; Shoemark, 2007). An example of these competencies (Shoemark, 2007) can be found in the Appendix for this chapter.

In many NICUs, recorded music is added to the NICU environment by staff and families (Field, Hernandez-Reif, Feijo, & Freedman, 2005; Graven, 2000; Kemper, Martin, Block, Shoaf, & Woods, 2004), but the nonprescribed use of recorded music is not always recommended due to the unknown and potentially negative effects on the neurosensory development (Graven, 2000). Music therapists are researching and practicing music-based interventions with premature infants, but many have not fully addressed some of the issues related to music and noise in the NICU. The sound effect on perinatal brain development

(Schwartz, 2004) and the effects of live music therapy on the sound environment (Stewart & Schneider, 2000) are essential areas of consideration for the NICU music therapist and will be addressed later in this chapter. Music therapists have a responsibility to educate caregivers in the most appropriate music incorporating both cultural, aesthetic sensitivity and preferences, while ensuring responsible choices in the music selections offered. Furthermore, music therapists should be educated about developmental rationale that informs their interventions. Developmental neuroscience, familiarity with research protocols, understanding the rationale behind interventions, as well as caregiver cultural sensitivity and careful observation of the infants themselves are all parameters that inform clinical practice

Developmental neuroscience can inform practice with an understanding of fetal and premature infant neurobehavioral development, behavior state development, the auditory environment, and how music therapy has been applied to the premature infant, enhancing musicality in infancy. Understanding of a broad knowledge base of fetal, premature, and infant development is necessary for the efficacious neonatal music therapy program. A comprehensive overview of the relevant literature is beyond the scope of this chapter; however, the information below provides a brief summary of relevant information.

Premature Infant Developmental Overview
(Summarized by Hanson-Abromeit, 2006)

- Neurobehavioral functioning is on a continuum with gestational age (Mouradian, Als, & Coster, 2000). Inappropriate stimuli that are too complex and intense can have a negative impact on neurobehavioral development (Als, 1986).

- Premature infants show decreased ability to habituate, greater defensive movements, difficulty calming and using self-soothing techniques when upset, and less autonomic stability than full-term infants. But premature infants (compared to full-term infants) were better at orienting to an auditory cue (Stjernqvist & Svenningsen, 1990).

- By 28–32 weeks, the fetus is demonstrating a slowing of activity, an indication of neural organization that allows for the regulation and integration of multiple neural systems (DiPietro, Hodgson, Costigan, Hilton, & Johnson, 1996). Fetal behavioral states demonstrate organization at 36 weeks gestational age (Nijhus, Prechtl, Martin, & Bots, 1982).

- As time passes, the fetus demonstrates longer transitions between sleep states than the neonate. The neonate has more frequent changes in eye movement and heart rate prior to, or with, the transitions between states. Neonates have smoother transitions than the fetus (Groome, Swiber, Atterbury, Bentz, & Holland, 1997).

- At approximately 34 weeks gestational age, the premature infant is capable of maintaining a quiet alert state, but continues to struggle with regulation and orientation when attending to a high demand task (e.g., nutritive sucking) (Medoff-Cooper, McGrath, & Bilker, 2000).

- Fetal response (20–28 weeks GA) is greater to low frequencies than to high frequencies (Rubel, 1984); sounds at 100 Hz and above are attenuated by at least 20dB in utero (Hepper, Scott & Shahidullah, 1993).

- As early as 25 weeks, fetal response to sound stimulus was immediate and occurred only during the stimulus presentation (Shahidullah & Hepper, 1993). Reliable heart rate responses are indicated at 29 weeks GA (Kisilevsky, 1995).

- Between 38–40 weeks, the fetus is beginning to habituate to a low frequency sound stimulus when in a quiet (1F) or active (2F) behavior state, indicating attention and orientation to the sound stimulus (Lecanuet, Granier-Deferre, Cohen, Le Houezec, & Busnel, 1986). Classic habituation and dishabituation has been confirmed (at full-term gestation) when presented with a repeated tone (Kisilevsky & Muir, 1991). Atypically developing neonates are inconsistent in their attention away from a strong competing stimulus (Gray & Philbin, 2004).

- Auditory learning to recorded music has been demonstrated in the fetus with post birth recognition as early as 2 days (Hepper, 1991). The duration of recognition is extended with repeated exposure post birth (Polverini-Rey, 1992). Infants exposed pre- and post-birth to the same song took less time to calm when presented with the song (Polverini-Rey, 1992).

- Neonates demonstrate a preference for prenatal exposed auditory stimulus, e.g., filtered maternal voice, maternal heartbeat, or story passage (DeCasper & Sigafoos, 1983; DeCasper & Spence, 1986; Spence & DeCasper, 1987).

- Fetus can discriminate and demonstrate a preference for the mother's normal voice over her speaking "motherese" and another female voice (normal and "motherese" speech) (Hepper et al., 1993). Preference for a familiar (prenatal exposed) melody suggests that preferences could be based on non-word information. The patterns of the maternal voice may be a potent reinforcer to engage the infant's attention (Panneton, 1985).

- There are more major triads in infant-intended songs than in adult-intended songs. Infants respond with greater attention to a wider range of intervals. They are also more attentive and have more positive affect to consonant music as compared to dissonant (Trehub & Trainor, 1990).

- Characteristics of infant-directed songs include higher pitch, greater rhythmicity, slower tempo, briefer utterances, simple pitch contours, flowing articulation, more energy, and lower frequencies, and they are described as emotionally engaging (Trehub & Trainor, 1990; Trehub et al., 1997). Infants listen longer to recorded versions of infant-directed singing than to speaking. There is greater attention to higher pitches than lower pitches (Trehub, 2001; Trehub & Trainor, 1990).

- Infants have a more inward response to infant directed lullabies than to play songs (Rock, Trainor, & Addison, 1999; Trainor, 1996; Trainor, Clark, Huntley, & Adams, 1997).

- Pauses within musical phrasing disrupt attention more than if a pause occurs between phrases (Trehub & Trainor, 1990).

- Auditory signals support the organization of intersensory coordination when the signal is predictable and familiar (Gray & Philbin, 2004).

- Infants tend to listen to everything; thus, they are more sensitive to unexpected sounds and find it challenging to focus on expected sounds that may be weak (Gray & Philbin, 2004).

Music Therapy in the NICU

As the survival rate of infants born prematurely increases, the needs of these infants are being addressed more seriously. Caregivers are using their knowledge of infant development across the prenatal and postnatal stages to structure the environment to provide supportive care. Interest in interventions that support the sensory experience of the infant includes a consideration of music and music therapy (Field et al., 2006). Music therapists and other professionals are examining the potential implications of music therapy interventions. However, the number of studies is limited and all have small participant numbers. The newness of this research area indicates that protocols are still being established (Cassidy & Ditty, 1998; Shoemark & Dearn, 2008). One such protocol, The Heather on Earth Multi-site NICU Study (Loewy & Stewart, 2008), is currently underway at The Louis Armstrong Center for Music & Medicine at Beth Israel Medical Center. This study involves clinical trials at 10 NICUs in the Northeast, where music therapy researchers are investigating the effects of live music on 240 neonates. Clinical trials that are diagnoses-specific and that can be conducted at a variety of NICUs may best inform clinical practice and at the same time provide evidence-based feedback potential for expansion of program practices.

Working with the Infant

A variety of concerns must be addressed when interacting with the hospitalized newborn infant. These include assessing the infant as an individual, examining and minimizing the stress factors in the environment, and providing cost-effective interventions that will encourage growth, promote lower weight loss and stress levels, as well as decrease the length of hospitalization. Collectively, the literature suggests that the use of music therapy with the premature infant is effective in addressing these concerns.

Compared to other environmental sounds, musical sound waves have organized structural characteristics of pitch, dynamics, timbre, and harmony. The *Merriam-Webster Online Dictionary* (n.d.) defines music as "the science or art of ordering tones or sounds in succession, in combination, and in temporal relationships to produce a composition having unity and continuity." Music is an agreeable sound that can be vocal, instrumental, or mechanical sounds that have rhythm, melody, or harmony. The structural characteristics of music should be introduced and assessed on a case-by-case basis and implemented at a level of complexity that each infant can handle. Music can be adapted to infants' patterns of behavior organization and ability to handle specific stimuli and can be modified in response to their behaviors. The extent of the benefits, however, must be determined through the use of culturally sensitive (Loewy, 2004) and appropriate clinical indicators within the control of the neonatal nursery (Hanson-Abromeit, 2003) and may vary depending on the presentation mode (live or recorded).

The environmental sounds of the newborn intensive care nursery may provide additional stress and overstimulation in the premature infant (Caine, 1991; Cassidy & Standley, 1995; Lorch, Lorch, Diefendorf, & Earl, 1994; Schwartz, 2004; Stewart & Schneider, 2000).

Studies on the effects of music have been conducted as a way to counteract these unpleasant and sometimes loud auditory stimuli (Stewart & Schneider, 2000). The effects of musical stimuli, consisting of lullabies and children's music, may reduce the hospital stay of premature infants (Caine, 1991), suggesting that music therapy can be a cost-effective intervention in the care of the premature infant (Standley, 1991). Improved feeding and physiological response (Cassidy & Standley, 1995; Cevasco & Grant, 2005; Collins & Kuck, 1991; Marchette, Main, Redick, & Shapiro, 1992; Moore, Gladstone, & Standley, 1994; Standley & Moore, 1995), lower initial weight loss, and lower stress levels (Caine, 1991) have also been demonstrated through the presentation of music stimuli with premature infants.

The effect of music on the physiological responses of premature infants has been examined in intensive care nurseries (Cassidy & Standley, 1995; Lorch et al., 1994). Music has been shown to affect the physiological responses of premature infants. Lorch et al. presented sedative and stimulative music to infants. The infant systolic blood pressure showed more variability when listening to the stimulative music, while the sedative music produced more variation in the infant heart rate recordings. The respiratory rates in these infants showed no significant variability between musical selections. When compared to the baseline measurement, all three physiological measures were significantly different for the music conditions. This study clearly demonstrates how varied types of music can have a different response and that the characteristics of the music selection may be important to the outcomes of the study. In 2002, Courtnage, Chawla, Loewy, and Nolan studied infant-directed singing with mothers and babies and found it had an impact on heart rate as compared to no singing with neonates. They found no significant difference in respiratory rate or oxygen saturation levels with these infants.

Cassidy and Standley (1995) alternated 4 minutes of recorded lullabies with 4 minutes of silence for premature infants in the experimental group. These infants had better oxygen levels and lower heart rates and were breathing with more stability than infants in the control group. Overall, infants in the experimental group were more stable, had fewer medically unacceptable responses, and appeared to be more relaxed and comfortable.

Burke, Walsh, Oehler, and Gingras (1995) conducted a descriptive study with four premature infants with bronchopulmonary dysplasia (BPD) who required frequent **suctioning**. Each infant served as his or her own control. The investigators wanted to discover whether music interventions could decrease negative behaviors, defined as "crying, facial grimacing, limb movement, rigid or startle responses," after suctioning (p. 41). They were also interested if music could affect heart rate and oxygen saturation levels, keeping them within acceptable parameters for longer durations. Finally, they wanted to determine if the pairing of vibrotactile stimulation with music reduced agitation and arousal levels more than music alone. The control condition did not involve auditory or vibrotactile stimulation. Each newborn responded slightly differently to each of the conditions. This strengthened the idea that consideration must be given to the individual needs of each infant.

Overall, Burke et al. (1995) found that both music conditions (taped music and vibrations paired with music via the Somatron™) improved oxygen saturation levels, decreased the time the infant spent highly aroused, and increased time spent sleeping. Heart rate improved during the music only condition. When music was paired with vibration, the time the infant was in a quiet alert state increased. A quiet alert state is important for development and stability in the premature infant and is conducive to improved oxygen levels and reduction in caloric use, both of which are needed for growth. Finally, infants had more limb movements during the control condition, indicating music can be a useful intervention to reduce energy consumption and decrease the negative effects of the stressful environment of the newborn intensive care nursery.

Through continued research and the development of protocols for the clinical applications of music therapy with premature infants, music therapists and medical staff may find music a useful and necessary intervention in NICUs. These studies have shown that music therapy can promote the physical and medical well-being of the premature infant, thus reducing the amount of time spent in the hospital. It is possible that music can affect the emotional state of the infant, providing a less traumatic transition between pre- and postnatal life. It can be advantageous for the music therapist to work with expectant parents, especially those who are defined as "high-risk" and are hospitalized in a neighboring maternity unit of the hospital. Music psychotherapy pre-birth can provide assurances for the parents as the therapist nurtures, relaxes, and builds confidence in what might otherwise be experienced as a traumatic time for these parents. Providing music therapy for the parents has inherent outcomes for their fragile infants (Lu, 2002). Music therapy has also been used as a way to encourage attachment and prolonged interactions between the parents and the premature infant (Charpie, 2002). It may also assist the parents in coping with this transition and may provide them with tools for interactions with their critically ill newborn (Cassidy & Standley, 1995), as well as providing an additional modality of support.

Music Preferences in Infancy

Infants' musicality is evident at birth as they use their voice to communicate their needs through crying and other simple vocalizations (cooing, gurgles, and other "baby talk"). Crying and comfort sounds are the first means of musical expression that later lead to interactive phonemes and babbles (Loewy, 1995, 2004). As they develop in their first year of life, infants have an advancing awareness of sounds and begin to respond more actively through movement and increased vocalizations. The emergence of their musicality is demonstrated through their rhythmic vocalizations that have definite pitch and contour and are differentiated from speech sounds (Brand, 1985).

Infants are able to discriminate singing that is directed intentionally to them (called infant-directed singing). When singing directly to the infant, the qualities of the singing change, differing from the singing qualities evident when the infant is not present. Infant-directed singing by both parents illustrates a higher pitch level, slower tempo, and is considered more emotionally engaging (Trehub et al., 1997). When mothers were recorded singing a playsong and lullaby, both in the presence and absence of their infants, there were noticeable differences in the songs. Both infant-directed lullabies and playsongs had a slower tempo, more energy at lower frequencies, and higher pitch. In the infant-directed playsongs, the pitch variability was higher and the rhythm more exaggerated. Adults also rated the infant-directed playsongs as being more brilliant, clipped, and rhythmic, having more "smiling" and prominent consonants. Infant-directed lullabies were characterized as being airy, smooth, and soothing.

The features of infant-directed singing are directly related to the development of musicality in the infant. Infant-directed singing has a heightened pitch of 3–4 semitones, falls into the infant's vocal production range, and encourages reciprocal vocalizations. Other features of infant-directed singing include an increased pitch range, greater rhythmicity, slower tempo, briefer utterances, simpler pitch contours, greater emotional quality, and a more flowing articulation (i.e., more slurred) than singing that is not infant-directed. Additionally, infants attend to the melodic contour of nonspeech sequences.

It is possible that the changes that occur in infant-directed singing may function as a way to attract the infant's attention and actually communicate an emotional message based on the context of the song (Rock et al., 1999; Trainor, 1996; Trainor et al., 1997). These stylistic changes in singing are noticed by infants. They become more inwardly focused (i.e., attention to their bodies, their clothing, or objects they were holding) when listening to infant-directed lullabies and more attentive to the external world (i.e., attention to the caregiver) during infant-directed playsongs (Rock et al., 1999).

Not only does infant-directed singing facilitate communication, but infants will also spend a longer time listening to singing than to speaking. They listen significantly longer to recorded versions of women singing in an infant-directed manner, and they have greater attention to higher pitched versions of the song than a lower pitched version. They attend longer and find their mother's singing voice more engaging than her speaking voice. There are also references to this with respect to recognition of the father's voice (Coleman, Pratt, Stoddard, Gerstmann, & Abel, 1997; Rock et al., 1999). These preferences indicate the potency of singing and may contribute to the infant's overall well-being in that it promotes reciprocal emotional attachment and bonding brought on by the positive outcomes of singing, such as lulling the baby to sleep or cessation of crying (Trehub, 2001; Trehub & Trainor, 1990). The emotional attachment and communication between the infant and parent, which occurs through singing, may also facilitate emerging language acquisition and the development of musicality in the young infant (Brand, 1985). The context of infant-directed singing in clinical practice informs how the musical selection relates to the therapeutic intent.

Lullabies are the most often cited stylistic category of auditory stimuli for infants (Hanson-Abromeit, 2003). Lullabies are typically a melody with a vocal line sung by the caregiver to calm an infant or put it to sleep. Lullabies have unique qualities that combine both lull and bye, meaning repetitive motion and separation that implies a transition of consciousness or awake to sleep state (Loewy & Stewart, 2008). The lullaby, as a song form, has naturally occurring salient features that are greatly representative across the category (Trehub & Unyk, 1991). Lullaby melody has more descending contours, fewer contour changes, and a higher median pitch than other songs (Unyk, Trehub, Trainor, & Schellenberg, 1992). The lullaby is rhythmically simple, with a lilting meter, often 3/4

(Loewy, Hallan, Friedman, & Martinez, 2005) or 4/4 (Hawes, 1974), as well as 6/8 (Loewy, in press) or 2/4. The text may also provide a cue to the identification of a song as a lullaby. Lullabies may demonstrate a preferred pattern of humming and nonsense syllables, possibly due to the fact that the singer cannot recall the lyrics (Hawes, 1974).

Lullaby singing has persisted for centuries in most cultures and may be a universally recognized aspect of caregiving. The longevity of lullabies may be related to the changes in the prosodic qualities present when singing directly to infants. Lullabies are repetitive, simple, and slow and possess a described quality of "soothing" and "soft" (Trehub, Unyk, & Trainor, 1993), suggesting that there is a biological significance in singing lullabies to infants. Loewy et al. (2005) have used culturally sensitive music from caretaker preference surveys and implemented these lullabies in a research study comparing them with chloral hydrate for sedation prior to EEG testing in infants through 4-year-olds. This study, designed by a music therapist, pediatric neurologist, nurse, and researcher, reflected the impact of lullabies as being especially significant in their inherent ability to adhere to a caregiver's intentions, ancestry, and/or heritage through honoring the caregiver's music and encouraging its use. The researchers entitle this sacred usage as "song of kin." Using songs of kin can provide infants with a recognizable melody that has the ability to calm, soothe, and sedate (Loewy, in press). Especially during circumstances of stress, songs of kin can serve as transitional objects (Winnicott, 1971), whereby the most invasive of experiences (EEG) or separations can be withstood with ease. Healthy infants process musical stimuli in a fashion similar to that of an adult. Their attentiveness and behaviors change in relation to the type of song sung, perhaps an indication that the infant's positive response to infant-directed singing is a factor in parent's singing behavior. This reciprocal interaction may contribute to the overall well-being of the infant, suggesting there is a biological propensity in mothers to sing and for infants to respond in a positive manner, creating a communicative continuum (Trehub, 2001, 2003).

There can be wide variation in the structural characteristics of the lullaby based on the instrumentation, performer interpretation (articulation and musicality), and overall quality of the voice or recording and playback equipment (if presenting recorded music). There has been little discussion in the literature of the relationship between infant outcomes and the musical characteristics of the stimulus, such as pitch, dynamics, timbre, and harmony. These structural characteristics can affect the responses of the infants. From a clinical perspective, a lack of consideration of the structural characteristics of the music on the physiological, psychosocial, and behavioral responses of the infant can be problematic in that they can potentially have a negative effect on the infant. Thus, in research and clinical practice, the musical selections themselves can be consequential.

Music-based stimuli appropriate for the NICU demonstrate preferred characteristics of limited accompaniments, simple rhythms, consistent dynamic levels, steady tempos, lilting melodies, and a structured and organized form that is soothing and comforting (Bates, Brez, & Kaplan, 2003; Hanson-Abromeit, 2003; Loewy, in press, Shoemark, 1999; Standley, 2001a, 2001b, 2002). Systematic tools that provide an objective way to carefully select recorded music for premature infants are in development (Bates, Kaplan, Reed, & Whitmer,

2005), but require a knowledge base and understanding of music terminology. Based on a review of the developmental science literature, music selected for use in the NICU, presented as a recording or sung/played by a person, should be culturally sensitive (Loewy, 2004) and simple—with few changes or pauses, organized, predictable, repetitive, smooth, soothing, stable, slow, flowing, and comfortable (Hanson-Abromeit, 2006).

Music Therapy Clinical Programs in the NICU

There are currently few comprehensive clinical music therapy programs in the NICU; those that exist value the services offered by music therapy. Neonatal music therapists provide direct and/or indirect clinical services and education to infants, their families, and staff serving the NICU. Some music therapists serve the NICU only when a referral is made, while others are assigned to the NICU as their primary practice area. This section of the chapter is written from the perspective of the music therapist whose primary role in the hospital is as a clinician on the NICU.

Referral for Services

Referral for music therapy services on the NICU will be dependent on a number of theoretical and contextual factors, such as the prevailing channels for referral in the hospital, the type of music therapy program that has been implemented on the unit, the relationship with the staff, the expertise of the music therapist, and the amount of clinical time the therapist has available or is allocated for services on the unit. Referral criteria reflect these factors in its detail. For example, the referral criteria at one Midwestern hospital reflected the developmental care practices of the unit, nursing and **neonatology** input, the clinical expertise of the music therapist, and the needs of the infants and families.

Referrals may be individually generated or based on predetermined criteria (e.g., all babies with a particular condition are referred). Individual referrals can be made by various professional caregivers (nurses, doctors, social workers, physical or occupational therapists, child life specialists), and by families. Typically, the neonatologist will sign the referral form, even when generated by someone else, although this may vary depending on the hospital protocol. In addition to physician-approved referral, some NICUs may encourage or require a parental consent for music therapy services.

Standing referrals indicate that music therapy is ordered for each infant that meets the established criteria in which case individual and physician-approved referrals are not necessary. Specific parental consent may also not be necessarily required with standing referrals. However, as family-centered practice emerges as a model of care, acknowledgment that nothing should happen to the infant without family involvement promotes consultation with the family prior to providing services. In fact, there may be times when the primary referral for music therapy may include one or more family members (parents, siblings, extended family). The relationship of the parent-infant dyad is important for development, and families are an integral part of the care of their infant. Their well-being is a primary consideration within a family-centered care approach.

In one clinical program, the referral process began as individually generated. Once the program was established and the efficacy of the services was evident, music therapy was added to nursing services developmental standards of practice for premature infants. Thus, in this program, the music therapist assesses each hospitalized infant at 29 weeks gestational age for some level of services. In this hospital the referral criteria is:

- At least 1 week old and a minimum of 29 weeks gestational age
- Medically stable (unless otherwise indicated)
- Need for prolonged or high percentage of supplemental oxygen
- Agitated and/or unorganized behaviors
- Prolonged hospitalization expected

In an overseas hospital, the reverse development has occurred. Early in the service, all infants who were deemed "old enough" were referred, whereas now the referring staff is well educated about referral criteria and think carefully about who should receive priority. In this case, priority is given for cases where:

- State issues exist—infant is irritable, has trouble making transition in state (wake to sleep, etc.)
- Limitation imposed by care regime means the infant has limited opportunities for appropriate developmental activity
- Family is unavailable either psycho-emotionally or physically
- Mother, father, or caregivers are in need of support to affirm their role as primary nurturer

In both of the above cases, the acknowledgment is that music therapy is a valuable service that plays a key role in the well-being of infants. The permutations for referrals will be many and varied and context-dependent.

In a third inner city hospital, music therapy expanded from a service for well-care term babies in Pediatrics. Music therapists began by attending NICU rounds and simply observing the infants for approximately 6 months before piloting a program of five cases. These cases were reviewed and discussed individually with each member of the team and then, collectively, the following Criteria for Referral was developed for babies >32 weeks (or younger in special cases when approved by the doctor on a case-by-case basis).

Initial referrals may be made informally via a phone call, conversation, or email, each followed by an official consult form. The hospital may have a standard referral or consultation form, or the music therapist may design a form relevant to the needs and referral criteria of the music therapy program. A music therapist and team designed referral form fitting the above established criteria serves to educate the staff to the various issues that can be addressed through music therapy. The referral form in Figure 1 is an example.

Music Therapy Referral Criteria
The Louis and Lucille Armstrong Music Therapy Program
Beth Israel Medical Center
(developed by J. V. Loewy, 2000)

I. Bonding: Parents and infants (identified by the team) that are in need of collaborative experiences may be referred. Incorporating Brazelton's Neonatal Behavioral Assessment Scale, musical focus will emphasize infant–parent attachment. Music and soft singing with skin-to-skin contact will be encouraged. Melodic (3–5 note) vocalizations will be modeled and simple lullabies will be encouraged for use by mom/dad/caretaker. The parent–infant dynamic will be strengthened as the use of soft sounds (repeated sung phrases) will be patterned for use during times of sleep, transitions, and/or separations.

II. Irritability/Crying (Intense high pitched): Music (lullabies and toning) will be offered as a means to contain the sound environment for the infant in distress. Toning will be provided as a blanket of steady sound to comfort and sustain a homeostatic environment. Tones enable the infant to trust his/her surroundings and offer an atmosphere of predictability. Human voice sounds made through vocal tones provide an atmosphere of safety, which induces sleep and assists in relaxation.

III. Respiratory Difficulties: The Gato box and breath sounds can be useful in helping the infant synchronize and regulate the rhythm of his/her breath. The Gato box provides a predictable rhythm that mimics the sound of a human heart.

The infant can entrain to the provided rhythm, which can lengthen and ease the meter of the breath. The breath voice is soothing and provides a flowing release of oxygen, which can enhance the breathing process. The ocean disc provides an interuterine sound environment that provides safety and familiarity, stimulating the infant's breathing process.

IV. Feeding/Sucking/Weight Gain: Comfort sounds may be a catalyst for inducing gurgles and vegetative sucking. Soft, rhythmic sound scaping prior to feeding may assist in the infant's coordination with sucking, swallowing, and breathing. Nutritive sucking with rhythmic reinforcement may help infants maintain steady mouth motion, which can be further sustained through melodic holding during feedings.

V. Sedation/Sleep/Pain: Music therapy can provide an environment of safety during painful procedures. Tonic tones that match the pitch of the infant's cry, entrained with the meter of the breath, can ease and alter the experience/perception of pain. Using the Attia (et al) infant pain scale, the music therapist can assess the level of pain and distract the infant from attending to the painful stimuli. Music can assist the infant in reconstitution at postprocedure time. Music therapy can be used in conjunction with (complementary) or as an alternative pharmacological sedation, depending upon the MD order.

For the infant who appears overstimulated and/or is in need of sleep, simple lullabies containing < 5-note melodies can provide an aural atmosphere of nurturance. Altering the tempo and meter of the lullaby can help the infant relax and shift gradually into a sleep state.

VI. Self Regulation: Central to the infant's development is his/her ability to self-regulate. Simple, consistent rhythms and melodies can help the infant organize and acclimate to the environment. Predictable, ordered aspects of music provide structure that assists in the development of self-nurturing behavior, physiological organization, and neurological pathways.

Music Therapy NICU Referral Form
Beth Israel Medical Center

Referrals may be made by the nurse practitioner, case manager, and residents but must have the consent of the attending physician and the parent/caretaker.

The age for referrals is >32 weeks unless approved on a case-by-case basis by the attending physician. If there are any questions or concerns, call Dr. Joanne Loewy at 420-XXXX or beeper XXXXX.

Infant's name_____

Gestational age_____ Chronological age_____

Diagnosis_____

Name of consenting Attending Physician: _____ Beeper_____

Family informed by _____ Beeper_____

Reason for Referral: (Check all of the following that apply and write in any comments).

_____Bonding: Caretakers and infants that are in need of collaborative experiences.

        Comments: _____

_____Psychosocial Issues: ACS hold, intrauterine exposure to drugs or alcohol, trauma, stress, violence, family illness, separation/divorce.
        Specify:_____

_____Respiratory difficulties: _____Crying/Irritability:

_____Feeding/Sucking/Weight Gain   _____Sedation/Sleep/Pain:

_____Difficulty sleeping   _____Requires music assistance for
                                                     sedation during procedure:
                                                     (date/time:)

_____Self-Regulation:

Comments:

_____   Beeper/extension:_____   Date:_____
        Person referring

Please place this form in music therapy referral box located at the nursing station.

Figure 1. **Music Therapy NICU Referral Form**

Assessment in the NICU

The dominant model of service provision in NICUs is developmental care. Based on the Neonatal Individualized Developmental Care and Assessment Program (NIDCAP) model, it informs all the treatment process and care procedures, including neonatal music therapy. Knowledge and understanding of NIDCAP informs assessment, the selection of stimuli, interventions, and evaluation of outcomes (Hanson-Abromeit, 2003). The cornerstones of NIDCAP indicate modified caregiving within the context of family-centered individualized interventions (Als, 1996). Based on the Brazelton Neonatal Behavioral Assessment Scale (BNBAS), the Assessment of Preterm Infants' Behavior (APIB) is an assessment tool designed for use specifically with premature infants, as well as high risk and healthy full-term infants (Als, 1982, 1986, 1996; Als, Butler, Kosta, & McAnulty, 2005). The APIB uses specific tasks to determine the regulation and balance of the infant's subsystems and identifies the infant's response in three ways: tasks that are already well integrated, tasks that stress the infant but can be handled with support, and tasks that are clearly not appropriate for the infant at a particular stage. These assessment tasks are "graded sequences of increasingly vigorous environmental inputs or packages, moving from distal stimulation presented during sleep to mild tactile stimulation, to medium stimulation paired with vestibular stimulation" (Als, 1986, p. 18). These are summarized in Table 1 for clarification.

It is through the behavioral subsystems that infants communicate their stress and disorganization, or their self-regulation that is balanced and competent for a particular task or stimulus (Fischer & Als, 2004). The APIB reports individual responses to the tasks through a classification of stress and defense behaviors and self-regulatory and approach behaviors allowing for the implementation of appropriate developmental goals. Behaviors are categorized by the autonomic, motor, and state subsystems. Autonomic stress and defense behaviors can include seizures, respiratory pauses, irregular breathing and holding of breath, color changes, spitting up, hiccoughing, gasping, coughing, yawning, sighing, startling, and sneezing. Motor stress signals can include flaccidity; hyperextensions of legs, arms, or trunk; fingers plays; facial grimacing or hyper flexions; as well as frantic activity and squirming. Stress signals for state-related behaviors could include sleeplessness, crying, irritability, hyper alertness, staring, and roving eye movements (Als, 1982, 1986, 1995).

Stability of the autonomic system can be indicated by smooth respirations and a pink, stable color. Motor stability indicators include regulated muscle tone, smooth movements, hand clasping, sucking, and hand-to-mouth actions. The infant has stable state and attention regulation when it demonstrates clear, robust sleep states, rhythmical crying, the ability to self quiet, alertness, animated facial expression, cooing, and smiling (Als, 1982, 1986, 1995). The goal of this assessment is to clearly understand the infant's observable behaviors in response to sensory stimulation. The basis of the APIB is that the infant will demonstrate behaviors that protect it from inappropriate stimuli in timing, complexity and intensity, and will be able to maintain a balanced integration of its subsystems, as well as an ability to attend to stimuli that are appropriately timed, complex, and intense (Als, 1986).

Table 1

Behaviors that Indicate Stress and Self-Regulation in the Premature Infant (Als, 1982, 1986; Klein, 2008)

Vital Signs	Indicators of Stress	Indicators of Self-Regulation
	Heart Rate < 120 or > 160	Heart Rate > 120 and < 160
	Respiration Rate < 40 or > 60	Respiration Rate > 40 and < 60
	SaO2 $\leq$ 95	SaO2 > 88 and < 95
	TcPO2 < 55 > 80	TcPO2 > 55 < 80
Respiratory Effect	Irregular	Regular
	Slow	
	Fast	
	Pause	
Color	Jaundice	Pink
	Pale	
	Webb	
	Red	
	Dusky (purple)	
	Cyanosis (blue)	
Visceral/Respiratory	Spit up	Visceral stability
	Gag	
	Burp	
	Hiccough	
	BM Grunt	
	Sounds	
	Sign (depending on frequency)	
	Gasp	
Attention	Fuss	Face Open
	Yawn	Frown (knits brows)
	Sneeze	Ooh Face
	Eye Floating	Cooing
	Avert	Speech Movement
Face	Tongue Extension	Hand on Face
	Gape Face	Smile
		Grimace (extend face)
		Mouthing (soft, relaxed, repeated)
		Suck Search
		Sucking

Table 1—Continued

Motor – Extremities	Finger Splay	Hand Clasp (at midline)
	Airplane (arms out shoulder level)	Foot Clasp (at midline)
	Salute (extended arms front)	Hand to Mouth
	Sitting on air (extended legs)	Grasping (active movements)
	Fisting (tight hold self)	Holding on (relaxed hold other)
Motor – Arms	Flaccid Arms	Smooth Movement Arms
	Active Extend Arms	Active Tucked Arms
	Posture Extend Arms	Posture Tucked Arms
Motor – Legs	Flaccid Legs	Smooth Movement
	Active Extend	Active Tucked
	Posture Extend	Posture Tucked
	Leg Brace (against something)	
Motor – Trunk	Stretch/Drown (panic with respiratory pause)	Smooth Movement
		Tuck Trunk
	Diffuse Squirm	
	Arch	
Motor – Other	Tremor (body)	
	Startle (jumping)	
	Twitch (isolated body parts)	

In addition to the neurobehavioral subsystems, it is also important for the music therapist to understand the development of sensory system organization. It has been established that the onset of the sensory systems develop in a sequence of tactile, vestibular, gustatory-olfactory, auditory, and visual (Gottleib, 1983; Lickliter, 1993). Furthermore, it is believed that the sensory systems are also reciprocal in their development, in that the maturity of early sensory systems influences the development of later systems. This is especially relevant to the infant in the NICU in that overstimulation of the earlier developing systems can have detrimental effects on the later developing systems (Lickliter, 1993). In fact, there is some speculation that premature birth alters the neurosensory sequence (Graven, 2000).

Practicing within a developmental care model and understanding the neurobehavioral and neurosensory system development informs the assessment process for music therapy. Due to the developmental changes normal to infancy, complicated by the medical intensity of prematurity or critical illness, assessment with these infants is ongoing. Selective assessment follows the referral and involves gathering of information related to history of the infant (prenatal care, birth, hospital course, medications) by reading the hospital charts and talking with the staff and family. Conversation with staff and family provides information on the family situation (challenges, coping, support systems); how the infant responds overall to sensory stimulation and the strategies family and staff have used to support the infant; and what the intended hospital course or prognosis is for the infant. The NICU Music Therapy Assessment Summary (Figure 2) can be used to gather and summarize the selective assessment information.

Observation of the infant in the nursery environment provides an infant-specific assessment. This observation period allows the music therapist to watch the infant for stress and self-regulatory behavioral responses to the environment and stimuli prior to the introduction of music-based stimuli. The behavioral observation also informs the therapist of the idiosyncratic behavioral cues of the infant helping the therapist identify and recognize the frequency of stress and self-regulatory behaviors in response to environmental and caregiving stimuli. These behavioral cues provide indicators useful to the music therapist of appropriateness for music therapy and communicate the necessity of adaptation during intervention. The Observation Sheet (Figure 3) from the NIDCAP Assessment of Preterm Infant Development (APID) (Als, 1999) can be used to gather and summarize the selective assessment information. With training and mentorship under a NIDCAP certified nurse, the music therapist can learn to identify specific stress and self-regulatory behaviors of the premature infant. It is important to note that the music therapist may need to practice multiple patient-specific observational assessments until behavioral markers are clearly and correctly interpreted with inter- and intra-rater reliability, prior to the implementation of any interventions.

The infant-specific observational assessment teaches the music therapist about the communicative behavioral cues of the individual infant. This allows the therapist to be alert to cues during the implementation of interventions and to assess the direction of the intervention. The running assessment allows for therapist adaptation and modification of the interventions in response to the behavioral and physiological cues of the infant. Ongoing observation is essential to evaluate the response to sensory (musical and other) stimuli.

Assessment in the NICU

Selective assessment: Reading of charts and talking with staff and family
NICU Music Therapy Assessment Summary

Infant-specific assessment: Observational assessment of infant behaviors in relationship to their environment and stimuli
Observation Form (NIDCAP Model)

Running assessment: Ongoing observation during MT sessions; therapist adapts and responds to observed behaviors
NICU MT Program Patient Intervention Tracking

NICU Music Therapy Assessment Summary

Name _____

Hospital # _____

Referral Date _____

INFANT BIRTH HISTORY

DOB _____ GA at birth _____

Mode of Delivery _____

Apgars _____ 1min _____ 5min

Birthweight _____ g

LBW   VLBW _____ ELBW

Length _____ cm

Head Circumference _____ cm

Diagnosis _____

_____

Complications of birth _____

_____

Other birth information _____

_____

Respiratory Assistance:

- ❏ HVF – settings _____
- ❏ CPAP – settings _____
- ❏ Nasal Canula – settings _____
- ❏ Room Air - settings _____
- ❏ Other – settings _____

Medications:

- ❏ *Sedatives:* Morphine (MS04)   Ativan
      Lozepan   Fentanyl   Other
- ❏ *Diuretics:*   Lasix   Other
- ❏ *Anticonvulsants:* Phenobarb   Idilamtin
           Other
- ❏ *Steroids:* Dexamethosone Decadron Other
- ❏ *Antibiotics:* Ampillician   Gentamyacin
      Vancomyocin   Pepracillian   Other
- ❏ *Other:*   Caffeine   Theophylline

FAMILY INFORMATION

Mother's Name _____

Mother's age _____

Father's Name _____

Father's Age _____

Sibling _____ Age _____

Sibling _____ Age _____

Sibling _____ Age _____

Sibling _____ Age _____

Family Availability/Restrictions: _____

_____

Date: _____

Location: _____

6/2003 D. Hanson-Abromeit

Assessment: _____

SOCIAL HISTORY

_____

_____

_____

MATERNAL HISTORY

Grava _____   Para _____

Prenatal Care/Complications: _____

_____

_____

Labor & Delivery: _____

_____

Medications: _____

_____

Other: _____

HOSPITAL COURSE

Current Respiratory Support:

- ❏ HVF – settings _____
- ❏ CPAP – settings _____
- ❏ Nasal Canula – settings _____
- ❏ Room Air - settings _____
- ❏ Other – settings _____

Current Medications:

- ❏ *Sedatives:* Morphine (MS04)   Ativan
      Lozepan   Fentanyl   Other
- ❏ *Diuretics:*   Lasix   Other
- ❏ *Anticonvulsants:* Phenobarb   Idilamtin
           Other
- ❏ *Steroids:* Dexamethosone Decadron Other
- ❏ *Antibiotics:* Ampillician   Gentamyacin
      Vancomyocin   Pepracillian   Other
- ❏ *Other:*   Caffeine   Theophylline

Current Feeding/Nutrition

Time _____   Type _____

Medical Problems:

Acidosis (pH<7.3)   Anemia   Apnea
Bleeding tendency   BPD   Bradycardia
Desaturations   Feeding difficulty
Hyperbilirubinemia (lights)   Hydrocephalus
Hypoglycemia   Hypotension   Hypoxic Events
IVH grade _____ R _____ L   NEC   Osteopenia
PDA   Pheumothorax RDS
Renal   ROP Stage _____ R _____ L
Seizures   Sepsis   Tracheostomy

Hearing Screen: Attempt _____ Passed _____

Figure 2. NICU Music Therapy Assessment Summary

OBSERVATION SHEET   Name:_____ Date:_____ Sheet Number:_____

	Time:	0-2	3-4	5-6	7-8	9-10			Time:	0-2	3-4	5-6	7-8	9-10
Resp:	Regular						State:	1A						
	Irregular							1B						
	Slow							2A						
	Fast							2B						
	Pause							3A						
Color:	Jaundice							3B						
	Pink							4A						
	Pale							4B						
	Webb							5A						
	Red							5B						
	Dusky							6A						
	Blue							6B						
	Tremor							AA						
	Startle						Face (cont.):	Mouthing						
	Twitch Face							Suck Search						
	Twitch Body							Sucking						
	Twitch Extremities						Extrem.:	Finger Splay						
Visceral/ Resp:	Spit up							Airplane						
	Gag							Salute						
	Burp							Sitting On Air						
	Hiccough							Hand Clasp						
	BM Grunt							Foot Clasp						
	Sounds							Hand to Mouth						
	Sigh							Grasping						
	Gasp							Holding On						
Motor:	Flaccid Arm(s)							Fisting						
	Flaccid leg(s)						Attention:	Fuss						
	Flexed/ Tucked Arms Act./Post.							Yawn						
	Flexed/ Tucked Legs Act./Post.							Sneeze						
	Extend Arms Act./Post.							Face Open						
	Extend Legs Act./Post.							Eye Floating						
	Smooth Mvmt Arms							Avert						
	Smooth Mvmt Legs							Frown						
	Smooth Mvmt Trunk							Ooh Face						
	Stretch/Drown							Locking						
	Diffuse Squirm							Cooing						
	Arch							Speech Mvmt.						
	Tuck Trunk						Posture:	(Prone, Supine, Side)						
	Leg Brace						Head:	(Right, Left, Middle)						
Face:	Tongue Extension						Location:	(Crib, Incubator, Held)						
	Hand on Face						Manipulation:							
	Gape Face							Heart Rate						
	Grimace							Respiration Rate						
	Smile							TcPO$_2$/SaO$_2$						

Reprinted with permission by the NIDCAP Federation International, Dr. H. Als, President. Training of the NICU Nurses at the University of Iowa Children's Hospital was completed in 1998 by Jean Gardner Cole, MS, Director/NIDCAP at Boston Medical Center. Als, H. (1999). Reading the premature infant. In E. Goldson (Ed.). *Nurturing the premature infant: Developmental interventions in the Neonatal Intensive Care Nursery* (pp. 18–85). New York: Oxford University Press.

Figure 3. **Observation Form (NIDCAP Model)**

Goals for Music Therapy in the NICU

There are three broad goal areas for music therapy practice in the NICU: to support the neurobehavioral and sensory system development of the infant; to increase developmental competence across domains (social/emotional, cognitive, motor, and communication); and to increase opportunities for culturally sensitive developmentally appropriate parent–infant interactions. These goal areas are specific to the developmental trajectory of the infant and are intentionally broad so that objectives can be individualized to the infant's changing needs.

Infants born prematurely, and those full-term infants demonstrating disorganized behaviors, will have a goal area focus on the neurobehavioral and sensory system development. Once an infant has reached full-term gestational markers and is able to handle multiple sensory stimuli in an organized and self-regulated manner, the goal focus can be enhanced to a goal that focuses on a normal infant development trajectory. Due to prolonged hospitalization and medical complications, infants may present an uneven developmental curve; that is, they may be more competent in one area than in another or may have varying levels of competence depending on the stimulation. Objectives will most likely have to scaffold to support developmental competency. Family-centered objectives are appropriate and necessary throughout hospitalization. Adaptations to the infant stability should be made in order to encourage positive and reciprocal parent-infant interactions.

Intervention Environments

Most interventions in the NICU are individualized to the infant and family. Infant follow-up and outpatient services may incorporate group experiences. During hospitalization, family support groups may be offered as part of the music therapy program. Family-centered care is the cornerstone of practice philosophies in the hospital setting.

Family-Centered Care in NICU

The Institute for Family-Centered Care (2007) defines *family-centered care* as "an approach to the planning, delivery, and evaluation of health care that is grounded in mutually beneficial partnerships among health care providers, patients, and families." This means that, during a hospital admission, care is planned for the whole family, not just the individual child (Shields, Pratt, Davis, & Hunter, 2007). Services that provide encouragement, respect, education, and active listening will offer containment and in turn help parents to contain and support their infant (Harris, 2005; Robertson, 2005).

While early hospitalization may have a long-term impact on the mother-infant relationship (Minde, 1999), family-centered care promotes the empowerment of parents to care and advocate for their infant (Shoemark, 2004). The music therapist calls on diverse methods to create an experience of music with infants and families, but first must create a context of respect and collaboration with the infant's family. Through reflexive discussions,

Shoemark and Dearn (2008) identified seven key themes, presented below, in providing family-centered music therapy service for families that include a hospitalized infant.

Key Themes of Family-Centered Music Therapy

(Shoemark & Dearn, 2008)

1. The essential character of the music therapist
2. Music therapy as a triadic relationship (parent, infant, and therapist)
3. Endurance of the relationship throughout the infant's admission
4. Parental joy during music therapy
5. Acknowledging the whole child
6. Music therapy as a context for a contingent relationship
7. Building memories in case life is short

Parents endure ongoing concern and uncertainty about their infant's survival (Hurst, 2001; Prentice & Stainton, 2003). The loss of choice and control about how to care for their infant as well as subsequent attachment difficulties may lead to feelings of intimidation, grief, and inadequacy (McGrath, 2001). Further, a lack of understanding of the different behaviors displayed by premature and medically compromised infants can impact their contingent relationship and may compromise the long-term attachment relationship so important to the infant's development (Van Beek & Samson, 1994; Vandenburg, 2000). The absence of traditional parental opportunities to bond can be difficult for caregivers of infants who are born prematurely. They often feel anxious, confused, guilty, and disempowered. Staff, as well, commonly report an experience of overwhelm paralleling that of the infants and notice how at times this can lead to desensitization to their work and to the environment. The profound sensory bombardment of the NICU directly correlates to current definitions of trauma as an overwhelming life experience. Kristen Stewart (in press), a music therapist who has advanced training and certification in trauma and a specialization in NICU music therapy, introduces an NICU music therapy model based on current trauma theory in her development of "PATTERNS" (Preventative Approach to Traumatic Experience by Resourcing the Nervous System). This model synchronizes multifaceted concepts of preterm infant development, the NICU care environment, music and music therapy practices, and trauma renegotiation principles, emphasizing the unique role of music and music therapy across the spectrum of traumatic experience for the preterm infant and his or her family of caregivers.

Family education about the naturally occurring musical nature of the parent-infant relationship and music as a therapy on the NICU contribute to the potential of a positive experience for families with their infants. Handouts and flyers placed at bedside, in the parent lounge, and as inserts in the parent information packet all provide opportunities to inform families about developmental uses of music for their infant. Information can also be provided on the value of music therapy for parent and sibling support.

One such group currently being developed is looking at improving secure attachment between the parent and child through an interdisciplinary parent education group. At the Children's Hospital of Iowa, it was recognized that parents would be interested in participating in an education group that facilitated education, normalcy, and emotional needs related to coping with hospitalization. The NICU music therapist, child life specialist, and social worker have coordinated the Parent Infant Attachment Group with the intention to decrease parent anxiety and facilitate parent confidence to interact with their infant. The desired outcome is to promote secure parent-infant attachment, despite the medical, physical, and emotional barriers of extended hospitalization. The Parent Infant Attachment Group provides education on various issues related to dealing with hospitalization and prematurity (e.g., sensory integration, appropriate developmental materials/toys, early infant development, noise vs. sound, safety), normalized parent activities, and parent self-nurturing. Weekly group sessions cover these concepts through creative, experiential, and educational-based interventions offered by a comprehensive multidisciplinary team (K. Hawkins, personal communication, July 8, 2008). At Beth Israel Medical Center, a weekly group on the maternity unit combines high-risk pregnancy couples-in-waiting with healthy newborn babies and parents and neighboring NICU babies and/or their parents. The group is called "Music and Your Baby." Inter-treating parents and caregivers at their varying levels of trauma, whether they are experiencing newfound joy (healthy newborn parents and babies) or are stuck within a traumatic (NICU parent) or apprehensive (high-risk pregnancy) waiting stage, can provide parents with a community of possibilities. Mixing healthy babies with their parents amidst apprehensive high-risk pregnant parents and fearful NICU parents, as well as nurses and doctors, provides a means of hope and inspiration for all involved. Music therapy, demonstrating specific aspects of bonding that foster emotional growth, is a valued service for these patients.

Beyond a general education process, some neonatal music therapy programs give focus in individualized services to the role that mother's emotional status plays in the development of attachment when the mother-infant relationship is at risk. This may include an assessment of how music therapy treatment might be most effectively pursued for both mother/ parent/caregiver and infant. An avoidance of this evaluation could pose significant threats to the fragile baby and growing relationship. If the mother has not recognized and addressed her own feelings of anxiety associated with having an infant prematurely or an infant who may be dangerously ill, her provision of music could be contraindicated. Themes of anxiety and separation may undermine the parents' attachment abilities (Harris, 2005) and distort contingent interaction.

Two European music therapists provided a valuable introduction to this important topic. Nöcker-Ribaupierre (2004) studied the short- and long-term effects of the maternal voice on the behaviors of very low birth weight infants in conjunction with their mothers and how this affected the attachment process. Lenz (1998) looked at interactional disorders in terms of aspects of bonding between mothers and infants. Staff may identify referrals in this domain as "psychosocial needs" of the mother. This may also be presented as parental occurrences, such as loss of a twin, previous birth trauma, drug use, domestic violence, and first-time parenting. There are several studies that recognize the importance of mother's voice and the infant's ability to recognize both mother's and father's voice (Coleman et al., 1997; Rock et al., 1999).

While the vast majority of NICU programs may retain a focus on the infant, some will have the opportunity to shift focus to the family and work primarily with the parents rather than the infant. After all, it is hoped that the relationship with the therapist is short-lived and that the family will go home with a healthy infant for a long life together. Therefore, providing a service that acknowledges the family as the therapeutic unit from the beginning preserves the natural relationship. The therapist is not "the expert" in a triadic relationship with the mother and infant, but rather a translator of knowledge, a facilitator, and a container for the experience. The potential of the expanded capacity in this partnership is to rebuild moments of joyful experience through attuned interplay (Shoemark, 2000).

Addressing the needs of the parent may be a primary modality of treatment prior to the music therapist working with the infant, or infant and parent together. The music provided for the struggling infant is most beneficial when therapists can address the music provider and how effective he or she is in creating an environment of **homeostasis** for the dyad. Additional understanding and supportive interventions in the family context are important areas for exploration in neonatal music therapy.

In all of this, it is important to remember that, at times, music therapy may be contraindicated. From basic stimulation through to harmful interplay, the music therapist must honestly assess the role of music for the infant and the family. If the service is not useful at the time, this must be explained carefully to ensure there is no sense of "failure" for the family. In some cases (e.g., the infant is too immature to make use of recorded music), the situation may be reviewed on a progressive basis, allowing an ongoing relationship of support to evolve in the meantime. Areas of for future consideration within this more music psychotherapeutic domain include how music therapists might work with postpartum depression, which can be exacerbated when one's infant is facing extremely fragile conditions; how bonding can occur when the mother's ability to provide touch and acoustic stimulation may be countertherapeutic; and how music therapy can address parent anxiety.

Co-treatment in the NICU

In addition to the medical and nursing staff, other adjunctive therapies provide services in the NICU. Due to the medical fragility of the infants, co-treatment is not regular on the NICU. However, coordinated treatment is necessary to ensure timely scheduling of interventions that foster an environment that is supportive and not overstimulating to the infant. For example, the NICU child life specialist, physical therapist, occupational therapist, and music therapist may all receive referrals for the same infant at, or around, the same time. It is important that these clinicians coordinate their visits to best meet the needs of the infant and family (Abrams et al., 2000).

Staff education is a vital component of the adjunctive therapies in the NICU to ensure appropriate referrals and support from the nursing staff. Neonatal nurses receive continuous education and training, and these therapies benefit from being part of the training and education schedule. A shared presentation can minimize the time commitment of the individual therapy staff, as well as inform and educate one another on the differing therapies in the NICU.

Interventions in the NICU

The environment of the NICU is constantly changing due to a variety of factors such as the time of day, staffing, infant development and medical stability, family needs and availability, and environmental influences. Each interaction with the infant and family must take into account these ever-changing factors prior to, during, and after an intervention. Before the music therapist begins a session, a brief assessment period should occur involving conversation with the nurse and family regarding changes and current status, observation of the infant's behaviors at that particular time, and determination of intervention appropriateness. Responsiveness to the infant is highly important and the music therapist must be aware of the infant's responses to the nuances of the stimulus being presented. Response and adaptation to the behaviors should be timely.

The "task" of the premature infant is to respond to the therapist-presented stimulus. Upon presentation of the stimulus, the therapist observes and responds to behaviors. If the infant handles the task in a well-integrated manner indicated by self-regulatory responses, the therapist could gradually increase the level of sensory stimulation. If the task appears stressful, indicated by minimal and subtle stress behaviors, the therapist will decrease the level of sensory stimulation and add supports (e.g., shift humming from song to repetitive phrase, add a hand on top of head, or finger to hold). If stress behaviors continue or intensify, then the infant is clearly not able to handle the task at this point. The stimulus should be stopped and the therapist should support the infant's return to homeostasis (e.g., provide a pacifier, gentle hold, or physical touch) and monitor for complications.

It is critical that the therapist recognize the infant's early stress behaviors and allow him or her to disengage in order to avoid overstimulation. Once a threshold is determined, a therapist should never push an infant to determine how much stimulation can be tolerated, as this could have potentially negative outcomes. The therapist should never hesitate to ask for support from the nursing staff to assist an infant who is struggling. Post-session observation and follow-up with the nursing staff and family are important components of the music therapy session.

A decision tree is available to guide how the music therapist directs the stimulation in response to the infant. The original decision tree was developed as part of a nursing protocol for multimodal stimulation (Burns, Cunningham, White-Traut, Silvestri, & Nelson, 1994). The nursing protocol was adapted to include humming as the auditory stimulation (Standley, 1998), and the decision tree was modified for use in the music therapy session (Shoemark, 1999).

Therapist Response to Infant Behaviors During Music Therapy

Infant handles task in a well-integrated manner.
Therapist gradually increases level of sensory stimulation.

Infant finds task is stressful, but can be handled with support.
Therapist decreases sensory stimulation and adds supports.

Infant behaviors indicate that task is clearly not appropriate for the infant at this stage.
Therapist stops intervention and supports infant's return to homeostasis; watches for complications.

Although premature infants exhibit a wide variety of behavioral responses by the time they reach term age, caregivers must be sensitive to the infants' physiological cues of overstimulation and their need for supportive comfort measures (Stjernqvist & Svenningsen, 1990). Minimizing behaviors that elicit stress and supporting behaviors that indicate self-regulation will encourage organization in the behavior states of premature infants and improve their medical and developmental outcomes (Als, 1986). Premature infant behavior state criteria are outlined in Table 2. Behaviors that demonstrate organization or disorganization are indicated for each behavior state (Als, 1995).

The Phases of Interplay (Shoemark, 2008) provides a framework for clinician decisions in response to infant cues. While outlined in response to work with full-term hospitalized infants, the framework can inform work with other infants and even other populations where interpretation of responses is needed (Shoemark, 2008). This framework recognizes the reality that when working the premature and medically fragile full-term infant, the interplay is often near or at the infant's threshold for stimulation. This means that, almost inevitably, interplay will exceed the infant's threshold. Therefore, while it is essential that the therapist understand how to adjust the quality and intensity of the interplay to keep the infant safe, it is just as important to understand how to reduce and support the infant when the threshold is traversed (Shoemark, 2008).

Music Therapy Intervention Techniques in the NICU

A myriad of techniques have been demonstrated, through research and clinical evidence, to be effective with infants in the NICU. Some NICUs use recorded music, either commercially available or family-created; others utilize live singing or accompaniment by a board certified music therapist. Current development of live entrained music techniques implementing instruments that replicate heart and womb sounds are being investigated (Loewy & Stewart, 2008). Several techniques will be only referenced in this chapter, as they

Table 2

Behaviors in the Premature Infant that Indicate State Modulation (Als, 1995)

Sleep States:

Deep Sleep	Disorganized	Breathing in rhythm with respirator, eyes closed, no eye movements, quiet facial expression, poor color, no spontaneous activity
	Organized	Regular breathing, eyes closed, no eye movements, relaxed facial expression, no spontaneous activity, occasional isolated startles
Light Sleep	Disorganized	Eyes closed, REM, disorganized movements, irregular respirations, sucking, grimacing, poor color
	Organized	REM, dampened startles, lower amplitude movements, regular respirations, mild sucking, infrequent sighs or smiles

Transitional States:

Drowsy	Disorganized	Eyes open or closed, eyelids fluttering or blinking in exaggerated fashion, variable activity level, startles, fussing, facial grimacing, vocalization
	Organized	Robustly drowsy, little vocalization or facial grimacing

Awake States:

Quietly awake	Disorganized	Low: Diffuse awakeness, quiet, minimal motor activity, eyes glazed or dull, little energy, looks through rather than at a subject High: Hyperalert, impression of panic, appears to be hooked to the stimulus, hard to break gaze
	Organized	Bright shiny eyes, animated facial expressions, able to process stimulation, minimal motor activity
Actively awake and aroused	Disorganized	Eyes may or may not be open, motor arousal, distressed facial expression, grimacing, vocal fussing
	Organized	Robustly actively aroused, eyes may or may not be open, well defined motor activity, may be fussy, but not hard crying
Highly aroused, agitated, upset, and/or crying	Disorganized	Intense upset, grimace and cry face; cry sound may be strained, weak or absent, high intensity of upset
	Organized	Robust high arousal with rhythmic, intense, lusty, vigorous crying

are reported in detail in another American Music Therapy Association publication (Standley, 2003). It is important to note that interventions should be tailored to the individual responses of the infants, rather than strictly adhering to a prescribed protocol or written task analysis. Techniques utilizing live or recorded music are implemented only after an assessment has been completed and the infant has been carefully observed prior to implementation (refer to the section above on assessment). The selection of methods may also reflect the philosophical and theoretical stance of the individual music therapist.

- **Music and Multi-Modal Stimulation**—See Standley, 2003, pp. 92–93.

- **Individual Sustained Music** (Recorded or Live)—See Standley, 2003, pp. 76–77.

- **Prescriptive Recorded Music Listening**—See Hanson-Abromeit, 2003, 2006; Shoemark, 1999; Standley, 2001a, 2001b, 2002, 2003, for related literature on the guidelines for the appropriate use of recorded music in the NICU.

- **Multi-Sensory Stimulation with Live Singing** (MSSLS) (Hanson-Abromeit, 2002; Shoemark et al., 2007)—An adaptation of the music and multi-modal stimulation technique (Standley, 2003) that does not involve taking the infant out of the bedside. This technique has been used clinically for the more medically fragile and younger infant who is not ready for music and multi-modal stimulation. Sensory stimulation is offered in a variety of forms dependent on the infant's stability and self-regulatory responses. For example, the therapist may first offer low intensity tactile stimulation by placing his or her hands in a cupped fashion around the infant's head and feet or offering a finger for the infant to hold. Auditory stimulation would be introduced as humming that progresses to soft singing as indicated by infant's receptiveness. Infant will be engaged in eye contact as appropriate.

- **Low-Stimulus Humming** (e.g., descending minor third), progressing to singing at bedside. No other stimulation is provided.

- **Developmental Interventions** for full-term and older infants as indicated by a developmental assessment.

- **Environmental Music Therapy** (EMT) incorporates the sounds within the NICU environment into the construction of live musical themes performed by a skilled music therapist. EMT must be carefully implemented with strict consideration for the timbre, attack, dynamics, contour, and harmonic sophistication of the music, as well as the location of the musician to the infants. Most importantly, the infants must be continuously monitored during EMT for adverse responses, as does the unit to ensure decibel decreases. For more information see Stewart and Schneider, 2000. Guidelines for EMT in the NICU have been devised in a careful process of collaboration and thematic analysis with elite musicians from the Melbourne Symphony Orchestra (Shoemark, 2007, available from the Music Therapy Unit, the Royal Children's Hospital, Melbourne). These give priority to choice of repertoire, location of musicians on the ward, intention, soloist/duets, multiple visits, and the need for direct support.

- **Family Vocal Recordings**—Parents and siblings are provided with materials and directions to make vocal recordings to leave at the bedside when they are unable to be present. Singing is encouraged. Supports for recordings include lullaby books, nursery rhymes, and lyric sheets. In optimal care, the music therapist may cater the construction of the theme-based recording with the mother or father, fostering harmonic or melodic support that enhances their strength in music making for the baby's recording. This can build parental self-confidence.

- **Therapist Vocal Support Recordings**—Therapist records singing voice to support parent singing at bedside.

- **Reflective Instrumental Support**—Using instruments (e.g., small Remo ocean disc) that reflect an interuterine environment with supportively toned breath sounds in the case of the infant referred for respiratory distress may be effective in assisting the regulation of breath. The gato box may be helpful in providing a consistent contour within the environment, much like a heartbeat, that the fetus acclimates to when in the womb. This instrument may also provide an entraining rhythmic repetitive beat necessary to support the feeding action required for an infant who cannot sustain a suck response.

- **Music as Controlled Motion**—The sensation of soothing motion, provided through musical phrasing, that can induce a sense of homeostasis for the infant in a very short period of time. Such an effect is achieved through principles of entrainment (Bradt & Dileo, 1999; Rider, 1997). The notion that premature infants seek rhythmic stimulation is not new. Thoman, Ingersoll, and Acebo (1991) studied the effects and the experience of entrainment and how it facilitated neurobehavioral development. Entrainment was achieved through the use of a breathing bear device that reflected the infants' breathing patterns. Eventually, the infants with this device in their beds illustrated more regulated breathing patterns and improved oxygenation.

- **Singing as Entrainment**—A lullaby or song of kin can be offered, but is best simplified into an intervallic, vowel-toned rhythmic response. That is, the lyrics are removed and a holding meter of 3/4 or 6/8 is set to the infant's rhythm of exhibiting symptom. For instance, if the infant is exhibiting irritability through a high-pitched scream, the therapist may seek to frame this response to the root or tonic tone of the infant's voiced tone/pitched cry, on a perfect 5th root/tonic tone. Eventually the tone can be pulsed. It can start after an audible breathing-in (inhalation) is presented and the tone begins only as the infant commences. The therapist and infant release the vocal tone at immediately the same time. As the cry slows down, the therapist can pulse a triplet meter to create a feeling of motion for the infant, still exactly during the release of the infant's cry. In this way, the sound is surrounding and holding the infant, creating a feeling of balance and also one of being heard and supported. The cry will often become less accented and less pronounced, losing its severity. This method is particularly effective with infants with Neonatal Abstinence Syndrome (NAS) (Loewy, in press; Loewy et al., 2005).

Outcome Measures

Each visit with an infant can have completely different outcomes based on the infant's developmental and medical changes. An infant can be medically stable on one visit and within a matter of hours have a different prognosis. Tracking progress in both objective and subjective form session-by-session provides information for a summation of progress to report during interdisciplinary rounds, family meetings, and upon discharge.

Family outcomes are often observational and subjective. Parent satisfaction of their experiences during NICU hospitalization is a valued measurement. A visible and efficacious music therapy program that is integrated into the care of the infant and family can be influential on the satisfaction of parents. Unsolicited letters of support from family members can solidify the role of the music therapist in the NICU.

The documentation of outcomes is related to what is considered relevant to the medical staff and the requirements and regulations of the hospital and unit charting procedures. Reliable and valid measurement tools and techniques for music therapy are not well documented in the literature. Individual sessions can be tracked and documented using an intervention summary form. Some hospitals may incorporate such a form into their standard charting procedures. In other hospitals, it serves to inform the therapist's official patient record documentation and functions as a program-based data collection tool. The NICU Intervention Summary (Figure 4) allows the therapist to monitor behavioral markers and physiological changes across the intervention time period. Reporting a percent of change from baseline to the end of the intervention (percent of change = baseline average − intervention average ÷ baseline average × 100 = %) provides documented intersession outcomes, as well as consistency or change across the treatment period.

In addition to documenting infant physiological and behavioral changes, it is also important to note changes in the infant's mental health status and psychosocial interactions. These are not easily reduced to a number or other charting mechanisms. Clear narrative that conveys the potency of the infant's behaviors still offers the best picture of the experience.

Providing details of the music therapy intervention is also informative to the music therapist. There is still much to be learned about the relationship between music and the responses of premature and critically ill infants. Current intervention protocols provide guidance to the music therapist; however, the realities of the clinical environment do not always allow for strict adherence to the established protocols. Much of what music therapists still need to understand involves the relationship between the musical elements and the physiological, behavioral, and psychosocial responses of the infant. By illustrating the details of the intervention and what informed the decisions of the therapist, music therapists will create knowledge as to the therapeutic function of music with premature infants.

NICU Music Therapy Program Patient Intervention Tracking

Patient Name _____ Patient # _____ Unit _____ Rm/Bed _____

Date _____   GA _____   Adjusted Age _____

Pre-intervention Assessment:
Current Weight/Trend _____   Last Feeding _____
Comfort Items _____
Tolerance for nursing care _____
Concerns/Abnormalities Observed _____
Position restrictions _____   Family availability today _____
Environmental Stimuli
Lights: *High   Med   Low*   Noise: *High   Med   Low*   Activity: *High   Med   Low*

Goal_____ **+ / -**   Objective _____ **+ / -**

Physiological and Behavioral Response

	Base Start	Base 2 min	Base 5 min	Inter Start	Inter 5 mm	Inter 10 m	Inter 15 m	Inter 20 m	Inter End	Post 2 min	Post 5 min
HR											
RR											
O2											
FiO2											
Stress											
Reg											
% chng	Avg. base:		% chng	Avg. Int:						Avg. post:	% chng

Calculation of % change: Base average-intervention average÷base average X 100 = %

Environmental Stimuli During Intervention:
Lights: *High   Med   Low*   Noise: *High   Med   Low*   Activity: *High   Med   Low*
Session Summary _____
_____
_____
_____
_____
_____
_____
_____
_____

Post Session Environmental Stimuli
Lights: *High   Med   Low*   Noise: *High   Med   Low*   Activity: *High   Med   Low*

Rationale for Interventions/Musical Choices _____
_____
_____
_____

Other Comments/Observations _____
_____
_____
_____
_____

Page ___ of ___

Figure 4. **NICU Intervention Summary**

When parents are present for direct service, the music therapist should involve them in the treatment as much as possible. At the very least, descriptive comments about the process and the decisions made by the music therapist should be articulated to the parents at bedside. Frequently parents are unavailable when the therapist visits. Parent-friendly documentation, such as a small distinctive communication book left at the bedside, should communicate to the parents the nature of the therapy session, the infant's response, and documented outcomes. Communication with families, written or oral, should be presented in a manner that is appropriate to the cultural context of the family. Sometimes it is appropriate to arrange a regular telephone conversation with parents. This offers an additional interaction that acknowledges the parent's pivotal role in the care of the infant. The ability to document outcomes, both written and verbal, in sophisticated, professional-language and in more simplistic, nonprofessional language is critical for family-centered practice.

Music Therapy Note for the Parents of _____

Time _____   Date_____

Comments: _____
_____
_____
_____
_____
_____
_____
_____
_____

Deanna Hanson-Abromeit, MA, MT-BC   voice mail 3-XXXX
Monday, Wednesday and Thursday   pager XXXX
                                                                   email XXXXXXX@uihc.uiowa.edu

---

Some infants may be followed for several weeks or months before being discharged. Many of them will be discharged to home. The music therapist can provide a summary of the music therapy sessions for the family in addition to a discharge packet. The discharge packet contains standard music-based games, resources, and developmental strategies for all families, with specific recommendations for the individual infant.

Some will be discharged to their homes with their families but will still require continued nursing or developmental support through home health and governmental agencies. Still others may be transferred to another hospital, perhaps closer to home. In these cases, a discharge summary may be relevant to provide the home health or governmental agency with information about the progress and recommendations for services following hospital discharge. For the infant being discharged to another hospital, the discharge summary serves to inform the music therapist, child life, or other developmental specialist at the new hospital.

Discharge Summary for Baby J.
Music Therapy Program
Department of Rehabilitation Therapy
(discharge with need for continued developmental services)

J. was referred for music therapy services shortly after his transfer to The University of Iowa Hospitals and Clinics Intermediate Care Nursery. He was referred for developmentally appropriate environmental stimulation and early intervention due to his age and length of extended hospitalization. Goals for music therapy have evolved as J.'s medical condition has changed. His response to music therapy interventions has often been active, positive, and reciprocal. The following is an outline of the basic therapeutic goals established for J. and his response to the music therapy interventions.

Goal: Increase opportunities for reciprocal social interactions

J. is a highly social baby. He enjoys interacting with people and responds positively to appropriate stimuli in relation to his medical condition. Music therapy interactions were adapted to be more sedative when appropriate. These interventions tended to have a calming effect by lowering his heart and respiration rate. More active interventions were incorporated when his medical condition was more stable.

Prior to his tracheotomy tube placement, J. was frequently vocal. He appeared to be particularly vocal during interaction with people. He often vocalized with the therapist as she sang. A repetitive repertoire of songs was used to encourage familiarity. J.'s recognition of songs was indicated by his increased vocalizations, change in affect (smiles, brighter eyes), and movement. He clearly demonstrated recognition to the opening song, which consisted of lyrics that implied a social relationship ("Hello J., I see you; it's nice to see you today"). One song in particular encouraged singing together and offered J. an opportunity to vocalize in response to a sung request. Through positive reinforcement, he was able to vocalize at the request and on occasion seemed to match the therapist's pitch for very brief moments.

Following tracheotomy tube placement, J. obviously could not participate in vocal play. However, it should be noted that on several occasions he moved his mouth in response to the reciprocal song discussed above and experienced an increase in saliva during the music therapy session, possibly indicating a continued desire to vocalize. This therapist did note a decrease in the mouth movements in the last few sessions. However, secretions of the mouth continue to increase during music therapy sessions, requiring frequent suctioning. Reciprocal social interactions focused more on providing J. with a variety of sensory stimulation experiences and assessing his preference for such stimulation. For example, following his transfer to 2JCW, a greater variety of instruments was appropriate to introduce in this private atmosphere. J. seemed to demonstrate a clear preference for the guitar; therefore, it was incorporated at both the beginning and end of the session. Using a shaker instrument (chiquita) encouraged J. to track the sound with his eyes, thus encouraging eye contact by moving the instrument until he was directly looking at the therapist.

Goal: Increase opportunities for purposeful movement

During our initial interactions, it was noted that J. consistently moved his feet and hands at his own initiative in response to the live music stimuli (e.g., soft singing). To encourage his purposeful movement, interventions were designed to "warm-up" his muscles to the idea of movement. Musical instruments that were easy to elicit a pleasant sound were then introduced to J. The chime was the most successful instrument for J. in that he could produce a sound independently and he appeared to enjoy the sound indicated by his level of motivation to play for long periods of time (i.e., more than 15 minutes using both hands and feet). J. was most successful in playing the chime when it was within his visual range. Although he would continue to try to elicit a sound, he demonstrated more effort to move his arm and hand when he could also see the instrument. His eye gaze and increased motor movement when the chime was introduced to him, either visually or through sound, indicated his preference for this instrument.

J. has very limited grasp ability; however, an increase in his ability to grasp instruments has been noted and he is demonstrating a firmer grasp on the therapist's fingers. He also tolerates various tactile stimulation to his hands to encourage their use (e.g., using the cabasa, an instrument with metal beads wrapped around a cylinder to encourage an open position).

Recommendations for Continued Music Therapy Services

Much of J.'s care has centered on his medical needs. Music seems to provide J. with an enjoyable experience that is nonmedical in nature, yet is also therapeutic. Music is a normal and age-appropriate activity for an infant. Encouraging playful interactions through music to promote his nonmusical goals (i.e., motor development, communication, psychosocial, and emotional development) may be beneficial to both J. and his parents. J. has repeatedly demonstrated positive reactions to music therapy services. The provision of these services is unique for J. in that music therapy, provided by a qualified music therapist, can be flexible and adapted to meet his ever-changing medical conditions and developmental growth. Interventions can be adapted to be low stimulus or more active depending on his current stability, and continuous music therapy services will provide consistency in his early intervention program.

Community music therapy services are available in this area, and funding for such services, which J. may qualify for, is available through the Johnson County Department of Human Services. Contacts at DHS for these particular services are J. M. and S. M.

Respectfully submitted,

Deanna Hanson-Abromeit, MA, MT-BC
Music Therapist – Board Certified

Discharge Summary for Baby M.
Music Therapy Program
Department of Rehabilitation Therapies
(*transfer to a hospital in another state*)

M. was referred to music therapy due to increased concerns with her level of agitation and prolonged length of stay. Assessment indicated that M. was often overstimulated from environmental noises and interactions. Based on observation and conversations with medical and nursing staff and with parents, the following goals for music therapy have been addressed with M.

Goal 1: Decrease agitation and negative reactions to environmental stimuli

This therapist has noted that M. can present extreme sensitivity and variability to environmental stimuli. Environmental noises and activity have proved to be anxiety-provoking for M. indicated by her behavior cues (reflex startling, irregular respiration, exaggerated eye movements, and frantic head movements), inability to transition to a quiet-alert or sleep state, high heart rates, and low oxygen saturation levels.

Music therapy interventions have been able to assist M. to transition from an agitated or actively awake state to a quiet and drowsy state. Occasionally music therapy interventions were successful in helping M. transition to a sleep state. Interventions with this therapist were consistently able to lower M.'s heart rate and increase her oxygen saturation levels.

Goal 2: Increase opportunities for positive developmentally appropriate
social interactions

This goal has become increasingly important as M. has aged. Providing M. with developmentally appropriate stimulation and interaction can be challenging due to her medical conditions and ability to handle such interactions. Careful observation of M.'s behaviors is critical when addressing this goal, as she can indicate her acceptance of such interaction through subtle behavior cues. Her reactions to the same interventions, with a few exceptions, have been sporadic and unpredictable. For example, some days M. can handle the introduction of singing and touch, but on another day she may not tolerate the therapist's presence in her visual range. She also demonstrated a distinct preference for particular songs by calming at the onset, as well as demonstrating a dislike for a particular song by negative reactions (behavior and physiological) when this song was presented to her.

When addressing this goal, focus has been placed on following M.'s cues so that relationships and psychosocial development can have a positive impact on her ability to interact in reciprocal relationships.

Goal 3: Increase opportunities for quality of life experiences

Providing consistent and familiar interaction throughout M.'s hospitalization has been an important role for this therapist. This therapist has been able to follow M. between units on an ongoing basis, adapting the interventions as appropriate to her medical stability and development. For example, while M. was heavily sedated, therapist interventions were provided consistently on a receptive level so that she was still able to participate in a positive form of sensory stimulation.

Recommendations for Continued Music Therapy Services

Music therapy is an appropriate treatment modality for early intervention with M.. Encouraging reciprocal interactions through music to promote her nonmusical goals (i.e., motor development, psychosocial and emotional development) may be beneficial to M. and her parents. The music therapist can adapt interventions to be receptive or active, based on M.'s ability to handle such interactions and her medical stability. Music therapy sessions can continue to integrate the family into her developmental growth. Music therapy services, provided by a qualified music therapist, will provide flexible and consistent services in her early intervention program.

The following are recommendations for future music therapy services:
1. Increase ability to appropriately integrate a variety of sensory stimulation.
2. Provide consistency in environmental stimuli through music listening of familiar recorded music.

3. Increase opportunities for maintaining a quiet-alert state.
4. Increase early intervention programming to address developmental issues in a conservative manner based on M.'s ability to integrate these interventions into her behavior state development.
5. Increase opportunities for M.'s family to build reciprocal and playful interactions with her.

Respectfully submitted,

Deanna Hanson-Abromeit, MA, MT-BC
Music Therapist – Board Certified

Discharge Summary for Baby R.
Music Therapy Program
Department of Rehabilitation Therapies
(*discharge to family home*)

Music therapy services have been following R. for the last five months (August 15, 200X through December 19, 200X. Upon assessment, music based interventions focused on supporting developmental progress during extended hospital stay with the following primary objectives:

1. Provide positive sensory stimulation.
2. Enhance cognitive, communication, and social/emotional development.

R.'s mom was present for the majority of the music therapy sessions.

Goal 1: Provide positive sensory stimulation
The type and duration of sensory stimulation has varied depending on R.'s medical stability. Responses varied based on how he was feeling on a particular day; however, he consistently demonstrated awareness to the stimulation presented.

Goal 2: Enhance cognitive, communication, and social/emotional development
Cognitive development: R. responds to sounds and voices demonstrated by his positive affect and direct eye contact. He will turn his eyes towards the sound of voice but resists turning his head to the left side. He actively inspects his own hands and brings them together at midline. He enjoys repeating an activity if it is familiar, touching the instrument when he recognizes it to restart or continue the activity. R. is observant of objects and people in his environment and shows awareness to novel objects; however, he is contemplative about purposeful reaching towards an object. His desire to reach is demonstrated by a progression of movements (i.e., active movements of legs, bringing hands together at midline and then releasing, followed by attempts at reaching before making contact with the object). Given enough time (> 2 minutes on 12/18/0X), he will tentatively reach for an object of interest and engage actively with it. R. seems to be cautious of tactile stimuli from a source other than his mother, demonstrated by his slight resistance when hand-over-hand manipulation is attempted.

Communication: Initially, R. was being encouraged to respond to sound stimulation (i.e., singing) by vocalizing. He shows active interest in the therapist for greater than 1 minute and would mimic oral movements modeled by the therapist. He was beginning to participate in reciprocal vocal interactions. Prior to his trach placement, primary vocalizations observed by this therapist were soft fussing in response to being uncomfortable or unhappy. Following the trach placement, nonverbal communication has been encouraged by modeling simple signs (e.g., music, more, thank you, bye-bye). Hand-over-hand modeling has been attempted, but R. seems to be resistive to this type of physical contact from the therapist.

Social/Emotional: R. is a highly social infant. He quickly responds with a bright smile on approach and smiles when he enjoys an activity. He shows anticipatory excitement by kicking his legs and actively plays with his own hands. He enjoys repeating familiar games/activities and establishes direct eye contact. As mentioned above, R. seems to show a slight tendency to withdraw from tactile stimulation; however, he enjoys physical contact, cuddles and relaxes when with his mother (this therapist has not had the opportunity to observe interactions with Dad).

Recommendations for Continued Music Therapy Services

R. is a joyful infant, with a supportive family environment. He appears to be organized in his behaviors and in his ability to transition between behavior states. However, it is recommended that R. be monitored for developmental delays due to his prolonged hospitalization. Based on this therapist's interactions with R., the following are recommended:

1. Encourage active participation/engagement with playful activities.
2. Continue to introduce new sounds, sights, and textures for exploration. These may be initially introduced within the context of a familiar activity to increase their successful acceptance by R. and to decrease his hesitation.
3. Integrate simple signs into communications with R. to encourage language development and a method of expressive communication.

It has been a pleasure to interact with R. and his mother during his hospitalization.

Respectfully submitted,

Deanna Hanson-Abromeit, MA, MT-BC
Music Therapist – Board Certified

Follow-up Services

There is a need and interest in providing music therapy services in the NICU follow-up clinics. Infants discharged from the NICU are followed and tracked for developmental outcomes in an outpatient clinic. Infants identified as at-risk can receive recommendations and provisions for additional services. Music therapy, as an early intervention strategy, is well recognized (Abad & Williams, 2007; de l'Etoile, 2006a, 2006b; Hanson-Abromeit, Crump, & Eakin, 2007; Walworth, 2008) with limited evidence to substantiate structured group music activities (Walworth, 2008). Music therapists should be encouraged to implement services in the NICU follow-up clinics for individual infants, as well as group-based services for infants and their families. For those music therapists trying to begin programming in the NICU, outpatient services may be a good place to start.

Competencies for Clinical Practice

Clinical practice as a neonatal music therapist is not an area for the entry-level music therapist. The board certified music therapist should have clinical experience in the hospital setting, as well as experience with healthy full-term infants. Knowledge and experience in early intervention is also advised. The music therapist who plans to provide safe and appropriate therapeutic interventions in the NICU should receive training, mentoring by an experienced NICU music therapist and neonatal nurse or developmental specialist, and supervision. Specialized training is currently offered through Tallahassee Memorial HealthCare and The Florida State University's Infant and Child Medical Music Therapy Institute (http://otto.cmr.fsu.edu/memt/institute) and at The Louis Armstrong Center for Music & Medicine at Beth Israel Medical Center. Portions of the Tallahassee training are offered at the annual national conference of the American Music Therapy Association as a preconference institute.

At this time, there is no defined quality assurance for clinical practice competence in the NICU. Until such a time, music therapists are encouraged to be ethically responsible and practice within these recommendations. Minimal competence should be demonstrated in the following areas:

- Identify pertinent information from the patient charts, nursing and medical staff.
- Demonstrate knowledge of commonly used equipment (e.g., monitors, respiratory support systems).
- Understand fetal neurobehavioral and sensory system developmental sequence, including infant musicality.
- Understand the developmental sequence for the sensorimotor, communication, cognitive, social-emotional systems for infants, preterm to 1 year of age.
- Demonstrate ability to monitor and interpret vital signs.
- Demonstrate ability to identify stress and self-regulatory behaviors.
- Based on assessment criteria, demonstrate ability to determine appropriateness for therapeutic intervention.
- Demonstrate ability to adjust interventions based on vital signs and behavioral responses (stress and self-regulatory behaviors).

For a comprehensive outline of recommended competencies for the clinical music therapist in the NICU, refer to the Appendix of this chapter.

The Future of Music Therapy in the NICU

Concerns for the use of music in the NICU are being raised in the literature. An expert panel organized by the Center for the Physical and Developmental Environment of the High-Risk Infant has raised concerns for the use of music in the NICU. The Study Group on Neonatal Intensive Care Unit Sound does not recommend the use of recorded voice or music, even though they are widely used (Graven, 2000). The concern is that there are not enough studies that examine the neurosensory development and the possible negative effects of the listening experience. Music-specific studies are criticized for the method of subject selection and grouping, data collection and analysis, as well as interpretation of the results. These concerns lead to clinical practice recommendations that minimize the use of recordings (music or voice) with the premature infants due to a lack of established benefits and long-term impact found in the literature (Philbin, 2000).

As a reasonably young area of clinical practice, there is vast potential for future development. Currently, music therapists rely on the available research literature to direct appropriate interventions. Practice techniques are formed based on the music therapy literature (Standley, 2003). However, the protocols driven by research may be different than the reality of clinical practice (Shoemark & Hanson-Abromeit, 2005). In addition, there is little recognition of the musical characteristics (e.g., rhythm, timbre, melody, dynamics) and their effect on the premature and high-risk infant (Shoemark & Hanson-Abromeit, 2005).

Randomized, controlled studies on the impact of music on the developing premature infant are unmistakably justified. It is also clear that clinical outcomes may be validating the use of music in NICU, as it has been noted that music continues to be used despite recommendations to the contrary. Contraindications for live music therapy have not, as of yet, been indicated. Music therapists are acting responsibly by taking a conservative approach in their clinical interventions, particularly in using a sound meter (Stewart & Schneider, 2000), as well as exerting caution in their selections of recorded music. One study has demonstrated that carefully selected recorded music did not incur harmful outcomes to 34-week gestational age premature infants, in that there was no effect on the cardio-respiratory systems or behavioral states. However, the clinical applications of recorded sedative music that followed the study indicate possible positive effects for regulation of cardio-respiratory systems, supporting transitions to organized behavior states and masking adverse environmental noise (Calabro, Wolfe, & Shoemark, 2003).

Evidenced-based practice is a focus area for music therapists, particularly driven by research protocols. Due to the fragile nature of the premature infant and limited knowledge of long-term outcomes, it is recommended that clinical practice be approached thoughtfully and meticulously. Clinicians in the NICU should have received specialized training, education, and mentorship in music therapy practice in the NICU as a minimal requirement. Ongoing mentorship and interdisciplinary collaboration will further these clinicians' specialization in neonatal music therapy. For music therapists, it is the music that distinguishes these services from others. A broader knowledge of the music and its relationship to the outcomes will provide a greater understanding of, and direction for, the clinical methodology of neonatal music therapy. Therefore, it is important that clinicians and researchers have a much richer description of the music and its impact on immediate and long-term development. This will generate solid hypotheses for further research, as well as the development of sound clinical practices (Shoemark & Hanson-Abromeit, 2005). Clearly, research addressing behavior changes in premature infants based on the elements of the musical characteristics is warranted.

Additionally, it has been recommended that only those interventions that are developed and researched be implemented into clinical practice. While this is a wise and safe recommendation due to the fragile nature of the infants, it can also prevent future development of effective interventions. Substantiating clinical practice and research protocols with well-supported theoretical constructs is critical. Collaborative initiatives between neonatal music therapy clinicians and researchers, and their interdisciplinary counterparts (nurses; neonatologists; developmental specialists; physical, occupational, and speech therapists; and child life specialists) will be essential to the future of music therapy in the NICU.

References

Abad, V., & Williams, K. E. (2007). Early intervention music therapy: Reporting on a 3-year project to address needs with at-risk families. *Music Therapy Perspectives, 25*(1), 52–58.

Abrams, B., Dassler, A., Lee, S., Loewy, J., Silverman, F., & Telsey, A. (2000). Instituting music therapy in the NICU: A team centered approach. In J. V. Loewy (Ed.), *Music therapy in the neonatal intensive care unit* (pp. 21–37). New York: Satchnote Press.

Als, H. (1982). Toward a synactive theory of development: Promise for the assessment and support of infant individuality. *Infant Mental Health Journal, 3*(4), 229–243.

Als, H. (1986). A synactive model of neonatal behavioral organization: Framework for the assessment of neurobehavioral development in the premature infant and for support of infants and parents in the neonatal intensive care environment. *Physical and Occupational Therapy in Pediatrics, 6*(3/4), 3–53.

Als, H. (Ed.). (1995). *Manual for the naturalistic observation of newborn behavior: Newborn Individualized Developmental Care and Assessment Program (NIDCAP).* (Available from Harvard Medical School, 320 Longwood Ave., Boston, MA 02115)

Als, H. (1996). *Program Guide for Newborn Individualized Developmental Care and Assessment Program (NIDCAP): An education and training program for health care professionals.* (Available from National NIDCAP Training Center, Harvard Medical School, Children's Hospital, Boston, 320 Longwood Ave., Boston, MA 02115)

Als, H. (1999). Reading the premature infant. In E. Goldson (Ed.), *Nurturing the premature infant: Developmental interventions in the Neonatal Intensive Care Nursery* (pp. 18–85). New York: Oxford University Press.

Als, H., Butler, S., Kosta, S., & McAnulty, G. (2005). The Assessment of Preterm Infants' Behavior (APIB): Furthering the understanding and measurement of neurodevelopmental competence in preterm and full-term infants. *Mental Retardation and Developmental Disabilities Research Reviews, 11*, 94–102.

American Academy of Pediatrics, American College of Obstetricians and Gynecologists. (2005). *Guidelines for perinatal care* (5th ed.). Elk Grove Village, IL: American Academy of Pediatrics.

Attia, J., Amiel-Tison, C., Mayer, M. N., Shnider, S. M., & Barrier, G. (1987). Measurement of postoperative pain and narcotic administration in infants using a new clinical scoring system. *Anesthesiology, 67,* A532.

Bates, D., Brez, C., & Kaplan, R. (2003, November). *Sink or swim: Wading through the literature to develop music therapy protocols in the NICU.* Concurrent session at the annual meeting of the American Music Therapy Association, Minneapolis, MN.

Bates, D., Kaplan, R., Reed, A., & Whitmer, C. (2005). *The Premature Infants' Lullaby Rating Scale (PILRS).* Unpublished manuscript.

Bowlby, J. (1988). *A secure base: Parent child attention and health bonding.* New York: Basic Books.

Bradt, J., & Dileo, C. (1999). Entrainment, resonance, and pain-related suffering. In C. Dileo (Ed.), *Music therapy and medicine: Theoretical and clinical applications* (pp. 181–188). Silver Spring, MD: American Music Therapy Association.

Brand, M. (1985). Lullabies that awaken musicality in infants. *Music Educators Journal, 71*(7), 28–31.

Burke, M., Walsh, J., Oehler, J., & Gingras, J. (1995). Music therapy following suctioning: Four case studies. *Neonatal Network, 14*(7), 41–49.

Burns, K., Cunningham, N., White-Traut, R. C., Silvestri, J. M., & Nelson, M. N. (1994). Modification of an infant stimulation protocol based on physiologic and behavioral responses. *Journal of Obstetric, Gynecologic, and Neonatal Nursing, 23,* 581–589.

Caine, J. (1991). The effects of music on the selected stress behaviors, weight, caloric and formula intake and length of hospital stay of premature and low birth weight neonates in a newborn intensive care unit. *Journal of Music Therapy, 28*(4), 180–192.

Calabro, J., Wolfe, R., & Shoemark, H. (2003). The effects of recorded sedative music on the physiology and behaviour of premature infants with a respiratory disorder. *The Australian Journal of Music Therapy, 14,* 3–19.

Cassidy, J. W., & Ditty, K. M. (1998). Presentation of aural stimuli to newborns and premature infants: An audiological perspective. *Journal of Music Therapy, 32*(4), 208–227.

Cassidy, J. W., & Standley, J. M. (1995). The effect of music listening on physiological responses of premature infants in the NICU. *Journal of Music Therapy, 32*(4), 208–227.

Cevasco, A. M., & Grant, R. E. (2005). Effect of the Pacifier Activated Lullaby on weight gain of premature infants. *Journal of Music Therapy, 42*(2), 123–139.

Charpie, M. (2002). *A magical play of love: Music therapy as a bridge between mother and baby in the NICU.* Unpublished master's thesis, New York University, New York, NY.

Clinical Core Competency Training Manual, Premature Infant Course and Exam. (2005). (Available from the Louis & Lucille Armstrong Music Therapy Program, Beth Israel Medical Center NICU Music Therapy Training, First Avenue at 16th Street, New York, NY, 10003.)

Coleman, J. M., Pratt, R. R., Stoddard, R. A., Gerstmann, D. R., & Abel, H.-H. (1997). The effects of the male and female singing and speaking voices on selected physiological and behavioral measures of premature infants in the intensive care unit. *International Journal of Arts Medicine, 5*(2), 4–11.

Collins, S. K., & Kuck, K. (1991). Music therapy in the neonatal intensive care unit. *Neonatal Network, 9*(6), 23–26.

Courtnage, A., Chawla, H., Loewy, J., & Nolan, P. (2002). Effects of live infant-directed singing on oxygen saturation, heart rates and respiratory rates of infants in the neonatal intensive care unit [Abstract 2346]. *Pediatric Research, 51*(4), 403A.

de l'Etoile, S. K. (2006a). Infant behavioral responses to infant-directed singing and other maternal interactions. *Infant Behavioral & Development, 29*(3), 456–470.

de l'Etoile, S. K. (2006b). Infant-directed singing: A theory for clinical intervention. *Music Therapy Perspectives, 24*(1), 22–29.

DeCasper, A. J., & Sigafoos, A. D. (1983). The intrauterine heartbeat: A potent reinforcer for newborns. *Infant Behavior and Development, 6*(1), 19–25.

DeCasper, A. J., & Spence, M. J. (1986). Prenatal maternal speech influences newborns' perception of speech sounds. *Infant Behavior & Development, 9*(2), 133–150.

Department of Rehabilitation Therapies. (2003). *Department of Rehabilitation Therapies Competency Program, Special Care Nurseries.* Iowa City, IA: University of Iowa Hospitals and Clinics/Children's Hospital of Iowa.

DiPietro, J. A., Hodgson, D. M., Costigan, K. A., Hilton, S. C., & Johnson, T. R. (1996). Fetal neurobehavioral development. *Child Development, 67*, 2553–2567.

Field, T., Hernandez-Reif, M., Feijo, L., & Freedman, J. (2006). Prenatal, perinatal and neonatal stimulation: A survey of neonatal nurseries [Electronic version]. *Infant Behavior and Development, 29*(1), 24–31.

Fischer, C. B., & Als, H. (2004). Trusting behavioral communication: Individualized relationship-based developmental care in the newborn intensive care unit—A way of meeting the neurodevelopmental expectations of the preterm infant. In M. Nocker-Ribaupierre (Ed.), *Music therapy for premature and newborn infants* (pp. 1–19). Gilsum, NH: Barcelona.

Gardner, S. L., & Lubchenco, L. O. (1998). The neonate and the environment: Impact on development. In G. B. Merenstein & S. L. Gardner (Eds.), *Handbook of neonatal intensive care* (4th ed., pp. 197–242). St. Louis: Mosby.

Gottlieb, G. (1983). The psychobiological approach to developmental issues. In P. H. Mussen (Ed.), *Handbook of child psychology* (4th ed., pp. 1–26). New York: John Wiley & Sons.

Graven, S. N. (2000). Sound and the developing infant in the NICU: Conclusions and recommendations for care. *Journal of Perinatology, 20*, S88–S93.

Gray, L., & Philbin, M. K. (2004). Effects of the neonatal intensive care unit on auditory attention and distraction. *Clinics in Perinatology, 31*, 243–260.

Groome, L. J., Swiber, M. J., Atterbury, J. A., Bentz, L. S., & Holland, S. B. (1997). Similarities and differences in behavioral state organization during sleep periods in the perinatal infant before and after birth. *Child Development, 68*(1), 1–11.

Hanson-Abromeit, D. (2002, November). *Recorded and live music presented to premature infants: Outcomes of behaviors and physiological responses.* Research Poster Session, 4th Annual conference of the American Music Therapy Association Conference.

Hanson-Abromeit, D. (2003). The Newborn Individualized Developmental Care and Assessment Program (NIDCAP) as a model for clinical music therapy interventions with premature infants. *Music Therapy Perspectives, 21*(2), 60–68.

Hanson-Abromeit, D. (2006). Developmentally based criteria to support recorded music selections by neonatal nurses for use with premature infants in the neonatal intensive care unit. *Dissertation Abstracts International, 67*(4-A), 1143.

Hanson-Abromeit, D., Crump, J., & Eakin, H. (2007, November). *A pilot program for preventative music-based interventions for at-risk infants and toddlers.* Paper presented at the annual meeting of the American Music Therapy Association, Louisville, KY.

Harris, J. (2005). Critically ill babies in hospital—Considering the experience of mothers. *Infant Observation, 8*(3), 247–258.

Hawes, B. L. (1974). Folksongs and function: Some thoughts on the American lullaby. *The Journal of American Folklore, 87*(344), 140–148.

Hepper, P. G. (1991). An examination of fetal learning before and after birth. *The Irish Journal of Psychology, 12*(2), 95–107.

Hepper, P. G., Scott, D., & Shahidullah, S. (1993). Newborn and fetal response to maternal voice. *Journal of Reproductive and Infant Psychology, 11*, 147–153.

Hurst, I. (2001). Mothers' strategies to meet their needs in the newborn intensive care nursery. *Journal of Perinatal and Neonatal Nursing, 15*(2), 65–83.

Institute for Family-Centered Care. (2007). *Definition of family-centered care.* Retrieved July 25, 2007, from http://www.familycenteredcare.org/

Kemper, K. J., Martin, K., Block, S. M., Shoaf, R., & Woods, C. (2004). Attitudes and expectations about music therapy for premature infants among staff in a neonatal intensive care unit. *Alternative Therapies, 10*(2), 50–54.

Kisilevsky, B. S. (1995). The influence of stimulus and subject variables on human fetal responses to sound and vibration. In J.-P. Lecanuet, N. A.. Krashegor, W. P. Fifer, & W. P. Smotherman (Eds.), *Fetal development: A psychobiological perspective* (pp. 263–278). Mahwah, NJ: Laurence Erlbaum and Associates.

Kisilevsky, B. S., & Muir, D. W. (1991). Human fetal and subsequent newborn responses to sound and vibration. *Infant Behavior and Development, 14*, 1–26.

Klein, J. (2008). Pulse oximetry. *Iowa neonatology handbook: Pulmonary.* Retrieved October 13, 2008, from http://www.uihealthcare.com/depts/med/pediatrics/iowaneonatologyhandbook/pulmonary/pulseoximetry.html

Laws, P., Abeywardana, S., Walker, J., & Sullivan, E. (2007). *Australia's mothers and babies 2005*. Sydney, Australia: AIHW National Perinatal Statistics Unit.

Lecanuet, J.-P., Granier-Deferre, C., Cohen, H., Le Houezec, R., & Busnel, M.-C. (1986). Fetal responses to acoustic stimulation depend on heart rate variability pattern, stimulus intensity and repetition. *Early Human Development, 13*, 269–283.

Lenz, G. (1998). Music therapy and early interactional disorders between mother and infants. In R. Pratt & D. Grocke (Eds.), *Music Medicine 3, Musicmedicine and music therapy: Expanding horizons* (pp. 162–174). Melbourne, Australia: Melbourne University Press.

Lickliter, R. (1993). Timing and the development of perinatal perceptual organization. In G. Turkewitz & D. A. Devenny (Eds.), *Developmental time and timing* (pp. 105–123). Hillsdale, NJ: Lawrence Erlbaum Associates.

Loewy, J. (1995). The musical stages of speech: A developmental model of pre-verbal sound making. *Music Therapy, 13*(1), 47–73.

Loewy, J. (2004). A clinical model of music therapy in the NICU. In M. Nöcker-Ribaupierre (Ed.), *Music therapy for premature and newborn infants* (pp. 159–176). Gilsum, NH: Barcelona.

Loewy, J. (in press). Musical sedation: Mechanisms of breathing entrainment. In R. Azoulay & J. Lowey (Eds.), *Music the breath and health: Advances in integrative music therapy* (pp. 209–216). New York: Satchnote Press.

Loewy, J., Hallan, C., Friedman, E., & Martinez, C. (2005). Sleep/sedation in children undergoing EEG testing: A comparison of chloral hydrate and music therapy. *Journal of Perianethesia Nursing, 20*(5), 323–331.

Loewy, J., & Stewart, K. (2008). *The Heather on Earth NICU multi-site study* (IRB #413-06). New York: Beth Israel Medical Center.

Lorch, C. A., Lorch, V., Diefendorf, A. O., & Earl, P. W. (1994). Effect of stimulative and sedative music on systolic blood pressure, heart rate, and respiratory rate in premature infants. *Journal of Music Therapy, 31*(2), 105–118.

Lu, M. (2002). *The effects of fetus-directed singing on at risk pregnant women*. Unpublished master's thesis, Drexel University, Philadelphia.

March of Dimes (n.d.). *Preterm birth overview*. Retrieved February 6, 2006, from http://www.marchofdimes.com/peristats

March of Dimes (2007, February). *Fact sheet: Preterm birth*. Retrieved July 8, 2008, from http://www.marchofdimes.com/professionals/14332_1157.asp

Marchette, L., Main, R., Redick, E., & Shapiro, A. (1992). Pain reduction during neonatal circumcision. In R. Spintge & R. Droh (Eds.), *MusicMedicine* (pp. 131–141). St. Louis, MO: MMB.

Martin, J. A., Hamilton, B. E., Sutton, P. D., Ventura, S. J., Meancker, F., Kirmeyer, S., & Munson, M. L. (2007). *Births: Final data for 2005*. (National Vital Statistics Reports, No. 56-6). Hyattsville, MD: National Center for Health Statistics.

McGrath, J. (2001). Building relationships with families in the NICU: Exploring the guarded alliance. *Journal of Perinatal and Neonatal Nursing, 15*(3), 74–84.

Medoff-Cooper, B., McGrath, J. M., & Bilker, W. (2000). Nutritive sucking and neurobehavioral development in preterm infants from 34 weeks PCA to term. *MCN American Journal of Maternal Child Nursing, 25*(2), 64–70.

Merriam Webster Online Dictionary (n.d.). Music. Retrieved December 14, 2004, from http://www.merriam-webster.com/dictionary/music

Minde, K. (1999). Mediating attachment patterns during a serious medical illness. *Infant Mental Health Journal, 20*(1), 105–122.

Moore, R., Gladstone, I., & Standley, J. (1994, November). *Effects of music, maternal voice, intrauterine sounds and white noise on the oxygen saturation levels of premature infants.* Poster session presented at the annual meeting of the National Association for Music Therapy, Orlando, FL.

Mouradian, L. E., Als, H., & Coster, W. J. (2000). Neurobehavioral functioning of healthy preterm infants of varying gestational ages. *Developmental and Behavioral Pediatrics, 21*(6), 408–416.

Nijhuis, J. G., Prechtl, H. F., Martin, C. B., Jr., & Bots, R. S. (1982). Are there behavioral states in the human fetus? *Early Human Development, 6,* 177–195.

Nöcker-Ribaupierre, M. (2004). The mother's voice—A bridge between two worlds. In M. Nöcker-Ribaupierre (Ed.), *Music therapy for premature and newborn infants* (pp. 97–113). Gilsum, NH: Barcelona.

Panneton, R. K. (1985). Prenatal auditory experience with melodies: Effects on postnatal auditory preferences in human newborns (Doctoral dissertation, University of North Carolina at Greensboro, 1985). *Dissertation Abstracts International, 47*(09), 3984B. (UMI No. 8701333)

Philbin, M. K. (2000). The influence of auditory experience on the behavior of preterm newborns. *Journal of Perinatology, 20,* S77–S87.

Philbin, M. K., & Evans, J. B. (2006). Standards for the acoustic environment of the newborn ICU. *Journal of Perinatology, 26,* S27–S30.

Polverini-Rey, R. A. (1992). *Intrauterine musical learning: The soothing effect on newborns of a lullaby learned prenatally (prenatal learning)* [CD-ROM]. Abstract from ProQuest File, Dissertation Abstracts Item 9233740.

Prentice, M., & Stainton, C. (2003). Outcomes of developmental care in an Australian neonatal intensive care nursery. *Neonatal Network, 22*(6), 17–23.

Rider, M. (1997). *The rhythmic language of health and disease.* St. Louis: MMB.

Robertson, J. (2005). A psychoanalytic perspective on the work of a physiotherapist with infants at risk of neurological problems: Comparing the theoretical background of physiotherapy and psychoanalysis. *Infant Observation, 8*(3), 259–278.

Rock, A. M. L., Trainor, L. J., & Addison, T. L. (1999). Distinctive messages in infant-directed lullabies and play songs. *Developmental Psychology, 33*(2), 527–534.

Rubel, E. W. (1984). Ontogeny of auditory system function. *Annual Reviews of Physiology, 46*, 213–229.

Schwartz, F. (2004). Medical music therapy for the premature baby—Research review. In M. Nöcker-Ribaupierre (Ed.), *Music therapy for premature and newborn infants* (pp. 85–96). Gilsum, NH: Barcelona.

Shahidullah, S., & Hepper, P. G. (1993). The developmental origins of fetal responsiveness to an acoustic stimulus. *Journal of Reproductive and Infant Psychology, 11*, 135–142.

Shields, L., Pratt, J., Davis, L., & Hunter, J. (2007). Family-centred care for children in hospital. *Cochrane Database of Systematic Reviews* (Issue 1), Art. No.: CD004811DOI: 004810.001002/14651858.CD14004811.pub14651852.

Shoemark, H. (1999). Singing as the foundation for multi-modal stimulation. In R. Pratt & D. Grocke (Eds.), *Music Medicine3, Musicmedicine and music therapy: Expanding horizons* (pp. 140–152). Victoria, Australia: The University of Melbourne.

Shoemark, H. (2000). The use of music therapy in treating infants with complex bowel conditions. In J. V. Loewy (Ed.), *Music therapy in the neonatal intensive care unit* (pp. 101–109). New York: Satchnote Press.

Shoemark, H. (2004). Family-centered music therapy for infants with complex medical and surgical needs. In M. Nocker (Ed.), *Music therapy for premature and newborn infants* (pp. 141–157). Gilsum, NH: Barcelona.

Shoemark, H. (2007). *Competencies for the clinical music therapist in the neonatal unit.* Melbourne, Australia: Royal Children's Hospital, Music Therapy Unit.

Shoemark, H. (2008). Mapping progress within an individual music therapy session with full-term hospitalized infants. *Music Therapy Perspectives, 26*(1), 38–45.

Shoemark, H., & Dearn, T. (2008). Keeping the family at the centre of family-centred music therapy with hospitalised infants. *Australian Journal of Music Therapy, 19*, 3–24.

Shoemark, H., & Hanson-Abromeit, D. (2005, July). *Building practice wisdom in neonatal music therapy: Considerations for ontology, epistemology and method.* Paper presented at the 11th World Congress of Music Therapy, Brisbane, Queensland, Australia.

Shoemark, H., Malloch, S., Newnham, C., Paul, C., Prior, M., Črnčec, R., & Coward, S. (2007). An investigation of intersubjectivity: Music therapy and hospitalised infants (Abstract). *Journal of Paediatrics and Child Health, 43*(Suppl.1), A135.

Spence, M. J., & DeCasper, A. J. (1987). Prenatal experience with low-frequency maternal-voice sounds influence neonatal perception of maternal voice samples. *Infant Behavior and Development, 10*(2), 133–142.

Standley, J. M. (1991). The role of music in pacification/stimulation of premature infants with low birthweights. *Music Therapy Perspectives, 9*, 19–25.

Standley, J. M. (1998). The effect of music and multimodal stimulation on physiologic and developmental responses of premature infants in neonatal intensive care. *Pediatric Nursing, 21*(6), 532–539.

Standley, J. M. (2001a). Music therapy for premature infants in neonatal intensive care: Physiological and developmental benefits. *Early Childhood Connections, 7*(2), 18–25.

Standley, J. M. (2001b). Music therapy for the neonate. *Newborn and Infant Nursing Reviews, 1*(4), 211–216.

Standley, J. M. (2002). Music therapy in the NICU: Promoting the growth and development of premature infants. *Zero to Three, 23*(1), 23–30.

Standley, J. M. (2003). *Music therapy with premature infants: Research and developmental interventions*. Silver Spring, MD: American Music Therapy Association.

Standley, J. M., Cevasco, A., Walworth, D., Nguyen, J., Whipple, J., Jarred, J., & Abromeit, D. (2005, November). *Music therapy and premature infants*. Preconference institute conducted at the annual meeting of the American Music Therapy Association, Orlando, FL.

Standley, J. M., & Moore, R. S. (1995). Therapeutic effects of music and mother's voice on premature infants. *Pediatric Nursing, 21*(6), 509–574.

Standley, J. M., Whipple, J., & Abromeit, D. (2003, November). *Music therapy and premature infants*. Preconference institute conducted at the annual meeting of the American Music Therapy Association, Minneapolis, MN.

Stern, D. (1995). *The motherhood constellation: A unified view of parent infant psychotherapy*. New York: Basic Books.

Stewart, K. (in press). Music therapy, the preterm infant, and the spectrum of traumatic experience. In K. Stewart (Ed.), *Music therapy and trauma: Bridging theory and clinical practice*. New York: Satchnote Press.

Stewart, K., & Schneider, S. (2000). The effects of music therapy on the sound environment in the NICU: A pilot study. In J. V. Loewy (Ed.), *Music therapy in the neonatal intensive care unit* (pp. 85–101). New York: Satchnote Press.

Stjernqvist, K., & Svenningsen, N. W. (1990). Neurobehavioral development at term of extremely low-birthweight infants (< 901g). *Developmental Medicine and Child Neurology, 32*, 679–688.

Thoman, E. B., Ingersoll, E. W., & Acebo, C. (1991). Premature infants seek rhythmic stimulation, and the experience facilitates neurobehavioral development. *Journal of Developmental and Behavioral Pediatrics, 12*, 11–18.

Trainor, L. J. (1996). Infant preferences for infant-directed versus noninfant-directed playsongs and lullabies. *Infant Behavior and Development, 19*, 83–92.

Trainor, L. J., Clark, E. D., Huntley, A., & Adams, B. A. (1997). The acoustic basis of preferences for infant-directed singing. *Infant Behavior and Development, 20*(3), 383–396.

Trehub, S. E. (2001). Musical predispositions in infancy. In R. J. Zatoree & I. Peretz (Eds.), *The biological foundations of music: Annals of the New York Academy Sciences, 930*, 1–16. New York: New York Academy of Sciences.

Trehub, S. E. (2003). The developmental origins of musicality. *Nature Neuroscience, 6*(7), 669–673.

Trehub, S. E., & Trainor, L. J. (1990). Rules for listening in infancy. In J. Enns (Ed.), *The development of attention: Research and theory* (pp. 87–119). Amsterdam: Elsevier.

Trehub, S. E., & Unyk, A. M. (1991). Music prototypes in developmental perspective. *Psychomusicology, 10*(2), 73–87.

Trehub, S. E., Unyk, A. M., Kamenetsky, S. B., Hill, D. S., Trainor, L. J., Henderson, J. L., & Saraza, M. (1997). Mothers' and fathers' singing to infants. *Developmental Psychology, 33*(3), 500–507.

Trehub, S. E., Unyk, A. M., & Trainor, L. J. (1993). Adults identify infant-directed music across cultures. *Infant Behavior and Development, 16*, 193–211.

Unyk, A. M., Trehub, S. E, Trainor, L. J., & Schellenberg, E. G. (1992). Lullabies and simplicity: A cross-cultural perspective. *Psychology of Music, 20*, 15–28.

Van Beek, Y., & Samson, J. F. (1994). Communication in preterm infants: Why is it different? *Early Development and Parenting, 3*(1), 37–50.

Vandenburg, K. (2000). Supporting parents in the NICU: Guidelines for promoting parent confidence and competence. *Neonatal Network*, *19*(8), 63–64.

Walworth, D. (2008, Summer). Ongoing infant and toddler research. *American Music Therapy Association Early Childhood Newsletter, 14*, 6.

Winnicott, D. W. (1971). *Playing and reality.* London: Routledge.

Wolke, D. (1998). Psychological development of prematurely born children. *Archives of Disease in Childhood, 78*, 567–570.

Appendix

 Royal Children's Hospital, Melbourne

Flemington Rd., Parkville, Victoria 3052, AUSTRALIA

Music Therapy Unit
Tel: 61 3 9345 5421 Fax: 61 3 9345 5090

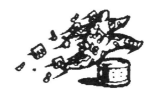

Competencies for the Clinical Music Therapist in the Neonatal Unit*

(Neonatal Unit incorporates the NICU and Special Care Nursery)*

Preliminary statements

The Neonatal Music Therapist must hold <u>current</u> registration as a Music Therapist with the Australian Music Therapy Association Incorporated. This qualification attests to a set of appropriate foundation competencies as a music therapy clinician.

The clinical application of music in a Neonatal Intensive Care Unit or Special Care Nursery requires a range of sophisticated and subtle skills as a musician and therapist. Therefore it is strongly recommended that the Music Therapist seeking to work in Neonatology is experienced in working with families, children, toddlers or pregnant women.

Criteria are listed according to the three main strands of the current RCH program, which include:

❑ Family support – verbal interaction with families, particularly primary care-givers, to inform and support their efforts to sustain a nurturing role with their infant. The main focus is to empower the use of voice and touch.

❑ Face-to-face developmental music therapy – regular sessions of developmentally appropriate music experiences that support and enhance the infant's cognitive, motor and social development.

❑ Receptive music (music listening) – preparation of a program of recorded music for the family and infant to impact on the physical environment and thus indirectly affecting the infant.

The Music Therapy Unit welcomes the possibility of expanding strands to the program. These should be developed in consultation with the Senior Music Therapist.

Helen Shoemark, Music Therapy Unit, Royal Children's Hospital, Melbourne, Australia.© Original 13th Jan 2003, Revised April 20th 2007

Key Areas of Competency

Infant development

The music therapist should have:

- An understanding of normal newborn infant development (Als, 1982) with regard to:
    - Autonomic system – physiologic functioning and visceral behaviour
    - State organisation – range of states indicated by behaviour, transition between states, self-regulation
    - Sensory processing – ability to respond and process stimulation
    - Motor system – muscle tone, posture and movements

- An understanding of foetal development and the impact of preterm birth or congenital anomalies on the developing infant, particularly the auditory system.

- A working knowledge of behavioural and physiological indication of over-stimulation.

- An established understanding of older infant development with regard to musicality, interpersonal relationships, communication, motor skills and other cognitive processes.

Music

Music listening

The music therapist must:

- Understand the musical elements of stimulative and sedative music and their impact on infant physiology.

- Using appropriate assessment to ensure that the infant is developmentally able to benefit from the experience of music.

- Understand and utilise the family's music history. The potential of their music listening as a social, recreational and emotional experience may be employed to support the infant as part of his/her family.

- Be able to assemble and utilise the resources to provide an individualised program of recorded music that is informed by the family preferences.

- Be informed and able to give an opinion about commonly reported music listening experiences such as intrauterine heart beat ('womb sounds'), instrumental Mozart music and lullabies.

Helen Shoemark, Music Therapy Unit, Royal Children's Hospital, Melbourne, Australia.© Original 13th Jan 2003, Revised April 20th 2007

Technical implementation of recorded music

The music therapist will:

- Utilise parameters for listening to recorded music including modes of presentation, volume levels, duration of stimulus and frequency of presentation in a 24-hour period (Cassidy & Ditty, 1998).

- Implement Infection Control practices as required by the hospital's Infection Control Department.

- Abide by the legal requirements of all copyright agencies.

Developmental music therapy

The music therapist should:

- Utilise those methods that have been shown to be safe for premature and medically fragile full-term infants (Standley, 1998; Standley & Moore, 1985; Whipple, 2005).

- Have a strong, adaptive voice for singing and speaking.

- Be skilled in 'recreative song' and 'improvised singing' (Shoemark, 1999, 2000).

- Understand and implement the principles of Infant-Directed Speech and Infant-Directed Singing (Bergeson & Trehub, 2002; de l'Etoile, 2006; Trainor, 1996; Trehub, Unyk, & Trainor, 1993).

- Be skilled in shaping shared musical experiences for fragile newborns (Shoemark, 2006).

- Employ safeguard systems for ensuring infant's physical and psychological stability with regard to over-stimulation (e.g., White-Traut's multi-modal protocol; Burns, Cunningham, White-Traut, Silvestri, & Nelson, 1994; White-Traut et al. 1999).

- Be aware of psychological models of infant development pertaining to sensory processing (Stern, 1985; Trevarthen & Malloch, 2000) which inform the interpersonal and therapeutic relationship.

Interpersonal

The music therapist must be able to:

- Understand and truly implement family-centred care (Peebles-Kleiger, 2000; Steinberg, 2006), including an understanding of the cultural implications of giving birth to a sick child.

- Communicate effectively and sensitively with the family.

- Inform and support the family's potency of their active participation in nurturing their infant, principles of intervention, therapeutic activities and assessments associated with their infant (O'Gorman, 2006).

Helen Shoemark, Music Therapy Unit, Royal Children's Hospital, Melbourne, Australia.© Original 13th Jan 2003, Revised April 20th 2007

- Be an active member of the Neonatal Developmental Care or any other relevant team (Hanson-Abromeit, 2003).

- Take regular professional supervision as needed, as this work engenders many issues (particularly around attachment and parenting).

Context / Neonatal Unit environment

The music therapist should:

- Promote all positive sensory possibilities within the infant's current context.

- Be knowledgeable about the noxious aspects of the auditory environment in the Neonatal Unit and ways in which to ameliorate them (Philbin & Evans, 2006).

- Understand the impact of the Neonatal Unit environment on the developmental opportunities for the infant.

Medical

The music therapist will

- Develop a knowledge base of those conditions forming the common caseload for the Neonatal Unit.

- Develop an understanding of the clinical pathways of treatment for common conditions.

Other

The music therapist will:

- Prepare and maintain a range of useful resources for families and staff—this includes a brochure with key information, reading material, speaking material for education sessions.
- Educate other professionals about the role of music as a therapeutic intervention for sick newborns infants and their families.

Prepared by:
Helen Shoemark, MME, BMus, RMT (Aust.)
Senior Music Therapist – Neonate & Infant Program
Music Therapy Unit, Royal Children's Hospital, Melbourne

Contact
E-mail helen.shoemark@rch.org.au
Tel: 61 3 9345 4127
Fax: 61 3 9345 5090

Helen Shoemark, Music Therapy Unit, Royal Children's Hospital, Melbourne, Australia.© Original 13th Jan 2003, Revised April 20th 2007

References

Als, H. (1982). Toward a synactive theory of development: Promise for the assessment and support of infant individuality. *Infant Mental Health Journal, 3*(4), 229–243.

Bergeson, T., & Trehub, S. (2002). Absolute pitch and tempo in mothers' songs to infants. *Psychological Science, 13*(1), 72–75.

Burns, K., Cunningham, N., White-Traut, R., Silvestri, J., & Nelson, M. (1994). Infant stimulation: Modification of an intervention based on physiologic and behavioural cues. *Journal of Gynaecological and Neonatal Nursing, 23*(7), 581–589.

Cassidy, J., & Ditty, K. (1998). Presentation of aural stimuli to newborns and premature infants: an audiological perspective. *Journal of Music Therapy, 35*(2), 70–97.

de l'Etoile, S. (2006). Infant behavioral responses to infant-directed singing and other maternal interactions. *Infant Behavior & Development, 29*, 456–470.

Hanson-Abromeit, D. (2003). The Newborn Individualized Developmental Care and Assessment Program (NIDCAP) as a model for clinical music therapy interventions with premature infants. *Music Therapy Perspectives, 21*, 60–68.

O'Gorman, S. (2006). Theoretical interfaces in the acute paediatric context: A psychotherapeutic understanding of the application of infant-directed singing. *American Journal of Psychotherapy, 60*(3), 271–283.

Peebles-Kleiger, M. (2000). Pediatric and neonatal intensive care hospitalisation as traumatic stressor: Implications for intervention. *Bulletin of the Menninger Clinic, 6*(2), 257–280.

Philbin, M. K., & Evans, J. B. (2006). Standards for the acoustic environment of the newborn ICU. *Journal of Perinatology, 26*, S27–S30.

Shoemark, H. (1999). Singing as the foundation for multi-modal stimulation of the older pre-term infant. In R. R. Pratt & D. E. Grocke (Eds.), *Music Medicine 3: Musicmedicine and music therapy: Expanding horizons* (pp. 140–152). Melbourne, Australia: University of Melbourne.

Shoemark, H. (2000). The use of music therapy in treating infants with complex bowel complaints. In J. Loewy (Ed.), *Music therapy in the neonatal intensive care unit* (pp. 101–107). New York: Satchnote Press.

Shoemark, H. (2006). Infant-directed singing as a vehicle for regulation rehearsal in the medically fragile full-term infant. *Australian Journal of Music Therapy, 17*, 54–63.

Standley, J. M. (1998). The effect of music and multimodal stimulation on responses of premature infants in neonatal intensive care. *Pediatric Nursing, 24*(6), 532–538.

Standley, J. M., & Moore, R. S. (1995). Therapeutic effects of music and mother's voice on premature infants. *Pediatric Nursing, 21*(6), 509–512.

Steinberg, Z. (2006). Pandora meets the NICU parent or whither hope? *Psychoanalytic Dialogues, 16*(2), 133–147.

Helen Shoemark, Music Therapy Unit, Royal Children's Hospital, Melbourne, Australia.© Original 13th Jan 2003, Revised April 20th 2007

Stern, D. N. (1985): *The interpersonal world of the infant. A view from psychoanalysis and developmental psychology*. New York: Basic Books.

Trainor, L. (1996). Infant preference for the infant-directed versus non-infant-directed playsongs and lullabies. *Infant Behavior and Development, 19*, 83–92.

Trehub, S., Unyk, A., & Trainor, L. (1993). Adults identify infant-directed singing to infants. *Developmental Psychology, 3*, 500–507.

Trevarthen, C., & Malloch, S. (2000). "The Dance of Wellbeing: Defining the Musical Therapeutic Effect." *Nordic Journal of Music Therapy, 9*(2), 3–17.

Whipple. J. (2005). Music and multi-modal stimulation as intervention in neonatal intensive care. *Music Therapy Perspectives, 23*(2), 100–105.

White-Traut, R. C., Nelson, M. N., Silvestri, J. M., Patel, M., Vasan, U., Han, B. K., Cunningham, N., Burns, K., Kopsihke, K., & Bradford, L. (1999). Developmental intervention for preterm infants diagnosed with periventricular leukomalacia. *Research in Nursing Health, 22*(2), 131–143.

Helen Shoemark, Music Therapy Unit, Royal Children's Hospital, Melbourne, Australia.© Original 13th Jan 2003, Revised April 20th 2007

CHAPTER 3

Pediatric Intensive Care Unit (PICU)

Claire Ghetti
Ann Hannan

General Characteristics and Definition of Population

Historical Perspectives of Pediatric Intensive Care

The first hospital units specifically created to address the needs of critically ill and injured pediatric patients emerged in the late 1950s. These earliest pediatric intensive care units were associated with improved management of life-threatening conditions, especially acute respiratory failure (Downes, 1993). Since that time, advances in the understanding of life-threatening disease processes and improvements in the technologies that allow for the monitoring and treatment of these processes have led to the continued development of pediatric critical care medicine (American Academy of Pediatrics, 1993). Pediatric critical care has developed into a recognized medical subspecialty, serving approximately 20 out of every 10,000 children each year (Zimmerman, as cited in Melnyk et al., 2004).

The pediatric intensive care unit (PICU) itself has evolved along with advances in medical practice. In 1993, guidelines for the creation and implementation of PICUs were revised to include two levels of pediatric critical care. According to the American Academy of Pediatrics (AAP), the Level I PICU must be able to provide "definitive care for a wide range of complex, progressive, rapidly changing, medical, surgical, and traumatic disorders, often requiring a multidisciplinary approach, occurring in pediatric patients of all ages, excluding premature newborns" (AAP, 1993, p. 166). Level II PICUs exist in geographic areas that are distant from Level I facilities and do not have enough of a population base to support the specialized requirements of a Level I facility. Patients served in Level II PICUs display medical conditions that are less complex, more stable, and typically more predictable in their course (AAP, 1993). PICUs may also be referred to as pediatric critical care units (PCCU).

The environment of the Level I PICU reflects the complexity of the monitoring and life-saving processes that occur within it. Pediatric patients are admitted to the PICU due to acute trauma or critical medical illnesses that affect one or more body systems, or for stabilization after complex surgeries. Due to the fragility of their medical status, critical care patients require constant **hemodynamic and respiratory monitoring**, with administration of medication carefully adjusted based on subtle patient responses (Stouffer & Shirk, 2003). Nurse-to-patient ratios in the PICU are high, ranging from 2 to 1 to no more than 1 to 3 (AAP, 1993). To facilitate this intense monitoring, PICUs may be designed as clusters of small, partially glass-enclosed rooms, with small nursing stations located within each. Curtains around individual beds are provided for privacy. Separate single rooms with air exchange and pressurization systems are provided for patient isolation and can effectively produce consistent airborne isolation conditions. A specialized staff made up of pediatricians, pediatric surgical subspecialists (e.g., **surgeons**, **neurosurgeons**, or **orthopedists**), pediatric subspecialists (e.g., **intensivists**, **cardiologists**, or **endocrinologists**), pediatric anesthesiologists, radiologists, **pathologists**, psychiatrists/psychologists, respiratory therapists, social workers, child life specialists, music therapists, physical therapists, occupational therapists, nutritionists, pharmacists, chaplains, patient care technicians or nursing aides, and radiology technicians are available to work with nursing staff to provide the gamut of critical care services.[1] The volume of personnel and equipment required to complete critical care results in a potentially frenetic environment. Background noise levels from monitoring equipment alarms and the bustle of activity in the PICU can approach levels similar to that of normal urban traffic and street activity (Stouffer & Shirk, 2003). This continuous auditory stimulation contributes to disturbances in a patient's daily sleep/wake cycles, which may result in sleep deprivation.

In attempt to minimize extraneous noise, access to the PICU is controlled and visitation policies are enforced. Patients are typically given options to dim their individual overhead lights and to use curtains to decrease stimulation from the unit. Some PICU units use individual glass-enclosed isolation pods that help assure continued monitoring and isolation precautions, but help decrease sound pollution. Due to the amount of equipment required for intensive care, physical space around a patient's bed is often quite limited (Stouffer & Shirk, 2003). However, with the increasing emphasis on family-centered care, some pediatric critical care units provide rooming-in options for at least one family member at bedside. Given the potentially negative impact of environmental stressors on the patient, clinical measures for decreasing patient anxiety become vital in the intensive care setting.

---

[1] Pediatric intensivists are physicians who have completed subspecialty fellowship training in intensive care. The attending intensivist is the head physician in the PICU. PICU fellows are pediatricians that are training to become attending intensivists. The PICU medical team also includes residents that are physicians who have completed medical school and are training to become pediatricians.

Music Therapy in Pediatric Intensive Care

The use of music with adult critical care patients has demonstrated positive results for decreasing anxiety and pain, increasing positive mood, and improving physiological outcomes (Chlan, 1998; Updike, 1990; Wong, Lopez-Nahas, & Molassiotis, 2001). Many of the studies referring to the use of music therapy in the ICU consist of sedative music listening programs that are implemented by nurses during research protocols. Though these studies have produced evidence that supports the use of music within the intensive care environment, their authors generally make no differentiation between the therapeutic use of music by medical professionals and the implementation of music therapy methods by a trained therapist. Some of these research and clinical articles even define music therapy as a nursing procedure, while citing sources and methods from actual music therapy literature (Johnston & Rohaly-Davis, 1996; Updike, 1990). Recent interdisciplinary research efforts investigating the use of music therapy within intensive care settings have the potential to optimize quantitative inquiry regarding the effectiveness of music therapy within this setting. Combining the strengths of music therapists' training in the effects of music upon the individual with nurses' expertise in measuring physiological outcomes will lead to more efficacious scientific inquiry.

Though documented less frequently, outcomes of the use of music therapy with pediatric critical care patients appear to be similarly beneficial. Pediatric subjects requiring **mechanical ventilation** demonstrated improved maintenance of desired levels of sedation when given a listening program of sedative music combined with the mother's voice (Stouffer & Shirk, 2003). A secondary outcome of this study was the creation of a clinical protocol based on the study's research method for the use of a specific music therapy intervention to maintain optimal sedation for ventilator-dependent pediatric patients.

The use of intensive music therapy to facilitate emergence from coma and improve orientation for pediatric patients with severe traumatic brain injury has also been explored (Rosenfeld & Dun, 1999). Progressively more interactive live musical stimulation was employed within this approach to facilitate the comatose patient's awareness of self and others and support eventual responsiveness to the environment. Similarly, clinical examples have described the use of music therapy with two pediatric patients who were slowly emerging from coma (Kennelly & Edwards, 1997). Music therapy was used to promote relaxation, provide normalized sensory stimulation, facilitate basic communication responses, and structure supportive social interactions with family and caregivers as the patients became semiconscious. Music therapy methods to reduce stresses resulting from cardiac PICU hospitalization for both patient and family have also been described (Dun, 1995). Music therapy was discussed as a technique for providing normalization, increasing feelings of mastery, facilitating compliance with physical therapy requirements, and empowering parents. Interdisciplinary research outcomes in pediatric critical care music therapy will help provide justification for clinical programs. Preliminary results from current studies are informative and help guide practice, but additional investigation into the use of specific music therapy techniques for particular critical care populations is needed to demonstrate consistency of outcomes.

Common Characteristics of Pediatric Critical Care Patients

Although each hospital develops specific criteria for admission to the PICU, the American Academy of Pediatrics offers guidelines for the admission process (AAP, 1999). The AAP suggests that "severe or potentially life-threatening disease" in any of the following areas could warrant admission to the PICU (AAP, 1999, p. 840). A patient admitted to the PICU may experience dysfunction in any one or a combination of these body systems:

- **Respiratory system** (e.g., respiratory failure, severe asthma)
- **Cardiovascular system** (e.g., cardiovascular disease, shock)
- **Neurologic** (e.g., seizure disorder, meningitis, traumatic brain injury, neurosurgical conditions, progressive neuromuscular dysfunction)
- **Hematology/oncology** (e.g., life-threatening complications related to disease, life-threatening bleeding)
- **Endocrine/metabolic** (e.g., severe electrolyte abnormalities)
- **Gastrointestinal** (e.g., unstable gastrointestinal disease, severe gastrointestinal bleeding, acute hepatic failure)
- **Surgical** (e.g., organ transplantation, multiple trauma, major surgeries)
- **Renal system** (e.g., renal failure or insufficiency)
- **Multiple organ system failure** (e.g., toxin ingestions, electrical injuries)

While some patients are admitted to the PICU solely for respiratory issues such as specific pulmonary disease or **endotracheal intubation**, others require critical care due to respiratory distress secondary to a primary diagnosis (Randolph, Gonzales, Cortellini, & Yeh, 2004). For example, in a pediatric specialty hospital, a **hematology/oncology** patient will receive standard treatment on a designated hematology/oncology unit. If the patient suddenly requires mechanical breathing assistance or higher supplemental oxygen, he or she will be transferred to the PICU where the lower nurse-to-patient ratio and specialized training can provide specific respiratory support for this patient. Likewise, if the same patient undergoes an intense surgical procedure, he or she may be admitted to the PICU for special observation and support prior to returning to the specialty unit.

Pediatric patients admitted to the intensive care unit are at higher risk for experiencing negative emotional, behavioral, and academic outcomes as compared to patients in general inpatient units (Jones, Fiser, & Livingston, 1992). Thus, intensive care patients tend to exhibit higher levels of anxiety, apprehension, agitation, detachment, sadness, and crying (Jones et al., 1992; Stouffer & Shirk, 2003). Psychological and behavioral outcomes are influenced by the patient's severity of illness, duration of hospitalization, number of previous hospitalizations, and presence of a preexisting anxiety or mood disorder (Jones et al., 1992). As pediatric critical care patients are at risk for adverse psychological reactions to hospitalization, psychosocial interventions and support systems play an important preventive role in improving patient outcomes. Recent research has demonstrated that psychological and psychosocial outcomes for pediatric critical care patients may be improved when an educational–behavioral intervention program that aims to enhance parental coping abilities is implemented (Melnyk et al., 2004). Music therapy is a cost-effective intervention that may help improve coping skills for both patients and family, thereby reducing potential deleterious psychosocial outcomes of the critical care hospitalization.

Current Treatment Modalities/Approaches for PICU Patients

Patients in pediatric critical care settings receive continuous hemodynamic and respiratory monitoring. Common forms of monitoring include:

- **Cardiac monitor (EKG)**—displays child's heart rate and rhythm
- **Pulse oximeter (pulse ox)**—monitors the concentration of oxygen in blood (a.k.a. O_2 sat. monitor)
- **Body temperature monitoring**
- **Arterial or central venous pressure monitoring (A-lines and CVPs)**—measures blood pressure
- **Respiratory monitoring**—monitors respiratory rate and alerts of problems during mechanical ventilation

In addition to intensive monitoring, critical care patients may require several types of procedures to achieve stabilization of body systems while in the PICU. Some of the most common procedures and accompanying apparatus required for stabilization include:

- **Mechanical ventilation**—provides mechanical assistance for patients who cannot breathe independently; requires intubation
- **Endotracheal intubation**—process of placing an endotracheal (ET) tube through the nose or mouth into the trachea to maintain an open airway and permit mechanical ventilation and removal of secretions
- **Sedation**—required for certain life-saving procedures such as endotracheal intubation and mechanical ventilation; used to induce sleep, control agitation/anxiety, induce amnesia during paralysis or painful procedures to avoid unnecessary recall, and potentiate analgesia
- **Intravenous catheter (IV)**—tube placed in several different locations, including veins in the arm, neck, leg or groin, or the scalp in small infants; delivers medications, glucose, or other electrolyte solutions.
- **Feeding tube**—tube placed through nose to deliver **total parenteral nutrition** (TPN) to the digestive system
- **Nasogastric tube (NG tube)**—tube placed through the nose to the stomach to remove or administer medications or fluids

- **Foley catheter**—placed into the bladder to drain urine
- **Chest tubes**—tubes inserted through the skin, into the space around the lungs to drain fluid or air
- **Suctioning**—removal of mucous and fluid from the nose, mouth, or endotracheal tube

> (Bavdekar, Mahajan, & Chandu, 1999; New York Presbyterian Hospital, 2000)

PICU patients may also experience various types of scans, including MRI and CT scans, or biopsies to monitor their condition, pinpoint abnormalities, or assist in diagnosis. Successful placement of IV **catheters** may require several attempts, which can result in significant pain and anxiety for a child who is conscious and alert. The music therapist can help the pediatric critical care patient cope with the stress of intensive monitoring, as well as with the pain and anxiety related to required medical procedures.

Assessment

Determination of Eligibility for Services

Despite the tenuous medical status of pediatric patients encountered in intensive care, patients may benefit from music therapy methods. The music therapist faces the challenge of efficiently assessing a patient's current level of functioning and immediate needs, and choosing the appropriate intervention strategy to effectively address those needs. The level of patient participation in music therapy intervention will vary widely according to differences in level of alertness; sedation; active cognition; physical restriction due to injury, medical equipment, or restraint; the type and extent of injuries present; and developmental level.

In pediatric intensive care, music therapy is generally indicated for patients needing pain and anxiety management, especially during medical procedures; patients displaying emotional or behavioral problems; patients emerging from coma; and patients requiring nonpharmacological assistance in weaning from mechanical ventilation (Stouffer & Shirk, 2003). Music therapy is also indicated for improving developmental outcomes of patients requiring long-term hospitalization.

Occasionally the use of music therapy methods may be contraindicated for specific patients at certain points in time. The music therapist must be sensitive to when music therapy is having a negative impact upon a critical care patient. Auditory stimulation may occasionally negatively influence the desired level of sedation for a patient, leading to increased agitation. The music therapist may avoid overstimulating the patient by obtaining nursing staff's assessment of a patient's previous responses to sensory stimulation and by being attentive to patient responses during implementation of music therapy. During periods of high stress, even the most well conceived supportive music therapy interaction might be perceived as overwhelming to patients or parents. Music therapists must know when to give patients or parents space and time and learn how to re-approach patients or offer support to parents at a later opportunity.

As many critical care patients can benefit from some form of music therapy intervention, the therapist needs to create a method for prioritizing patients. Patients who lack consistent social supports should receive high priority for music therapy. Patients aged 7 months to 4 years are most at risk for experiencing psychological upset related to hospitalization and separation from parents (Thompson & Stanford, 1981); therefore, they should be given precedence. Patients who must undergo repeated invasive procedures, patients experiencing their first hospitalization, and patients with impaired communicative functioning due to the presence of endotracheal tubes should also receive priority. Patients who are not responding to other forms of treatment should receive higher priority than patients who are exhibiting positive response to other therapies.

Prioritization of Patient Referrals in the PICU

- Lack of consistent social supports
- At risk for psychological upset related to hospitalization and separation from parents (e.g., patients 7 months to 4 years)
- Repeated invasive procedures
- Experiencing their first hospitalization
- Impaired communicative functioning due to medical interventions (e.g., endotracheal tubes)
- Not responding to other forms of treatment

Referral Process

When implemented consistently, a clear and concise referral process may assist the music therapist in identifying patients who could benefit from services, and it may facilitate the assessment process. Referral procedures will vary by hospital, and the initiation of a formal referral system may require a lengthy review process by the Patient Care Board. Some hospitals may require a physician's order for music therapy services. This is especially true for settings where music therapy is partially or fully funded by third party reimbursement. Most commonly, referrals are made by a variety of staff including physicians; nurses; psychologists/psychiatrists; child life specialists; social workers; recreational, physical, occupational, or speech therapists; and chaplains. Referrals may consist of a completed written form that is directed to the music therapist, a referral note in a patient's electronic or paper chart, an emailed referral that maintains patient confidentiality, or a verbal referral. A sample PICU Music Therapy Referral Form is included in Figure 1. The music therapist may also receive referrals while participating in medical or psychosocial rounds on the intensive

---

Music Therapy Referral Form
Pediatric Intensive Care Unit

Patient Information:

Patient Name: _____   Room #: _____

Age: _____

Diagnosis: _____

Referring Person:

Name: _____   Department: _____

Extension: _____   Date of Referral: _____

Reason for Referral to Music Therapy (check all that apply):

❑   pain management (specify: _____)

❑   anxiety management (specify: _____)

❑   procedural support (specify: _____)

❑   non-pharmacological sedation required

❑   patient weaning from mechanical ventilation

❑   patient weaning from paralytic or sedative medication

❑   arousal from coma desired

❑   expressive difficulties (i.e. patient is withdrawn, aggressive, nonverbal)

❑   affective difficulties (i.e. patient appears depressed, hopeless)

❑   non-compliance with treatment regimen

❑   patient with repeated or long-term intensive care hospitalization

❑   patient requires prolonged isolation

❑   developmental or sensory stimulation needed

❑   social support needed

❑   family support needed

❑   end-of-life care

❑   other: _____

Additional Comments:

_____

_____

_____

_____

Figure 1. **PICU Music Therapy Referral Form**

care unit. Formal referrals are ideal, as they assist the music therapist in prioritizing patients, as well as educate staff as to the availability and scope of practice of music therapy. Referral source, even when the referral was given verbally, should be documented in the assessment form or summary note. A music therapist in a newly developed program may find that referrals from staff are infrequent, which may necessitate that the music therapist initially assess all patients superficially to determine priority of need.

Assessment Procedure

Assessment of patients in the pediatric intensive care setting relies on information from a variety of sources. Music therapists may employ a combination of assessment methods, including chart review, to assess medical history, social history, and treatment progress; patient and/or family interview; and observation of patient and family during both the presence and absence of musical interaction. Due to the variability of patients' medical status in the PICU, frequent re-assessment of patient needs and strengths will be required to assure appropriate goal and intervention planning.

Best practice methods would indicate the completion of a formal music therapy assessment document to be included in the chart of each patient that receives services. However, just as a formal referral form may require lengthy review by a Patient Care Board, a formal music therapy assessment will need to be reviewed and approved by such a board prior to its inclusion as a part of the patient's legally binding chart. Music therapy assessments for any population evaluate functioning in psychological, cognitive, physical, communicative, and social domains, as well as document the client's music history, preferences, and responses to music. Assessments for pediatric intensive care patients should also include information regarding diagnosis, patient's awareness of diagnosis and prognosis, infection control precautions, allergies, the patient's medical regimen and possible side effects, medical equipment precautions, restrictions to activity or movement, and an evaluation of coping tendencies. The patient's and family's cultural and spiritual background may also have implications for intervention and may be included in the assessment. The format and length of this assessment form may be altered depending on the logistical needs and document requirements of the setting in question. A sample PICU Music Therapy Assessment Form is included in Figure 2.

In cases where the inclusion of a formal music therapy assessment in the patient's chart is not permissible, a summary note is advised. The frequent turnover of patients in the PICU can also make a lengthy formal assessment process unmanageable. The documentation of a summary assessment note, or the inclusion of an assessment summary in the first session/progress note, is acceptable in these cases. A sample music therapy assessment summary note is presented on page 81.

PICU Music Therapy Assessment 10/2003 C. Ghetti

Patient Name: _____   Date: _____   Admit Date: _____
D/O/B and Age: _____
Primary Diagnosis: _____
Secondary/admitting Diagnosis: _____
Pt. aware of diagnosis/prognosis? Yes   No   Not determined
First Admission? Yes   No

| Isolation Precautions: |
| Allergies: |
| Medical Equip. Precautions: |

Referred by: _____
Reason: _____

Medical Regimen and Possible Side Effects: _____

Cognitive:
Level of alertness/sedation/coma:_____
Approximate developmental level (specify, suspected/reported): _____

Pain/Physical/Communicative:
Pt.'s current level of pain (0-10 Wong/Baker Faces Rating Scale for verbal; FLACC 1-3 for nonverbal): _____
Observed behaviors indicating pain: _____ Pain tolerance level: _____
Observed behaviors indicating anxiety: _____
Activity Status/Restrictions:_____
Limits to ROM: _____ Postural restrictions: _____
Sensory Impairments: _____
Receptive communication limitations: _____
Expressive communication limitations: _____

Emotional/Psychosocial:
Mood/Affect: ❑ Appropriate affect ❑ Flat affect ❑ Incongruent affect Comments: _____
          Self-reported current emotional state (use faces scale): _____
          Observed behaviors r/t mood: _____
Level of stranger anxiety: ❑ minimal ❑ moderate ❑ pronounced Comments: _____
Level of separation anxiety: ❑ normal for age ❑ moderate anxiety ❑ pronounced anxiety ❑ not determined
Familial support: ❑ consistent ❑ inconsistent ❑ not determined Comments: _____
Parental/familial anxiety: ❑ low ❑ average ❑ high   Comments: _____
Compliance w/treatment regimen: ❑ good   ❑ fair   ❑ needs improvement   ❑ not determined
          Comments: _____
Attitude towards medical procedures/diagnosis/prognosis: _____
Observed coping strategies: _____
Past coping strategies: _____
Level of engagement in Child Life services: ❑ consistent ❑ minimal ❑ n/a   Referred to CL: Yes No, for: _____

Music preferences: _____
Past uses of music: _____
Responses to music: _____

Recommended goals of MT intervention:
❑ pain management (specify: _____)   ❑ provide nonpharmacological sedation
❑ anxiety management (specify: _____)   ❑ preparation for medical procedures
❑ procedural support (specify: _____)   ❑ facilitate supportive interaction w/family
❑ increase range of motion (ROM)   ❑ decrease parental anxiety
   (recommend co-treat w/OT/PT: Yes   No)   ❑ accomplish developmental tasks
❑ increase expressive communication   (specify: _____)
❑ identify fears r/t hospitalization/diagnosis   ❑ other: (specify: _____)

Recommended MT intervention: ❑ Individual ❑ with Family   ❑ Other: _____
❑ music-assisted relaxation (MAR) (specify: _____)   ❑ songwriting
❑ alternate engagement during medical procedures (MAE)   ❑ dramatic play
❑ instrument playing (specify: _____)   ❑ music listening
❑ singing   ❑ other (specify: _____)

Summary and Plan:
_____
_____

Name: _____   Title: _____   Date: _____

Figure 2. PICU Music Therapy Assessment Form

Sample Music Therapy Summary Assessment Note
Pediatric Intensive Care Unit

Date: 8/2/04
Time: 4:00 pm

History and Assessment:
Patient is a 3.5-year-old female with single ventricle, admitted to the PICU on 7/26/04 for monitoring status-post reconstructive heart surgery. Pt. was referred to music therapy by Child Life for developmental stimulation and to improve coping with possible long-term hospitalization. Pt. presents as alert, with suspected mild developmental delay as evidenced by expressive communication frequently limited to single-word responses, poor diction, echolalic responses to questions, and difficulty following two-step commands. Pt. currently reports no pain, though has demonstrated poor pain tolerance during medical procedures as evidenced by screaming and avoidant behaviors. Pt. demonstrates improved coping when caregiver (e.g., parent or sibling) is present and provides physical support. Pt. makes frequent demands for needs fulfillment, often requesting caregiver or nurse to be continuously present at pt.'s bedside. Pt. typically presents flat affect and is quiet and calm, but exhibits anxious behavior when caregiver is not present. Pt.'s family supports are inconsistent (parents are separated and argue when together at bedside), and pt. demonstrates marked difficulty separating from caregiver. Pt. is resistant to nursing interventions and has cried, appeared fearful, and demonstrated avoidant behaviors when presented with nursing procedures.

Pt. demonstrates positive affect when presented with familiar songs, instrument play, and the inclusion of family members in music interactions. Pt. sings along to familiar songs, approximating words, and actively engages in music making when not anxious. Music intervention is less effective when pt. is already anxious due to medical procedures.

Summary and Plan:
Pt. faces long-term admission status-post cardiac surgery and complications, has inconsistent social support, and demonstrates significant separation anxiety and possible developmental delay, which together negatively affect pt.'s compliance with medical interventions. Recommend use of active music engagement (e.g., singing familiar songs, instrument playing, music-facilitated dramatic play) 2x per week to decrease separation anxiety, improve independent coping skills, and facilitate developmental gains.

Goal 1: To decrease separation anxiety

Objective 1: Given prior preparation and opportunities for closure at the end of music therapy sessions, pt. will return instruments when cued, say good-bye, and choose an independent transitional activity without displaying stress behaviors for each session across 3 consecutive sessions.

Approach to Patients

Prior to approaching a patient in the PICU, it is important to consult with the patient's nurse to determine any patient restrictions in activity or stimulation, or to confirm current infection control requirements. This consult is often a very brief verbal exchange, but can be critical in preventing the music therapist from introducing contraindicated interactions. Occasionally a nurse may be unfamiliar with music therapy practices, and this brief consult may be used to reduce misconceptions that may be at the core of a nurse's resistance to music therapy intervention. Also, consulting with nursing staff prior to sessions may help them feel respected and partially invested in the intervention process. In the rare occasions when music stimulation is contraindicated, the music therapist may choose to use an initial session to provide support to parents and/or interview parents to assist in the assessment process.

When first approaching a patient in the PICU, it is important to assess and acknowledge the patient's current physiological, cognitive, and emotional status. Patient-reported levels of pain and discomfort may be used to prioritize goals for immediate interaction. The initial session is often a combination of formal or informal assessment, immediate goal setting, and corresponding intervention. Needs of the moment are addressed first, and the therapist takes note of long-term or secondary goals to be addressed in following sessions. When a patient is unconscious due to sedation or coma, parent interview may be necessary to determine the patient's musical preferences and past responses to music.

Typical Treatment Goals and Objectives for Pediatric Critical Care Patients

Upon completion of the music therapy assessment, the music therapist develops a treatment plan for the PICU patient. Table 1 lists common goal areas and objectives for PICU patients and their families. This list serves as a representative sample of possible goal areas and patient objectives, both of which will be individualized according to a patient-centered process during the development of the music therapy treatment plan. For each targeted goal area, the music therapist identifies one or more objectives that represent concrete steps towards the accomplishment of that goal. For each objective, the music therapist may develop criteria to specify duration and frequency of patient responses, such as how long the patient will maintain a particular rate of respiration or how many times the patient will verbally respond to the music interaction. These determinations are made based on the patient's needs and strengths.

In addition to patient-specific goal areas, several general goal areas are naturally addressed during most music therapy interventions. Music therapy helps provide normalization within the PICU environment for the patient. For example, the use of familiar music, inclusion of family members and friends, and opportunities for the patient to make choices all affect the patient's level of comfort with his or her hospital stay. These aspects of the normalizing music interaction also lead to feelings of competence and mastery over the environment. Music therapy can effectively create a supportive context that elicits improved responsiveness from the patient and fosters positive coping responses (Robb, 2003). Music therapy interactions affirm the patient's musical and nonmusical skills, highlighting abilities instead of disabilities. This is especially important for a patient who has experienced loss of previous functioning due to illness, injury, or surgery. Music therapy also facilitates improved verbal or nonverbal communication, which frequently leads to increased emotional expression. Improved communicative effectiveness and the supported release of emotions can help the pediatric patient experience feelings of empowerment, thereby improving his or her coping skills.

Table 1

Common Goal Areas and Objectives for PICU Patients and Families

Patient Goal Areas	Music Therapy Implementation Goals	Patient Objectives
ALL (The patient objectives included in this row are appropriate for all music therapy goals developed for patients in the PICU. Additional specific objectives are provided with each goal area.)		a. Patient's vital signs will remain in therapeutically acceptable range. b. Patient's vital signs will move into a therapeutically acceptable range. c. Patient will respond physically to music stimuli. d. Patient will make eye contact with the music therapist, other staff members, or family members in the room.
Alleviate Anxiety Related to: • Hospitalization • Ventilator use • Separation anxiety • New diagnosis • Fear of medical providers • Upcoming procedures and surgeries • During procedures	1. Music therapist will provide opportunities for creative expression through singing, songwriting, and playing instruments. 2. Music therapist will provide opportunities for relaxation through the use of live music.	a. Patient will identify hospital-related fears. b. Patient will verbalize one adaptive skill for coping with hospital-related anxiety. c. Patient will exhibit signs of relaxation as evidenced by release of physical tension.
Promote Relaxation and Decrease Agitation/ Combativeness Related to: • Ventilator dependency • Emergence from coma • Withdrawal from sedative medication • Children with developmental delays • Infant/toddler response to critical care environment	1. Music therapist will provide opportunities for relaxation through the use of live music. 2. Music therapist will provide opportunities for relaxation through the use of recorded music.	a. Patient will exhibit signs of relaxation as evidenced by release of physical tension. b. Patient will decrease frequency or intensity of combative behavior. c. Patient will fall asleep.

Table 1—Continued

Patient Goal Areas	Music Therapy Implementation Goals	Patient Objectives
Improve Pain Management • Chronic pain • During procedures	1. Music therapist will teach relaxation techniques (e.g., progressive muscle relaxation) with music. 2. Music therapist will provide opportunities for alternately engaging patient's attention through singing, songwriting, and playing instruments. 3. Music therapist will provide opportunities for patient to nonverbally or verbally express the pain.	a. Patient will exhibit signs of relaxation as evidenced by release of physical tension. b. Patient will verbalize decreased perception of pain. c. Patient will indicate decreased pain score using FACES (Wong, Hockenberry-Eaton, Wilson, Winkelstein, & Schwartz, 2005) pain scale. d. Patient will qualitatively describe the pain perception with words or sounds.
Increase Sensory Stimulation for Patients: • In isolation • With long-term stays • With developmental delays	1. Music therapist will provide **multisensory stimulation** through the use of touch paired with singing or humming. 2. Music therapist will provide multisensory stimulation through the use of instruments with appealing visual qualities. 3. Music therapist will pair music with tactile stimulation provided by family member or other healthcare worker (e.g., PT, OT, nurse)	a. Patient will initiate physical movement. b. Patient will tolerate sensory stimulation without exhibiting stress behaviors. c. Patient will demonstrate auditory and/or visual tracking given sensory prompts.

Table 1—Continued

Patient Goal Areas	Music Therapy Implementation Goals	Patient Objectives
Improve Active Cognition for Patients: • In isolation • With long-term stays • With developmental delays • Emerging from sedation or coma	1. Music therapist will provide cognitive stimulation through the use of live music. 2. Music therapist will provide cognitive stimulation through the use of conversation about musical material or ideas. 3. Music therapist will incorporate reality-oriented prompts within musical or verbal interaction.	a. Patient will sing with music therapist. b. Patient will respond verbally to music stimuli. c. Patient will initiate musical interaction. d. Patient will make musical and nonmusical choices. e. Patient will display long-term memory as evidenced by verbal comments or musical responses. f. Patient will display short-term memory as evidenced by verbal comments or musical responses. g. Patient will respond to prompts with reality-oriented answers.
Alleviate Depression Related To: • Diagnosis/prognosis • Lengthy hospitalization • Frequent invasive procedures • Decreasing required pain or sedative medications	1. Music therapist will provide opportunities for creative expression through singing, songwriting, and playing instruments.	a. Patient will verbalize one skill for coping with hospital-related depression. b. Patient will exhibit elevated mood as evidenced by smiles, positive comments, and by engaging in preferred activities.
Develop Therapeutic Environment for Palliative Care	1. Music therapist will provide live music to create a soothing environment based on patient and family preferences. 2. Music therapist will provide recorded music to create a soothing environment based on patient and family preferences.	a. Patient will exhibit signs of relaxation as evidenced by release of physical tension. b. Patient will exhibit decreased amount of agitation when using recorded music per nursing report when music therapist is not present.

Table 1—Continued

Patient Goal Areas	Music Therapy Implementation Goals	Patient Objectives
Increase Range of Motion • Fine motor skills • Gross motor skills • Facilitate compliance during PT/OT	1. Music therapist will support physical goals through playing instruments and singing. 2. Music therapist will use music as motivation and accompaniment for goals such as ambulation and positional changes.	a. Patient will maintain or increase functional movement. b. Patient will complete physical tasks when music is used as a timekeeper or for motivation.

Family Goal Areas	Music Therapy Implementation Goals	Family Objectives
Increase Family Support	1. Music therapist will provide live musical interaction and songwriting for creative expression. 2. Music therapist will provide supportive listening and verbal validation of family's emotional expression.	a. Family members will verbalize feelings and fears related to patient's hospitalization. b. Family members will provide information about patient and family musical preferences. c. Family members will identify their goals for patient during hospitalization. d. Family members will identify coping skills. e. Family members will create musical "gifts" or "mementos" for the patient.
Normalize Family Interaction	1. Music therapist will provide opportunities for family to be involved in making decisions about patient's care. 2. Music therapist will provide opportunities for family to interact with patient musically. 3. Music therapist will provide resources of family's preferred recorded music when possible.	a. Family members will initiate suggestions and make choices for patient's care. b. Family members will participate in musical interaction at each member's comfort level.

Several factors will affect the frequency and duration of music therapy sessions for the PICU patient. The number of sessions per week is determined by the patient's ability to tolerate the interventions, the patient's daily schedule, and the availability of the therapist. The duration of each session is affected by the patient's tolerance of the music stimulation and the length of time needed to complete tasks or reach goals.

Intervention Environment

Patients may be admitted to the PICU from the emergency department or a different pediatric unit of the hospital, transferred from a different medical facility, or admitted for monitoring or stabilization following major surgery. Patients may receive care and constant monitoring in the PICU for several days after major surgery or trauma. For patients with extensive medical conditions affecting more than one body system or for those whose condition is worsened by complications, a stay in the PICU may last for several weeks. Patients with chronic disease or disabilities may experience multiple admissions to the PICU over time with varying lengths of stay. The course of stay for a PICU patient will vary depending upon the patient's level of physiological stability, response to medication, and the need for additional procedures/surgeries.

The first priority upon admission to the PICU is stabilization of the patient. Occasionally parents are asked to wait in a family area during this process. Immediate goals of nursing care include minimizing complications and providing physical and psychological care and support. Once the patient has stabilized, efforts are made toward restoring maximum health potential and reducing health risks.

Patients are considered for discharge once they achieve stability in hemodynamic parameters, respiratory status, and neurological status, and do not require complex intervention, or have experienced a reversal in the disease process (AAP, 1999). Very few patients are discharged directly from the PICU to home. Once their condition becomes more stable and they require less intense monitoring, most patients transfer to a step-down unit or step-down beds within the PICU. Patients transferred to a regular inpatient unit will receive continued, but less intense, monitoring and follow-up care until they are ready to be discharged home.

Due to the logistical challenges of the intense monitoring that is used in critical care, almost all patients receive music therapy services at bedside. Thus, the vast majority of patient sessions are individual in nature, with the inclusion of siblings, parents, and other friends and family members as appropriate. Occasionally the music therapist may facilitate peer interaction between two or more patients who are roommates, when feasible and developmentally appropriate. As sessions occur at bedside, the music therapist must create a workable system for transporting equipment to the patient and for using instruments in a very limited amount of space. The monitoring and life-saving equipment surrounding each PICU bed leaves very little open room. Mobile computer stations, small bedside tables, sleeper chairs, and family effects may also be located around the bedside, further decreasing available space. The music therapist who uses a guitar must consider which side of the patient's bed allows enough room for the instrument, as well as which side would be most appropriate in terms of the patient's physical or sensory limitations. The use of portable keyboards may be hampered by a lack of table space. Often there is only a small, adjustable bedside tray table available to hold instruments or equipment in front of the patient. This tray table space is frequently covered with items used for nursing care or meal trays. Battery-powered electronic instruments are useful, as access to outlets may be limited in the PICU, and most hospitals require three-prong grounding for all electronic devices that are plugged into outlets. Infection control policies for proper cleaning and sanitization of musical instruments should be established through consultation with the facility's infection control or epidemiology department and should be strictly followed.

Group Work in the PICU

Due to the extensive monitoring and life-supporting measures of critical care, it is rare for a group of patients to be assembled for group work. Instead, music therapists working in the PICU may offer groups to parents, siblings, or staff members. Support groups for parents are often offered as part of family-centered care efforts and aim to reduce parental stress, provide a support network comprised of other parents, and improve parental coping with demands of the intensive care environment. These groups may meet weekly and may be led by social workers or child life specialists. Music therapists may consult at these groups and offer stress management, emotional outlets, and suggestions for improving interaction between parent and child. Music therapists may also provide supportive groups for siblings of PICU patients. Music therapy may be used within a sibling group to facilitate communication, decrease misconceptions, address siblings' fears, and provide support and validation for siblings who may be starved for individual attention. Music therapists may provide wellness services for staff on the intensive care unit either by setting up a relaxation protocol within a timeout room, or by offering brief stress management groups for nurses to engage in during breaks.

Follow-up Services on Other Inpatient Units

Many patients will transfer from the PICU to other inpatient units prior to being discharged from the hospital. Some patients will transfer to several different units during hospitalization. The music therapist serves a unique and important role for these patients. The music therapist can create a familiar and consistent environment for these patients through music interaction. When transferred, the PICU patient will meet new nursing staff members, residents, physicians, respiratory therapists, and social workers. If the music therapist has the flexibility to follow the patient to his or her new unit, the music therapist can assess the patient's adjustment to the changes in the care environment. The music therapist can adjust goals and objectives to allow the patient to explore his or her new environment from the familiar and supportive structure of the music therapy session.

Co-treatment in the PICU

The success of music therapy interventions in the PICU depends on the coordinated effort of the patient's entire treatment team. In the PICU, fatigue, sedation, and grave medical condition can affect the patient's ability to endure extended periods of stimulation. These situations can warrant co-treatment sessions to meet the patient's needs in a time-efficient manner. Music therapists can assist nursing staff in the PICU in several ways. Live music in the PICU atmosphere not only benefits the patients, but also serves to reduce stress for staff members. When patients' vital signs are in therapeutically acceptable ranges without signs of distress or agitation, nursing staff members report increased feelings of calm or relaxation. One author has received the following feedback from PICU nurses:

- "I wasn't here during your sessions last week and missed hearing the music."
- "We have had several stressful incidents today. May I participate in this music therapy session?"
- "The music from your sessions calms everyone down: doctors, family members, patients, and us nurses."

First and foremost, music therapy sessions focus on the needs of the patient and the patient's family. In addition, the music therapist can meet the needs of treatment team members by co-treating with other staff members to address multiple goals simultaneously. The music therapist can serve as a consultant to other treatment team members about patient preferences and abilities, while gleaning important information from these treatment team members about their interactions with the patient.

Co-treating requires advanced planning by both sets of medical professionals. At the very least, each specialty should have an opportunity to communicate its goals and objectives for the patient. This might occur during a care conference or medical rounds. For medical staff members who are unfamiliar with music therapy, the board-certified music therapist (MT-BC) should plan an in-service for each department. In addition to providing information about music therapy, the music therapist should also reserve time to discuss how MT-BCs and other medical staff can interface during a patient session. By seeking information about the patient goals determined by other medical staff members, the music therapist can gain greater insight into the overall needs of the patient. The music therapist can also serve as a consultant to other medical staff members by providing suggestions of how to incorporate music into treatment sessions when it is appropriate and beneficial for the patient.

The Child Life Council describes a child life specialist as one who "use[s] play, recreation, education, self-expression, and theories of child development to promote psychological well-being and optimum development of children, adolescents, and their families" (Child Life Council, n.d.). Many music therapists in the hospital setting are affiliated with the hospital's child life department. Others work closely with child life specialists assigned to inpatient units and outpatient clinics or centers. Child life specialists (CLS) can assist the medical music therapist by identifying patients who are appropriate candidates for music therapy assessment. CLSs formally or informally assess each patient on their units. The PICU CLS may also receive specific referrals for individual patients. The CLS presence and interaction with each patient and family provides valuable information for the music therapist to triage patient referrals.

Certified Child Life Specialists (CCLSs) are nationally certified professionals who help pediatric patients cope with hospitalization and positively adjust to illness. Child life specialists provide normalizing play and peer interaction opportunities for patients, developmentally appropriate preparation for medical procedures, and procedural support for a variety of invasive and noninvasive medical procedures. These professionals also work with siblings and parents to provide support and education and to improve patient–family interactions.

A music therapist may also identify patient issues during the course of the music therapy interaction that might be resolved through subsequent follow-up sessions with a child life specialist. Frequently, a patient will express a specific fear or medically based misunderstanding during expressive music play. The music therapist may then share this information with child life staff that can provide additional opportunities for medical teaching and the lessening of fears through medical play. Often the music therapist and child life specialist address similar goals through differing media, or address similar issues along a continuum. Child life specialists can work in tandem with music therapists, either simultaneously or sequentially, to prepare patients for procedures, to normalize medical equipment, to address a particular patient's phobia, or to implement a behavior management plan.

In addition to child life specialists, many child life programs employ schoolteachers, librarians, and special events coordinators. In one author's experience, co-treatment with child life specialists and other members of the child life department does not occur as a simultaneous presence at the patient's bedside. Rather, the music therapist and child life specialist discuss PICU patients at bi-weekly child life rounds. Together, they determine the best method of intervention for each patient's needs. In order to best utilize staff resources, the music therapist conducts sessions independently with the patient if members of the child life department determine that the patient's needs are best met by music therapy interventions.

For the school-aged PICU patient, the schoolteacher acts as a liaison between the patient's school and the hospital. The PICU patient may or may not be able to complete traditional schoolwork during admission. The music therapist has a unique opportunity to design an alternative music or fine arts curriculum (in consultation with the educational liaison) for the PICU patient. An intervention as simple as learning how to sing or play particular instruments can be applied as school credit for these nontraditional students. In this way, a music therapist can address goals such as chronic pain management or maintaining a functional range of motion while assisting the patient with his or her coursework. The music therapist may also reinforce academic concepts during music therapy interventions.

Music therapists may also co-treat with recreation therapists in the hematology/oncology setting. Recreation therapists aim to improve a patient's functional skills as they relate to play and leisure and to help facilitate the development of healthy leisure outlets. A music therapist may co-treat with a recreation therapist during a group music or movement activity to promote stress release, improve mood, and improve quality of peer interaction. Adolescent hematology/oncology patients often bond most easily while engaging in preferred recreational activities. The music therapist can collaborate with the recreation therapist to facilitate active participation and verbal or nonverbal expression during these activities. The two disciplines may also collaborate to assure a patient can engage in preferred leisure activities upon discharge, such as the initiation of music lessons or participation in music ensembles.

Next to child life department members, nursing staff can be the greatest advocates for music therapy. Bedside nurses can observe, firsthand, the benefits of music therapy interventions with PICU patients. They are most likely to read documentation provided by the music therapist and are valuable sources of undocumented information about the patient. Nursing staff can serve as the liaison between the music therapist and the physicians. The music therapist will not always have an opportunity to interact with the physicians depending on their availability, scheduled rounds, and patient caseload. Because nurses typically work 12-hour shifts and are unit-based, they interact with the physicians on a daily basis. They can request music therapy referrals and provide feedback to the physicians about the patient's progress during music therapy sessions.

Other disciplines such as occupational, physical, and speech therapies are typically impressed by accomplishments of patients when music therapy is involved in co-treatment. Patient responses to other therapies may be more positive with the involvement of music therapy. For example, the music therapist can co-treat with the physical therapist (PT) or occupational therapist (OT) to address physical range of motion (ROM) to maintain baseline levels of functioning. The addition of music interventions to PT/OT sessions can decrease the amount of time needed to provide passive ROM exercises. The music therapist can address the patient's possible need for pain management or relaxation during these exercises. This decreases the patient's resistance to such exercises, thereby decreasing the amount of time needed for such interventions. The music therapist can also provide structure and enjoyment by utilizing the patient's musical preferences and strengths to execute the exercises. This could include the live or recorded use of the patient's preferred music to create a natural timekeeper. This could also include the use of instruments to simulate movements prescribed by the PT or OT.

Speech pathologists may also be amenable to co-treatment. As it is difficult for disciplines to schedule time to provide simultaneous co-treatment, music therapy may be used independently to reinforce progress towards speech therapy goals. For instance, after reading documentation or consulting with a speech pathologist, the MT-BC learns that a child is having difficulty with articulation of initial and final consonants. The music therapist may write a silly song where the patient could practice repeated nonsense syllables in a safe musical context. Patients can also sing or say words to "fill-in-the-blank" within songs, guess answers to musical riddles, as well as rhyme words in order to practice articulation.

Music therapists may also work closely with social workers and chaplains to address the psychosocial and spiritual needs of long-term pediatric hematology/oncology patients. A patient may reveal certain preexisting psychosocial problems during the course of music therapy interaction, either through verbal or nonverbal expressive means. A pediatric patient may demonstrate evidence of prior abuse or familial conflict during musical play, improvisation, or songwriting experiences. The music therapist should discuss these issues with the unit social worker to determine the need for and nature of appropriate follow-up intervention. Occasionally during the course of music therapy intervention, parents will evidence the need for additional psychosocial support beyond the level that can be appropriately addressed by the music therapist. In these cases, the music therapist should notify the social worker of this potential need, which may ultimately result in referrals for individual psychotherapy, couples therapy, or domestic violence intervention. The social worker may also co-treat with the music therapist to provide supportive end-of-life services for patients, siblings, and parents when appropriate. In turn, the music therapist may collaborate with social workers and chaplains to provide music during patient memorial services on the unit, or for an annual memorial service to honor all pediatric patients who have died.

Family-Centered Care

According to the Institute for Family-Centered Care (n.d.), family-centered care is characterized by four principles:

1. People are treated with dignity and respect.
2. Health care providers communicate and share complete and unbiased information with patients and families in ways that are affirming and useful.
3. Patients and family members build on their strengths by participating in experiences that enhance control and independence.
4. Collaboration among patients, family members, and providers occurs in policy and program development and professional education, as well as in the delivery of care.

While the Institute for Family-Centered Care suggests that these principles be employed with all patients, regardless of age, this approach has had a special impact on pediatric settings throughout the United States. The design of music therapy interventions facilitates the process of family-centered care. The music therapist can consult with the patient's family during the assessment and treatment planning process. This is a symbiotic relationship for the therapist and family. The therapist obtains valuable information about the patient's preferences and needs from the "experts" about the patient. Families are the best sources of information about a patient since they are the patient's primary caregivers. The music therapist can provide tangible opportunities for family members and the patient to make choices about the patient's course of treatment.

As previously mentioned, pediatric patients requiring intensive care are at risk for experiencing short-term and long-term negative emotional, behavioral, and academic outcomes (Jones et al., 1992). Parents of these patients are likewise at risk for experiencing negative outcomes, including depression, anxiety, and post traumatic stress disorder (PTSD) (Melnyk et al., 2004). The stress of acute illness, trauma, or long-term hospitalization can affect all members of the family unit. Often, parents who are stressed cannot give full support to their children, leaving patients and siblings without essential social and emotional support when they need it most (Dun, 1995; Robb, 1999).

Policies and practices that support families in their role of promoting the well-being of their children are seen in the pediatric critical care environment. Many PICUs do not limit visiting hours for parents in order to make parental support available to patients at all times; however, parents may be asked to momentarily step out of the room during procedures, physician rounds, nursing shift changes, or emergencies. Most frequently, accommodations are available for one parent or parental designee to sleep in a reclining chair or cot at bedside, or in a designated quiet room adjacent to the PICU. Some PICUs have created family-friendly glass-enclosed patient areas that will accommodate one parent. Overnight accommodations for a minimal charge may also be arranged at a nearby Ronald McDonald House for families who live more than 50 miles from the hospital. Extended family and friends are able to visit children in the PICU, with most units enforcing a two-person limit at bedside. School-age children can visit a sibling in the PICU, but they generally meet with a nurse prior to their first visit to prepare them for what they will encounter in the PICU. Many PICUs offer a parent lounge that includes bathroom facilities, telephones, Internet access, and vending machines. Interfaith chapels and quiet rooms offer refuge for parents who may be taxed by the demands of the critical care setting.

The recent emphasis on family-centered care is especially relevant to the pediatric critical care environment. The family is typically the pediatric patient's main source of support. Family-centered care acknowledges this strength and seeks to use this natural source of support to improve patient outcomes. Families are supported and empowered to excel in their caregiving and decision-making roles, even within the intensive care setting. Family-centered care has been associated with the following benefits: improved patient outcomes, increased patient and family satisfaction, improved use of family resources, increased staff satisfaction, decreased health care costs, and more effective use of health care resources (AAP, 2003). Parents supporting children through medical procedures, patients and families contributing to plans of care, patients participating in the management of their own health care, families participating in formal or informal support groups, and parents serving on family advisory councils to improve operational issues in hospitals are all realities within a family-centered approach.

Parents and siblings, along with the patient, are considered part of the treatment team in family-centered care. As such, families are encouraged to take part in decision making and to engage in caretaking to the greatest extent possible (e.g., feeding, diaper changing, bathing). Chaplaincy services, parent support groups, and social work services offer additional emotional and social support for family members. Child life specialists may work with siblings to resolve misconceptions regarding the patient's status and treatment, provide suggestions for meaningful engagement with the patient, and give developmentally appropriate coping support. Music therapists may use their medium to facilitate normalized family-patient interactions (Dun, 1995) and provide additional support to parents and siblings. End-of-life services, including anticipatory bereavement services, may also be provided for families through social work, chaplaincy, child life or music therapy programming.

End of Life Care/Bereavement Services

Medical personnel are understandably reluctant to give up life-saving measures for a patient whose health status is deteriorating for fear that this cessation may be premature. The resulting postponement of considering the possibility of imminent death can mean that patients die before families have begun to prepare for such an event. Ideally, end-of-life services would be offered for the patient, when developmentally appropriate, and anticipatory grieving support given to siblings and family prior to the patient's death. Social workers are available to counsel parents as to what they might expect emotionally and practically surrounding the death experience. When patients die unexpectedly, families may be given a bereavement packet that gives supportive information as well as referrals for formal bereavement services outside of the PICU setting. Some PICUs have a policy allowing for the arrangement of a private room for families to spend a period of hours with their recently deceased.

Music therapy may be used as the intensive care patient's health declines prior to death, as well as during the period immediately following the death. The music therapist tends to shift focus away from the patient and towards the family as the patient becomes less alert and the family begins to face the reality of the child's impending death. Music therapists may provide patient-preferred, sedative, or religious songs based on family preferences. The music therapist may also improvise songs that incorporate words of love and support for the patient from family members and provide a supportive musical context within which family members may comfortably express their grief. Families who have appreciated the prior use of music therapy with their child may ask the music therapist to play a religious or personally meaningful song immediately after the child's death while family members are mourning.

Implementation of Interventions

Due to the intensity of critical care needs in the PICU, a patient's current level of functioning becomes more of a deciding factor than does a patient's developmental level when considering intervention strategies. For example, patients with very different pre-injury developmental levels may present at the same functional level when in a comatose state or when sedated. The music therapist focuses more on the patient's current states of alertness and active cognition when choosing interventions, rather than making decisions based on typical developmental stages. However, music, instruments, and techniques should be selected with age-appropriate considerations in mind to convey respect for the patient's pre-injury age and developmental level.

Several music therapy interventions are used regularly in the PICU setting, with the therapist making individual modifications based on patient strengths and weaknesses. Music-assisted relaxation (MAR), music as alternate engagement during medical procedures (MAE), multisensory stimulation, structured or improvised songwriting, music-facilitated dramatic play, and instrument playing are all interventions that may be used in the critical care environment when appropriate. Task analyses of the first five of these interventions are included in the Resources at the end of this monograph. Readers are also encouraged to see Stouffer and Shirk (2003, p. 69) for a research-derived intervention protocol for the use of personalized sedative music with patients requiring mechanical ventilation.

The music therapist considers several factors when choosing which intervention to implement with a patient. Based on the results of patient assessment, the therapist chooses interventions that will most likely provide opportunities for the successful attainment of identified goals and objectives. The therapist must also consider the current cognitive, emotional, communicative, and physical functioning levels of the patient, along with the patient's music preferences, when choosing intervention strategies. Once the therapist selects an intervention that is likely to lead to desired outcomes and can accommodate the patient's abilities and disabilities, the therapist commences the initial approach.

During implementation, the therapist will make adaptations to the general intervention depending upon current patient needs and responses. Thus, a therapist may begin with a passively oriented intervention, such as music listening, and gradually increase the level of active participation as tolerated by the patient. All of the aforementioned interventions can be modified to match the patient's current functioning and developmental levels. For example, a school-aged child may participate in songwriting by offering single words to "fill-in-the-blank" during the rewriting of lyrics to a familiar song. Adolescents may successfully create complete original lyrics given the supportive structure of blues songwriting. A patient on mechanical ventilation who is unable to verbally communicate may indicate words or subjects to insert into a song using a pictorial communication board. The therapist will adapt individual interventions depending upon patient needs and will switch between interventions depending upon patient responses and outcomes.

Outcome Measures

Frequent evaluation of the effectiveness of music therapy interventions to achieve assessed goals and objectives is necessary when working with critical care patients. Changes in a patient's alertness, physical functioning, pain levels, and mood may be due to the occurrence of procedures, side effects of medication, disturbances in sleep patterns, presence of coma or sedation, or changes in a patient's overall health status. As these factors influence a patient's response to intervention, treatment approaches may also vary from session to session depending upon the abilities and responses of a patient on a particular day.

Pediatric Critical Care Case Examples

1. Short-term (single session): Procedural support for renal biopsy

H. was a 16-year-old patient admitted to the PICU with renal failure who required a renal biopsy. The biopsy was to be performed at bedside within the PICU. The patient's pediatric intensive care fellow made a verbal referral for music therapy to assist in anxiety management surrounding the procedure. The music therapist (MT-BC) approached the patient to offer music therapy as procedural support without knowing any of the patient's prior medical or personal history.

When the music therapist entered H.'s room, she was lying prone in bed awaiting an **ultrasound** that would identify the exact position for the biopsy. Three physicians and one nurse were moving around her bed, checking monitors, discussing matters related to her care, completing the ultrasound, and telling her to "relax." After introducing herself, the MT-BC explained how music could be used to help H. stay calm and feel more comfortable during the procedure. At this point, H. was alert and communicated verbally. H. reported a moderate level of anxiety and fear related to the upcoming procedure and stated that she had never experienced a biopsy before. Due to the patient's age-appropriate developmental level and moderate, but not pronounced, level of anxiety, the MT-BC decided to use music combined with imagery to facilitate a relaxation response. The music therapist then began slowly strumming a simple major chord progression on her guitar to approximate the rate of H.'s breathing, and gradually decreased tempo to encourage a calming response. The MT-BC used spoken and sung cues to facilitate deep breathing. The MT-BC asked H. to think of a place where she felt secure and calm, a place with relaxing associations. H. chose the beach, and the MT-BC directed H. to choose a place to sit or lay down at the beach where she would feel supported and secure. The MT-BC used prompts to provoke additional images related to sights, sounds, smells, and tastes of H.'s preferred scene. The MT-BC emphasized feeling calm and secure throughout. Gentle finger picking of chords on the guitar was used to structure deep and slow inhalations while the MT-BC quietly sang these prompts and incorporated H.'s imagery choices. As H. was demonstrating consistently sedated vital signs, the pediatric fellow decided to commence the administration of an anesthetic medication, but used significantly less than usual for the patient's size and age. The music-assisted relaxation sequence continued, with H. demonstrating continued sedation, until a sterile field was required. At that point, the MT-BC quietly faded out her improvisation and left the area while the fellow continued to give intermittent verbal prompts to facilitate maintenance of the beach scene. The biopsy was then performed with the physician administering one-fourth of the amount of Ketamine (an intravenous anesthetic agent with sedative and **analgesic** properties) usually used.

The music therapist followed up with H. two days later when H. had been transferred to the regular inpatient unit. H. remembered the beach scene and the "relaxing music" but had no recollection of the procedure itself or of any discomfort. The MT-BC verbally reviewed the music-facilitated imagery technique with H. so that H. might be able to use it independently with her own preferred relaxation music during painful procedures in the future. The fellow later commented to the MT-BC that H. had remained calm and sedated throughout the procedure and had asked him to "dry her feet off" as she was emerging from the sedation.

This case example demonstrates how patient assessment in the PICU sometimes occurs simultaneously with intervention. The music therapist offering procedural support must assess the patient's current levels of anxiety and pain, try to determine any specific fears or concerns, and identify and reinforce the patient's current adaptive coping skills. Music-facilitated imagery works well for older children and adolescents who are anxious but not yet overwhelmed with anxiety and fear. As this case study shows, the therapist must give careful attention to suggested images, as the imagery experience may be quite intense when coupled with sedative medication. The MT-BC emphasized images that provoked feelings of safety and security, along with calmness and relaxation. This was done intentionally to counter possible negative images that might arise within the same scene (e.g., a patient who imagines floating on water suddenly starts to imagine large waves or drowning). Images that evoke stability and security should be part of directives for relaxation imagery, especially during potentially anxiety-producing circumstances.

2. Long-term (multiple session): Developmentally appropriate multisensory stimulation during sedation weaning process

P. is a 23-month-old patient with hypoplastic left heart syndrome. This underdevelopment of the left side of the heart is typically treated with a series of three surgeries to reroute the flow of blood through the right side of the heart. Upon completion of this final surgery, P. was admitted to the PICU. He received IV fluids and sedative medications in addition to nutrition through an NG tube. P.'s clinical nurse specialist requested a music therapy consult for developmentally appropriate multisensory stimulation. The music therapist consulted with P.'s nurse and reviewed his medical chart prior to conducting a music therapy assessment.

Session #1: P. was sleeping when the music therapist (MT-BC) made initial contact. The MT-BC interviewed P.'s mother to determine P.'s baseline levels of functioning and personal preferences regarding music and play. According to P.'s mother, P. could walk, run, and verbalize prior to his most recent surgery. Per mother's report, P. was experiencing some withdrawal symptoms during the process of weaning P. from the sedative medication. P. had also begun to pull at his NG and IV tubes. As a result, P. was wearing socks on his hands to prevent him from removing his NG or IV tubing. The music therapist solicited information from P.'s mother about her goals for her child. P.'s mother wanted P. to have multisensory stimulation and socialization during the weaning process. The MT-BC scheduled a session for the following day in between respiratory therapy sessions and nap times.

Session #2: P. was seated in a tumbleform chair in his bed when the MT-BC arrived. The MT-BC used a Q chord (digital guitar) as an accompaniment instrument at the bedside and began with an opening song. The MT-BC introduced P., P.'s mom, the nurse, and herself to orient P. to the surroundings. P.'s eyes were closed throughout this session. He was actively pulling at his IV and NG tubing. When the music began, P. stopped moving and turned his head in the direction of the music. The MT-BC encouraged P.'s mom to use the stuffed animals she found in P.'s bed during "Down on Grandpa's Farm." P.'s mom made the animal sounds and placed the animals in P.'s lap. She provided hand over hand assistance to help P. stroke the fur. The MT-BC initiated hand motion songs such as "The Itsy Bitsy Spider" and "The Wheels on the Bus." The MT-BC invited P.'s mom to help P. approximate the hand motions. P. did not pull at his tubing during the music or whenever P.'s mom provided the hand over hand assistance.

Session #3: P. was sitting on his mom's lap when the MT-BC arrived. P.'s eyes were closed, but he was turning his head from side to side. The interventions used during session #3 were very similar to session #2. P. opened his eyes each time a new song began or each time a new voice was heard. This was a new behavior for P. during music therapy sessions. Per P.'s mom, P.'s heart rate and rate of respiration were more stable during music therapy sessions than before and after sessions.

Session #4: P. was lying in bed during this session. His father was present in the room. The MT-BC introduced P.'s father to music therapy and invited him to participate in the session. The MT-BC introduced simple percussion instruments for P. to touch and manipulate for tactile stimulation. P.'s father provided hand over hand assistance. Again, P. turned his head towards new sounds and voices. His eyes were open for the majority of the session until he became fatigued. P. became agitated when he was fatigued. He began pulling at his NG and IV tubing. The MT-BC sang lullaby style songs at the bedside while P.'s father provided soothing touch. By the end of the 30-minute session, P. stopped pulling on his tubing and showed no signs of physical agitation.

Session #5: P.'s mother, father, grandmother, and 3-year-old brother were present. P. was sitting on his mother's lap when the MT-BC arrived. Upon assessment of the situation, the MT-BC encouraged all the family members to participate in the session to provide appropriate socialization opportunities for P. In order to empower P.'s brother, the MT-BC encouraged him to make choices for the entire family about which instruments to play, which songs to sing, and which stuffed animals to use (due to hospital infection control policies, the MT-BC cannot use cloth animals or puppets with multiple patients, so the MT-BC utilizes toys and animals in the patient's room to enhance music interventions). P.'s mother, father, and grandmother took turns holding P. P.'s brother carried animals and instruments to P. and the other family members while the MT-BC encouraged music participation through the use of children's folksongs and blues songwriting. After the session, P.'s mom told the MT-BC that P.'s brother "usually takes a long time to warm up to new people." She said that it was special to her to see P.'s brother so involved in the session and with P. Since P. was walking, running, and playing with his brother prior to the surgery, P.'s brother wasn't sure how to play with him while he was in the hospital. Facilitating the interaction between P. and P.'s brother provided an opportunity for familiar and normalizing activity for P.

Session #5 was the last session for P. and his family. P. was transferred to the heart center the next week and was sleeping during the session time. P.'s family was not present, and the nursing staff requested that music therapy be postponed since P. had just fallen asleep. P. was discharged from the hospital prior to his next scheduled session.

This series of sessions illustrates the challenges a PICU MT-BC can face while facilitating developmentally appropriate multisensory stimulation for a patient in the PICU. Sedative medication and recuperation from surgery affects a patient's level of functioning. The PICU patient's family members are the most important sources of information about patient preferences and needs. P.'s parents were able to assist the MT-BC in developing objectives for P. This collaboration supports the tenets of family-centered care by including family members as treatment team members. Also, the family members assisted the MT-BC in the evaluation process by reporting P.'s behaviors and vital signs prior to and immediately following the session. As a result, the MT-BC was able to create a structured and familiar environment for P. through music interaction. This familiar environment at times facilitated auditory, tactile, cognitive, and visual stimulation. The music intervention also facilitated relaxation when P. became agitated or fatigued.

Techniques chosen to evaluate the efficacy of these interventions may also vary depending upon the type of intervention presented and the kind of behaviors being observed.

Intervention outcomes are noted periodically during the intervention itself, and the music therapist uses this information regarding patient responses to modify his or her methods in order to improve efficacy. The therapist may monitor patient reactions by observing physiological, behavioral, and psychosocial parameters. A music therapist can evaluate changes in physiological variables such as heart rate, respiratory rate, oxygen saturation levels, and blood pressure by periodically checking the patient's vital sign monitors. Stable decreases in heart rate and respiratory rate may indicate an improved relaxation response. Conversely, increases in heart rate in response to music may indicate that a patient who is sedated or in a coma perceives the auditory stimuli. Noting any changes in the level of required sedatives or analgesia for a patient undergoing a procedure is an additional physiological measure of intervention effectiveness.

Behavioral measures may include changes in the level of observable agitation and restlessness, or changes in the intensity of a patient's crying. Frequency and duration of eye contact, attending, visual or auditory tracking, and physical or communicative responsiveness are also behavioral outcome measures. Psychosocial variables include affective responses, self-concept, and changes in quality of social interaction. Mood may be measured informally by noting changes in positive affect, or formally by using patient self-report of current mood or visual analog mood scales. Visual analog scales consist of several drawn facial expressions from which the patient chooses the face that best matches his or her current mood. Patient attitudes related to self-image and overall self-esteem may be evaluated by documenting patient self-statements across sessions. Changes in level of social interaction may include frequency and quality of patient/caregiver interaction, peer interaction, and interaction with staff.

Level of perceived pain is frequently measured and documented in the intensive care setting. A visual analog pain scale, most commonly the **Wong-Baker FACES Pain Rating Scale** (Wong, Hockenberry-Eaton, Wilson, Winkelstein, & Schwartz, 2005), is often employed for pediatric patients. The patient points or verbally expresses which face indicates his or her current level of pain. Each face has a corresponding verbal descriptor and numeral indicating pain intensity (see Figure 3).

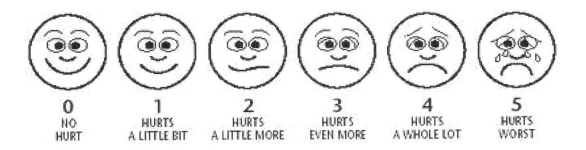

Figure 3. Wong-Baker FACES Pain Rating Scale

For children younger than 3 years old, or for nonverbal patients, the **FLACC Nonverbal Pain Scale** (Merkel, Voepel-Lewis, Shayevitz, & Malviya, 1997) is more appropriate and provides a pain rating system based on observable behaviors (see Table 2).

The Brief Behavioral Distress Scale (BBDS) (Tucker, Slifer, & Dahlquist, 2001) or **Observation Scale of Behavioral Distress** (OSBD) (Elliott, Jay, & Woody, 1987) are additional pain scales based on observable behaviors indicating pain or stress and work well for preschool and school-age children. Numeric rating of pain is also common for older pediatric patients. Other methods may provide qualitative information regarding the patient's pain experience, such as Loewy, MacGregor, Richards, and Rodriguez's (1997) Qualitative Color Pain Scale, in which pediatric patients use crayons to color on line-drawn human

Table 2

FLACC Nonverbal Pain Scale

Categories	Scoring*		
	0	1	2
Face	No particular expression or smile	Occasional grimace or frown, withdrawn, disinterested	Frequent to constant frown, quivering chin, clenched jaw
Legs	Normal position or relaxed	Uneasy, restless, tense	Kicking or legs drawn up
Activity	Lying quietly, normal position, moves easily	Squirming, shifting back and forth, tense	Arched, rigid, or jerking
Cry	No cry (awake or asleep)	Moans or whimpers; occasional complaint	Crying steadily, screams or sobs, frequent complaints
Consolability	Content, relaxed	Reassured by occasional touching, hugging, or being talked to; distractible	Difficult to console or comfort

*Each of the five categories—Face (F), Legs (L), Activity (A), Cry (C), and Consolability (C)—is scored from 0–2, which results in a total score of 0 and 10.

figures the areas where they feel pain. In addition to any qualitative pain measures chosen, the music therapist is encouraged to adopt the quantitative pain measurement scale currently used by his or her facility's PICU nursing staff in order to be consistent with treatment team standards.

Outcomes of music therapy intervention should be documented in a way that is consistent with the protocol for other members of the treatment team. Music therapy services may be documented in a patient's chart under the ancillary services section where social workers, child life specialists, physical/occupational/speech therapists, and chaplains enter notes. A music therapist may observe the documentation methods of these related disciplines and create a progress note format that includes pertinent assessment, goal, intervention, and evaluation information, while matching the writing style of these disciplines to facilitate ease in interdisciplinary communication. The music therapist aims to convey to the treatment team the goals of music therapy intervention; the methods employed; and specific, objective patient responses, indicating attainment of or progress toward the stated goals. Notes should be of a level of detail similar to other related disciplines and should generally avoid profession-specific jargon.

Many disciplines use a variation of the "SOAP" format to track progress during sessions, documenting *subjective, objective, assessment,* and *planning* information for each patient contact. A variation of this format might include a statement of the session goal(s), objective details of session content, objective patient responses, subjective patient responses, an assessment of whether goals were met, and a plan for future goals or interventions or a recommendation for further follow-up services. In contrast to session notes, progress notes track the aforementioned information across multiple sessions. Some facilities may require that each ancillary discipline include a brief summary of the patient's medical history at the beginning of a progress note to demonstrate that the clinician has an awareness of these issues. A sample pediatric intensive care music therapy progress note using this format is included below. Readers are also encouraged to consult Scalenghe and Murphy (2000) for additional information on documentation standards for managed care environments.

Sample Music Therapy Progress Note
Pediatric Intensive Care Unit

Date: 2/16/04
Time: 4:15 pm

M. is a previously healthy 15-year-old female with perforated duodenal ulcer who presented at an outside hospital on 12/14/03, condition progressed to acute respiratory distress syndrome and pt. was **intubated**. Pt. transferred to PICU on 12/29/03 for further management. Pt.'s condition has been complicated by sepsis, acute tubular necrosis, and acute renal failure.

M. has received music therapy sessions 2x/wk since 1/26/04 to improve expressive communication and improve mood while receiving mechanical ventilation and to facilitate adjustment to intensive care hospitalization. During 30-minute music therapy sessions at bedside, pt. has chosen to engage in music-assisted relaxation and song selection, preferring music-assisted relaxation when she is feeling nauseated or in pain. Pt. consistently demonstrates prolonged eye contact, communicates choices by mouthing words, and displays positive affect after music engagement. Pt. also mouths words as writer sings pt.'s chosen songs. Pt. displays affirmative head nodding given verbal support from writer, and has displayed tears on occasion during supportive verbal and musical interaction. Music-facilitated relaxation has helped divert pt.'s attention away from nausea/pain as per pt. report. Pt. has self-initiated sessions with assistance from caregiver to communicate pt.'s wants, and has declined sessions only when concurrently receiving peer visits

Pt. is making progress towards stated goals as demonstrated by increase in verbal (mouthing) communication during sessions, and improved mood exemplified by positive affect, reports of temporary relief from pain/nausea, and pt. self-initiating sessions. Pt. is beginning to use pictorial communication as gross motor skills improve to further enhance communication efforts. Recommend continued MT sessions 2x/wk to maintain pt.'s positive coping with intensive care hospitalization and mechanical ventilation.

It may not be feasible for the music therapist to document each session with a patient in the patient's chart. If the music therapist is not required to formally chart on each patient by the facility's standards, the therapist may determine a personal system for prioritizing patient charting. In such a case, the music therapist should prioritize documenting any sessions where a patient demonstrated a marked positive or adverse reaction, documenting sessions when patient responses were unusual for that patient, documenting patient progress over time for a patient who receives multiple sessions, and documenting when the music therapist believes that the patient needs follow-up care from a different discipline such as psychology, social work, or child life. If the facility requires that the therapist chart on each patient that is seen for services, ample charting time must be allotted in the therapist's schedule.

When a patient is discharged from the hospital, a Discharge Summary and Instruction Form is completed by a registered nurse. This form is a multidisciplinary discharge form that may be used by social work and dietary services in addition to nursing. A summary of the patient's status upon discharge is included, as well as written instructions for the patient regarding follow-up care. Music therapists may occasionally contribute to the multidisciplinary discharge summary in cases where follow-up music therapy services are recommended to address a particular goal that is identified by the treatment team. More commonly, music therapists write a final note in the patient's chart summarizing progress in music therapy and giving recommendations for future goal areas that may be addressed by music therapy providers, either during readmissions to the same setting or at a different institution.

The Future of Music Therapy on the PICU

The development of music therapy programs in PICUs may be realized by grants, endowments, or funds from the hospital budget. Grants may be research or clinical in nature and may require renewal on an annual basis. In both of the current authors' experiences, music therapy was brought to the PICU by grants awarded to the hospitals' child life programs. In one case, the child life director and hospital administrators contracted with a local music therapist to provide a consultation to determine the benefits of a hospital-wide music therapy program. The hospital administrator took this proposal to an in-house hospital auxiliary to request grant funding. This fundraising group offered a 3-year grant to cover a full-time music therapy position, and the hospital administration provided a budget for supplies and equipment from the general operating fund. This music therapist sees patients individually on a referral basis throughout the 247-bed pediatric specialty hospital. This includes two PICUs, for a total of 31 critical care beds. In the other author's experience, the child life coordinator submitted a proposal for music therapy services to a children's foundation. The resulting grant funds a per diem music therapy position servicing the PICU, general pediatric inpatient unit, neonatal intensive care unit (NICU), and pediatric patients in the burn center. The music therapist sees patients on the 20-bed PICU three times per week for one to two hours at a time. The grant must be renewed on a yearly basis, and funds from the hospital budget have not been available.

ICU physicians and staff continuously scrutinize the critical care environment. It is a carefully controlled setting, focused on the stabilization of seriously ill patients. As a result, new procedures and therapeutic support must be carefully researched before being accepted by the ICU staff. Though preliminary research efforts regarding the use of music therapy in the PICU have yielded encouraging results, additional inquiry related to music therapy's influence on specific stressors within the PICU environment is crucial. Future music therapy research should evaluate the effectiveness of using music therapy as procedural support during bedside and nonsurgical procedures for PICU patients. Music therapists are currently providing procedural preparation and support throughout the pediatric healthcare setting with successful outcomes (Edwards, 1999; Kallay, 1997; Loewy, 1999; Malone, 1996; Standley & Whipple, 2003; Turry, 1997; Walworth, 2003), but the instability of a pediatric ICU patient could present unique problems for the music therapist. The ICU patient's unique characteristics and responses should be formally studied and evaluated more thoroughly to develop appropriate clinical protocols for this population.

Patients in the PICU do not receive the same level or type of stimulation as they would in their home environments or even on a general or specialty floor. They are also at risk for sleep deprivation due to environmental stressors such as elevated noise levels, continuous lighting, and the occurrence of nursing activity during normal sleep periods. The combination of sleep deprivation and sensory deprivation may result in symptoms of disorientation, confusion, combativeness, hallucinations, and anxiety, which are often labeled as "**ICU psychosis**" (Dambro, 2004; Thomas, 2003). McGuire, Basten, Ryan, and Gallagher (2000) suggested that symptoms of ICU psychosis should actually be diagnosed and treated as a form of delirium. Regardless of the terminology, some patients experience severe physiological and behavioral responses to surgery and the ICU environment. Exploration and study of this phenomenon could lead to advances in the use of music therapy as a multisensory experience to provide normalized sensory stimulation and to promote more regular sleep patterns in an effort to prevent ICU psychosis in PICU patients.

Family involvement is recognized as an integral part of the patient's recovery. More research into how families can be empowered and involved in the patient's care through music therapy interventions could lead to the development of specific family-centered care protocols in music therapy. Such inquiry may also help identify how music therapy can be used to improve parental coping, which in turn may positively influence patient psychological outcomes.

Transfer from the PICU to a general pediatric unit, rehabilitation unit, specialty unit, or home can be an overwhelming and disorienting process for the PICU patient. Research regarding the PICU patient's specific transitional experience could be used to enhance music therapy protocols for supporting the PICU patient's transfer to a new care environment. Additional inquiry may then determine if music therapy can help smooth the patient's transition to a new care environment and facilitate improved coping skills within that new environment.

The presence of music therapy within the pediatric intensive care setting will increase in acceptance and esteem if clinicians, researchers, and educators continue to demonstrate its worth. Music therapists must illustrate how their services are cost-effective in terms of reducing length of PICU hospitalization and decreasing quantities of sedatives and analgesics required to keep PICU patients within desired physiological and behavioral parameters. Music therapists must demonstrate how their services are medically necessary to improve patient outcomes, and how these services also benefit families and the medical facilities themselves. Continued expansion and specification of research efforts, clinical practices, and documentation standards will assist in making the discipline of music therapy a more integral member of the interdisciplinary critical care team.

References

American Academy of Pediatrics (AAP), Committee on Hospital Care and Pediatric Section of the Society of Critical Care Medicine. (1993). Guidelines and levels of care for pediatric intensive care units. *Pediatrics, 92*, 166–174.

American Academy of Pediatrics (AAP), Committee on Hospital Care and Pediatric Section of the Society of Critical Care Medicine. (1999). Guidelines for developing admission and discharge policies for the pediatric intensive care unit. *Pediatrics, 103*, 840–842.

American Academy of Pediatrics (AAP), Committee on Hospital Care and Institute for Family-Centered Care. (2003). Family-centered care and the pediatrician's role. *Pediatrics, 112*, 691–696.

Bavdekar, S. B., Mahajan, M. D., & Chandu, K. V. (1999). Analgesia and sedation in paediatric intensive care unit. *Journal of Postgraduate Medicine, 45*, 95–102.

Child Life Council. (n.d.). *What is a child life specialist?* Retrieved September 30, 2004, from http:www.childlife.org

Chlan, L. (1998). Effectiveness of a music therapy intervention on relaxation and anxiety for patients receiving ventilatory assistance. *Heart & Lung, 27*(3), 169–176.

Dambro, M. (2004). *Griffith's 5 minute clinical consult—2004.* Philadelphia: Lippincott, Williams & Wilkins.

Downes, J. J. (1993). The future of pediatric critical care medicine. *Critical Care Medicine, 21*(Suppl. 9), S307–S310.

Dun, B. (1995). A different beat: Music therapy in children's cardiac care. *Music Therapy Perspectives, 13*, 35–39.

Edwards, J. (1999). Anxiety management in pediatric music therapy. In C. Dileo (Ed.), *Music therapy and medicine: Theoretical and clinical approaches* (pp. 69–76). Silver Spring, MD: American Music Therapy Association.

Elliott, C., Jay, S. M., & Woody, P. (1987). An observation scale for measuring children's distress during medical procedures. *Journal of Pediatric Psychology, 12*(4), 543–551.

Institute for Family-Centered Care. (n.d.). *Patient and family centered care core concepts.* Retrieved September 5, 2008, from http://www.familycenteredcare.org/pdf/CoreConcepts.pdf

Johnston, K., & Rohaly-Davis, J. (1996). An introduction to music therapy: Helping the oncology patient in the ICU. *Critical Care Nursing Quarterly, 18*(4), 54–60.

Jones, S. M., Fiser, D. H., & Livingston, R. L. (1992). Behavioral changes in pediatric intensive care units. *American Journal of Diseases of Children, 146*(3), 375–379.

Kallay, V. S. (1997). Music therapy applications in the pediatric medical setting: Child development, pain management and choice. In J. V. Loewy (Ed.), *Music therapy and pediatric pain* (pp. 33–43). Cherry Hill, NJ: Jeffrey Books.

Kennelly, J., & Edwards, J. (1997). Providing music therapy to the unconscious child in the paediatric intensive care unit. *The Australian Journal of Music Therapy, 8*, 18–29.

Loewy, J. (1999). The use of music psychotherapy in the treatment of pediatric pain. In C. Dileo (Ed.), *Music therapy and medicine: Theoretical and clinical approaches* (pp. 189–206). Silver Spring, MD: America Music Therapy Association.

Loewy, J., MacGregor, B., Richards, K., & Rodriguez, J. (1997). Music therapy pediatric pain management: Assessing and attending to the sounds of hurt, fear, and anxiety. In J. V. Loewy (Ed.), *Music therapy and pediatric pain* (pp. 45–56). Cherry Hill, NJ: Jeffrey Books.

Malone, A. B. (1996). The effects of live music on the distress of pediatric patients receiving intravenous starts, venipunctures, injections, and heel sticks. *Journal of Music Therapy, 23*, 19–33.

McGuire, B. E., Basten, C. J., Ryan, C. J., & Gallagher, J. (2000). Intensive care unit syndrome: A dangerous misnomer. *Archives of Internal Medicine, 160*(7), 906–909.

Melnyk, B. M., Alpert-Gillis, L., Feinstein, N. F., Crean, H. F., Johnson, J., Fairbanks, E., Small, L., Rubenstein, J., Slota, M., & Corbo-Richert, B. (2004). Creating opportunities for parent empowerment: Program effects on the mental health/coping outcomes of critically ill young children and their mothers. *Pediatrics, 113*, 597–607.

Merkel, S. I., Voepel-Lewis, T., Shayevitz, J. R., & Malviya, S. (1997). The FLACC: A behavioral scale for scoring postoperative pain in young children. *Pediatric Nursing, 23*(3), 293–297.

New York Presbyterian Hospital–Cornell Medical Center Pediatric Critical Care Center. (2000, September 1). *Information for parents: Parents' booklet for your child's PICU stay.* Retrieved October 1, 2004, from http://www-users.med.cornell.edu/~spon/picu/parents/prntbken.htm

Randolph, A. G., Gonzales, C. A., Cortellini, L., & Yeh, T. (2004). Growth of pediatric intensive care units in the United States from 1995–2001. *The Journal of Pediatrics, 144*(6), 792–798.

Robb, S. L. (1999). Piaget, Erikson, and coping styles: Implications for music therapy and the hospitalized preschool child. *Music Therapy Perspectives, 17*, 14–19.

Robb, S. L. (2003). Designing music therapy interventions for hospitalized children and adolescents using a contextual support model of music therapy. *Music Therapy Perspectives, 21*, 27–40.

Rosenfeld, J., & Dun, B. (1999). Music therapy in children with severe traumatic brain injury. In R. R. Pratt & D. E. Grocke (Eds.), *MusicMedicine 3: MusicMedicine and music therapy: Expanding horizons* (pp. 35–46). Parkville, Victoria, Australia: The University of Melbourne.

Scalenghe, R., & Murphy, K. M. (2000). Music therapy assessment in the managed care environment. *Music Therapy Perspectives, 18*(1), 23–30.

Standley, J. M., & Whipple, J. (2003). Music therapy with pediatric patients: A meta analysis. In S. Robb (Ed.), *Music therapy in pediatric healthcare: Research and evidence-based practice* (pp. 1–18). Silver Spring, MD: America Music Therapy Association.

Stouffer, J. W., & Shirk, B. (2003). Critical care: Clinical applications of music for children on mechanical ventilation. In S. Robb (Ed.), *Music therapy in pediatric healthcare: Research and evidence-based practice* (pp. 49–80). Silver Spring, MD: American Music Therapy Association.

Thomas, L. A. (2003). Clinical management of stressors perceived by patients on mechanical ventilation. *AACN Clinical Issues, 14*(1), 73–81.

Thompson, R. H., & Stanford, G. (1981). *Child life in hospitals: Theory and practice.* Springfield, IL: Charles C. Thomas.

Tucker, C. L., Slifer, K. J., & Dahlquist, L. M. (2001). Reliability and validity of the Brief Behavioral Distress Scale: A measure of children's distress during invasive medical procedures. *Journal of Pediatric Psychology, 26*(8), 513–523.

Turry, A. E. (1997). The use of clinical improvisation to alleviate procedural distress in young children. In J. V. Loewy (Ed.), *Music therapy and pediatric pain* (pp. 89–96). Cherry Hill, NJ: Jeffrey Books.

Updike, P. (1990). Music therapy results for ICU patients. *Dimensions of Critical Care Nursing, 9*(1), 39–45.

Walworth, D. D. (2003). Procedural support: Music therapy assisted CT, EKG, EEG, X-Ray, IV, ventilator, and emergency services. In S. L. Robb (Ed.), *Music therapy in pediatric healthcare: Research and evidence-based practice* (pp. 137–146). Silver Spring, MD: American Music Therapy Association.

Wong, D. L., Hockenberry-Eaton, M., Wilson, D., Winkelstein, M. L., & Schwartz, P. (2005). *Wong's essentials of pediatric nursing* (7th ed.). St. Louis, MO: Mosby.

Wong, H. L. C., Lopez-Nahas, V., & Molassiotis, A. (2001). Effects of music therapy on anxiety in ventilator-dependent patients. *Heart & Lung, 30*(5), 376–387.

CHAPTER 4

General Pediatrics Medical/Surgical

Ann Hannan

Around a bustling nurses station, a brightly colored activity room, and an aquatic-themed treatment room, 12 patient rooms line the hallways of a pediatric general medical surgical unit in one Midwest state's only comprehensive pediatric specialty hospital. Patients travel from throughout the state and from bordering states to receive specialized care for a multitude of medical conditions. In addition to specialized care areas for critical care, **hematology/oncology** care, neonatal care, and cardiac care, this hospital houses several general medical/surgical units. While nursing staff and physicians provide necessary medical care, these medical/surgical patients also receive therapeutic intervention provided by respiratory therapists, rehabilitation specialists (occupational therapy and physical therapy), child psychiatrists, social workers, child life specialists, and music therapists. Since the psychosocial effects of hospitalization often compound medical conditions, the pediatric medical/surgical patient should be treated by a combined effort of these clinicians.

Pediatric music therapy services are provided in one Midwest pediatric specialty hospital through grant funding from a hospital-affiliated auxiliary. Supplies, equipment, and instruments are funded through a general hospital contributions fund. The music therapist conducts combined weekly group sessions for four pediatric general medical/surgical units. Each unit can provide care for up to 25 patients. The music therapist also receives individual music therapy referral requests from all hospital general and specialty inpatient units.

For the pediatric medical/surgical patient, there is an increased exposure to uncertainty in diagnosis and course of treatment. Many medical/surgical patients are admitted to the general unit for **diagnostic testing**, and some patients exhibit symptoms without a clearly defined diagnosis. Once a patient is diagnosed with a particular medical condition, a course of treatment can be delineated. Until that time, the patient may experience an increased level of anxiety. Likewise, patients with a **chronic illness** may experience uncertainty with regards to treatment regimen. For many of these patients, there is no cure for their current conditions. Instead, patients receive treatments for symptoms for lifelong conditions. This lack of definition of treatment regimen has the potential for negative impact on patients' psychological and physical functioning (Bare, 1997).

Research in music therapy in the healthcare setting has historically addressed the needs of patients experiencing a particular course of treatment (e.g., mechanical respiratory assistance, dialysis) or a particular disease process such as **leukemia** or asthma. When working with a medical/surgical patient, the music therapist will encounter patients who are experiencing a multitude of different diagnoses and treatments. As a result, patient objectives and music therapy interventions should focus on physiological and psychological stressors that medical/surgical patients experience during hospitalization. General music therapy clinical objectives for pediatric patients have been categorized as follows:

golden

- Pain Reduction and Management
- Anxiety Reduction
- Infant Pacification
- Decreased Respiratory Distress
- Increased Coping Skills

Pain reduction
Anxiety reduction
Infant pacification
Decrease Respiratory stress
Increase Coping

Derived from current publications regarding pediatric music therapy, these categories may serve as a guideline for the delivery of music therapy services to the pediatric medical/surgical patient (Standley & Whipple, 2003).

General Characteristics and Definition of Medical/Surgical Population

same as cvicu

In a pediatric specialty hospital, patients who do not need critical care and cannot, by diagnosis, be admitted to a specialty unit will be admitted to a general medical/surgical (med/surg) unit. These patients may be preparing for surgery, recovering from surgery, or undergoing observation for the management of a chronic illness. Patients with an illness or symptoms of unknown etiology will also be admitted to a general unit for diagnostic testing and observation.

Common Diagnoses and Medical Conditions

Some common diagnoses and conditions treated by admission to a pediatric general medical/surgical unit include:

1. Major congenital anomalies
2. Malignancies
3. Major trauma
   a. Vehicular accident
   b. Near drowning
   c. Heavy machinery accident
4. Acute illnesses (Humes, 2000)
   a. **Gastroenterology** (e.g., appendicitis, small bowel obstruction)
   b. **Nephrology** (e.g., acute renal failure)

      c. Pulmonary medicine (e.g., pneumonia, acute respiratory distress syndrome)

      d. Endocrinology (e.g., diabetic ketoacidosis)

  5. Chronic illnesses (Humes, 2000)

      a. Gastroenterology (e.g., gastroenteritis, Crohn's disease, ulcerative colitis)

      b. Nephrology (e.g., chronic renal failure)

      c. Rheumatology (e.g., rheumatoid arthritis, **lupus**)

      d. Pulmonary medicine (e.g., asthma, cystic fibrosis)

      e. Endocrinology (e.g., diabetes mellitus)

      f. Neurology (e.g., epilepsy, depression)

  6. Infectious diseases (Humes, 2000)

      a. Bacterial meningitis

      b. Cellulitis

      c. Epstein-Barr virus

      d. HIV/AIDS

      e. Tuberculosis

      f. Chicken pox

      g. MRSA (**Methicillin-resistent** *S. aureus*)

      h. VRE (Vancomycin-resistant enterococci)

                         (American Academy of Pediatrics, 2002, p. 187)

Interaction with Medical Staff

The pediatric medical/surgical patient encounters many different caregivers and medical staff throughout the day. In a teaching hospital, physicians conduct patient rounds with fellows, residents, interns, and medical students on a daily basis. In some settings, nurse practitioners, social workers, case managers, and child life staff members may also participate in these rounds. After reviewing pertinent data about the patient, the physician assesses the patient and discusses treatment options with the patient and family. The physician may solicit questions from the patient and family at this time. Because some patients will see their physician only once per day, this visit is a central part of the medical/surgical patient's daily schedule.

If a patient is preparing for surgery, the **surgeon** may visit the unit prior to the scheduled surgery. If the surgeon is unavailable, a resident or fellow will assess the patient prior to surgery. The nursing staff typically prepares the patient for surgery by carefully monitoring the patient's physiological and psychological status. Ideally, the patient will participate in preoperative teaching prior to surgery. Ensuring the patient and family understand the surgical procedure helps to decrease anxiety (Brenn, 2003). Nursing staff, a social worker, a member of the surgical team, a child life specialist, or a music therapist may facilitate this teaching. A nursing staff member typically accompanies the patient and family to the operating room or preoperative area. The medical/surgical nurse has the greatest amount of direct contact with the surgical patient and therefore may develop an intimate rapport with the patient and family (Chase, 1995). This method of transfer (i.e., being accompanied by a trusted caregiver) is important to ensure low levels of **perioperative** anxiety for the patient and family members. Likewise, the patient and family may develop a similar rapport with another medical staff member (e.g., social worker, child life specialist, or music therapist). If this is the case, this trusted staff member may also accompany the patient to the preoperative area. The music therapist may have an opportunity to provide further preparation, distraction, or relaxation opportunities for the patient during this time.

Medical/Surgical Unit Daily Schedule

The morning and early afternoon hours on a medical/surgical unit can be noisy and chaotic. While patients will be assigned to a primary physician upon admission, many will see physicians from several different subspecialties. For example, a patient diagnosed with cystic fibrosis with positive cultures for MRSA (Methicillin-resistent *S. aureus*—antibiotic-resistant bacteria) is seen by the pulmonary team and the infectious diseases team. This creates a potentially chaotic and stressful environment for the pediatric medical/surgical patient. In addition to frequent consultations with medical staff, diagnostic tests such as CT (computed tomography) scans and MRIs (**Magnetic Resonance Imaging**) occur throughout the day as needed. Most prescheduled tests that require the patient to abstain from the consumption of solid foods occur early in the morning. Others may be scheduled as new symptoms occur or whenever previous diagnostic tests do not yield the desired results.

In between medical staff visits, diagnostic testing, surgery, and nursing intervention, the pediatric medical/surgical patient is faced with several unoccupied hours of time throughout the day. For the adolescent patient, these hours may extend late into the night as well. For very young patients, these daytime hours may be filled with anxiety and loneliness. While many patients have a family member or parent at the bedside at all times, some patients do not see their families until after siblings are out of school and parents are home from work. This is especially true for patients with chronic illnesses such as cystic fibrosis and Crohn's disease. Patients with cystic fibrosis are generally admitted for at least 2 weeks at a time. These admissions can occur several times throughout the year. Many working parents cannot afford to take several weeks off each year to stay with their children in the hospital. As a result, these children rely on trusted hospital staff members to fill this void by providing diversion and opportunities for developing ways to cope with anxiety, depression, loneliness, and uncertainty. The music therapist can develop a close rapport with, and create a supportive environment for, medical/surgical patients through music therapy intervention (Robb, 2000).

Physical Environment

While specific unit design varies greatly among pediatric hospitals, most pediatric general medical surgical units have several common characteristics. Most units are built around a primary nursing station. This area may include access to a secured medication room, storage of patient legal medical charts, storage of patient educational materials, and designated space and necessary equipment for documentation (i.e., computers, printers, cardo-plate machine, and preprinted forms). Smaller charting areas may be located directly outside patient rooms, and some units have nursing substations if patient rooms cover a large or uniquely shaped geographic area. Ideally, patient rooms are situated within view of the central nursing station to provide efficient response to patient needs.

Nonpharmacological medical supplies and patient linens are stored in clean utility rooms. Used linens, cleaning supplies and equipment, and used medical supplies are stored in dirty utility rooms to await appropriate disposal or transfer to laundry facilities. Miscellaneous storage closets may also be available for office supplies and unused medical equipment.

Nursing managers, social workers, and child life department members may have office space on the medical/surgical unit. Depending on the size of the unit, there may be a need for administrative secretarial support. Most nursing units have designated unit secretaries for each shift to coordinate patient admissions and discharges. These secretaries generally perform their duties within the physical space of the nursing station.

Most general pediatric units have a designated treatment room. Hospital admission generally requires at least one nonsurgical invasive procedure that can be performed on the unit. These can include intravenous (IV) line placement, venipuncture, **peripherally inserted central catheter** (PICC) line insertion, or **chest tube** insertion. These procedures occur in the treatment room to decrease the likelihood that the patient will associate negative procedural experiences with the general hospital environment.

The design of patient rooms varies greatly based on the age of the hospital, length of time since the most recent remodeling, and geographic location. Rooms tend to be private or semiprivate (i.e., two patient beds in one room). Some patient rooms include full bathrooms, while other units may have separate showers and tubs for general patient use. Most pediatric medical/surgical units provide at least one seating option at the patient's bedside. This may be a recliner or chair bed to provide an option for family members who wish to remain at the bedside overnight. Designated lockers or cabinets are provided for patient belongings and medical supplies. Most hospitals also provide a permanently mounted television and VCR and/or a DVD player for patient education and entertainment.

Pediatric patients generally have access to an activity room or designated play area. The hospital's child life staff may supervise the activity room during scheduled hours. In addition to regular group activities, the activity room may be available to patients when supervised by parents and nursing staff. These rooms generally include tables and chairs for participating in craft activities, completing schoolwork, and playing games. Some may include access to computers, game systems, televisions, CD players, stereo systems, and age-appropriate toys, books, and games. Many activity rooms are considered "safe areas," and child life staff members encourage physicians and nurses to perform necessary procedures in designated treatment areas.

Unit décor may be designed to appeal to the pediatric patient, especially in treatment rooms and activity rooms. The design of patient rooms, hallways, and waiting rooms often simulates the home environment. Some areas display patient artwork, letters, and photographs throughout the unit. Patients spend a majority of their hospital admission in their rooms or on their units; so ideally, the physical environment of the medical/surgical unit will enhance their comfort while facilitating the delivery of efficient medical care.

Current Treatment Modalities/Approaches for Medical/Surgical Population

Patients on the pediatric general medical/surgical unit receive a wide variety of treatments during their admission to the hospital. Medical/surgical patients may experience any of the following treatment interventions:

1. Monitoring of Vital Signs
   a. Heart Rate—can be monitored continuously or by a nursing staff member a set number of times during the day or per shift
   b. Blood Pressure—can be automatically monitored by a machine or by a nursing staff member during scheduled vital sign checks
   c. Temperature—is usually monitored on a set schedule by nursing staff
   d. Rate of Respiration—can be mechanically monitored on a continuous basis
   e. Pain Perception—can be monitored by patient report and by using a pain scale such as the **Wong-Baker FACES Scale** (Wong & Baker, 1988; Wong, Hockenberry-Eaton, Wilson, Winkelstein, & Schwartz, 2001)
2. Feeding Assistance
   a. Parenteral Feeds
   b. **Enteral Feeds**
   c. **Intravenous (IV) Nutrition**
   d. Restricted Oral Diet
      (i) Low salt
      (ii) Low fat
      (iii) Fluid restriction
3. Medication
   a. Oral
   b. Intravenous
4. Diagnostic Testing (Schwartz, 2003)
   a. **Complete Blood Count** (CBC)
   b. **Chemistry Panel**
   c. **Ultrasound**
   d. **Computed Tomography (CT) Scan**
   e. X-Ray
   f. **Magnetic Resonance Imaging** (MRI)
   g. Radiological Exams
   h. **Laparoscopy**
5. Surgical Procedures

6. Nonsurgical Procedures
   a. Intravenous (IV) start
   b. **Peripherally Inserted Central Catheter** (PICC) line
   c. Chest Tube

Since pediatric medical/surgical patients experience such extensive treatments, procedures, and tests, the music therapist must be knowledgeable about the procedural steps, psychosocial impact, and medical side effects associated with these interventions. This allows the music therapist to support the patient throughout the prescribed treatment regimen.

Determination of Eligibility for Services

Several factors affect the medical/surgical patient's eligibility for music therapy services. Depending on the specific hospital's music therapist-to-patient ratio, some patients who are referred to music therapy may not be seen by the music therapist on a one-to-one basis. In order to triage potential patients, the music therapist should first determine what services the patient is currently receiving. If the patient is exhibiting positive responses to other therapeutic interventions such as child life services, rehab services, or child psychiatry, he or she may not require music therapy services to the same extent as a patient who is not currently responding to other therapies. Aspects of music intervention, such as singing, may stimulate responses in those patients who are otherwise unresponsive to stimulation (Clair, 1996). A patient's lack of response to traditional social interaction may be due to severe developmental delay, psychological response to trauma, or side effects of medication. Although prior music experience is not necessary for patients to participate in music therapy interventions, a patient who has a significant positive response to music may be a particularly appropriate candidate for music therapy. This is especially true for a patient who is not responding to other therapies, is becoming agitated with other staff members, or is noncompliant with other treatment regimens.

Length of hospital stay varies greatly on a general medical/surgical unit. Admissions may last a few days up to several months. For a patient with an acute stay (4 or 5 days), the music therapist would need to determine if music therapy services would support the patient's short-term needs. These could include procedural support and preparation for discharge to home or a rehabilitation facility. For a patient whose admission will last 2 weeks or longer, the music therapist can assess the patient for short-term and long-term needs. Patients with chronic illnesses may have frequent hospital admissions throughout the year. Some of these patients receive referrals for music therapy at the onset of each admission. In this case, the music therapist can design treatment interventions to provide continuity across admissions. This could include detailed vocal or instrumental instruction, songwriting, or patient-directed music research. Long-term projects for patients with chronic admissions can decrease anxiety about hospitalization by providing the patient with a familiar and consistent experience during each admission.

Psychosocial adjustment

A child's psychosocial adjustment to hospitalization is an important and common area for a music therapist to assess and address. Research supporting the need for the development of coping methods for patients with a chronic illness such as **cancer** may be applied to the general medical/surgical population (Robb, 2003). Some medical/surgical patients exhibit signs and symptoms of depression, anxiety, regression, agitation, and altered sleep patterns due to the experience of hospitalization. The music therapist should gather information about the patient's psychosocial status as well as issues being covered by other medical disciplines to determine the appropriateness of music therapy intervention.

Many medical/surgical patients will need assistance learning to cope with loss of functioning due to surgery, chronic pain, chronic illness, or severe injury. Music therapy interventions can help patients maintain their current level of functioning or regain lost abilities while facilitating the development of coping mechanisms for the patients' new abilities.

The music therapist in a pediatric specialty hospital must take these and other patient needs into consideration when determining whether specific music therapy intervention can be provided for the medical/surgical patient. Some music therapists can address general medical/surgical needs for patients through group sessions, which maximize therapist-to-patient contact and can help prepare medical/surgical patients for return to their home environment. Group sessions can also provide a necessary opportunity for creative expression for patients who experience lengthy hospital stays.

If the music therapist determines that a patient is not an appropriate candidate for a group session (e.g., medical bed-rest, isolation precautions, complex psychosocial needs, or sensitivity to overstimulation), then the music therapist must determine the patient's eligibility for bedside interventions. Patients with needs that can be addressed only by a trained professional should receive private attention from the music therapist. Some medical/surgical patients would benefit from music interaction to normalize the environment, develop appropriate leisure skills, and participate in developmentally appropriate socialization, but do not necessarily have specific needs that should be addressed by a music therapist. Under the supervision of a music therapist, other musicians (i.e., volunteers or musically inclined patient care staff) may be able to provide quality music interactions to support the music interests of these patients. While this is not considered music therapy, the music therapist is still providing a valuable connection to musical expression for the patient by training volunteer and staff musicians to work with these patients.

Referral Process

Some hospitals require music therapy referrals to be initiated by physicians. Other hospitals allow the music therapist to design a referral process in conjunction with other healthcare staff members. Music therapists who are designing a new music therapy program should refer to the process used by other therapists for consults. For example, the music therapist could consult with the rehabilitation department, child life department, or social work department for information regarding hospital policy on the referral process. Some hospitals have an official, computerized referral system that can be used by physicians and nursing staff to request a consult for patient services. Although the process can be tedious to add music therapy to these systems, the music therapist should explore this option. The music therapist who works as a member of the hospital's child life program may be able to educate unit staff members to send an electronic consult for music therapy through the child life system by indicating "music therapy consult" in the comment section.

Even if a formal consult procedure is available, the music therapist should be open to other forms of referrals. This increases the likelihood that patients in need of music therapy intervention will be referred to the music therapist. Referrals could be received via phone, email, or pager. The music therapist could also receive verbal referrals from staff members on the unit or during medical, psychosocial, or departmental rounds. It is important for the music therapist to take formal and informal opportunities to educate medical colleagues about how music therapy can address the needs of the medical/surgical patient (Standley, 1986). Depending upon a music therapist's availability, he or she might also want to solicit referrals from unit staff or review patient charts to indicate potential candidates for music therapy.

Assessment Procedure

Prior to meeting the patient for assessment, the music therapist should gather as much information as possible about the patient from chart review, treatment team meetings, and consultation with the patient's physician or nurse. This background information prepares the music therapist for an active assessment session with the patient and the patient's family. During the initial assessment session, the patient's family may or may not be present. If they are, the music therapist must determine an appropriate amount of family involvement based on cues from the patient. The patient's comfort level with the music therapist and dependence on his or her family for security will affect this decision. Some patients need an opportunity to express thoughts or feelings that may be uncomfortable to express in front of family members. The music therapist may assess this need during the first session and request that family members be otherwise engaged during the next session. Generally, in a pediatric setting, family involvement is developmentally appropriate and important for the adjustment of the pediatric patient.

When first approaching a patient and family, the music therapist should introduce self and services to the family, which may be an informal verbal introduction. The music therapist may also choose to include printed materials and contact information for the patient and family. The music therapist should always give the patient and family the option to decline services after they are introduced to music therapy. If a family chooses to decline services, the music therapist should validate this choice and ask if he or she could return at a later time to follow up with the family. Some families and patients are overwhelmed by the many interactions with a large number of medical staff at the beginning of hospital admission. The music therapist can validate and support these feelings by offering these choices to the patient and family.

If the patient is not available during the first session (i.e., sleeping, sedated, recovering from same-day surgery, off the unit for diagnostic testing), the music therapist may be able to obtain important information from the patient's family members. The music therapist can educate the family members about music therapy interventions and involve the family in decisions regarding music therapy as a course of treatment. Family members can provide the music therapist with information about patient preferences and their perception of patient needs. Some medical staff will provide a referral for a medical/surgical patient without a specified need or goal area. The music therapist may also receive multiple referrals for the same patient with differing specified goal areas. In either case, the family members can assist the music therapist by identifying the areas they would like to see the music therapist address. This is especially important if the possible goals include transition to the home environment.

If the patient is available for the assessment session, the music therapist can conduct a music interaction based on the patient's current level of physical, cognitive, and social functioning. From this interaction, the music therapist will develop goals and objectives for the patient to accomplish during subsequent sessions.

Music therapists who work with patients during an acute length of stay (less than 2 weeks) may see the patient only once or twice during the hospital admission. The music therapist is then faced with the challenge of providing an intervention during the assessment process. This reiterates the importance of gathering information about the patient prior to the first session, since the music therapist may not have a second or third session to develop, address, and evaluate patient goals and objectives.

This author is currently developing an assessment to be used throughout the pediatric specialty hospital in collaboration with other music therapists in the hospital system (i.e., general pediatric floors and pediatric rehabilitation within a general hospital). At this time, a narrative assessment is documented in the patient's legal chart in the multidisciplinary history and progress section. In this author's experience, all nursing and patient care services staff members, including child life department members, are required to use the nursing focus note format:

D: Description of Event
A: Action
R: Response

To adapt this format to describe a music therapy assessment session, the following information should be included in each of the three sections.

Description of Event:
1. Referral date, referral source, referral reason (if available)
2. Basic patient information from chart review, patient/family interview, and medical staff consultation
3. Description of session environment

Action:
1. Type and duration of music therapy session
2. Brief description of music therapy assessment interventions

Response:
1. Description of patient behaviors, verbalizations, strengths, and needs
2. Music therapy goals and objectives, including method of outcome measurement
3. Plan for delivery of services (e.g., time, duration, and frequency of sessions)

A sample medical/surgical assessment narrative note is included below. Each medical facility develops protocols for assessment and progress notation in the patient chart. When developing a medical music therapy program, the music therapist should consult with other disciplines within the facility to determine the most appropriate method of documentation.

Sample Music Therapy Assessment Narrative Note

Pediatric General Medical/Surgical Unit

Date: 10/19/2004
Time: 18:05

D: Patient is a 4-year-old male with cystic fibrosis. Patient was admitted due to cystic fibrosis exacerbation. Patient lives with his father and his father's significant other who refers to herself as "mom." Patient was referred to music therapy by his child life specialist on this date. Referral reasons include:
1. Increased risk for depression due to barrier and respiratory isolation
2. Treatment regimen noncompliance

Patient was seated on his bed when the music therapist arrived. Patient's father and uncle were present at the beginning of the session. Patient's father's significant other exited the room as the music therapist entered the room. She returned 5 minutes into the session and stated to the patient, "You will receive a bolus feed if you do not eat your dinner."

A: Patient participated in a 30-minute bedside assessment session. The music therapist introduced self and services to the patient and his family. Due to the patient's immediate need to consume his dinner, the music therapist chose to conduct the music therapy assessment while assisting with this process. The music therapist engaged the patient in singing interactive children's folksongs. Patient initiated a game of catch with the music therapist. The music therapist suggested that the patient eat a bite of food after every five catches. The music therapist used improvisational singing to praise the patient's progress and transferred her role in the interaction to the patient's uncle at the end of the session.

R: Patient initiated clapping and dancing during the interactive folksongs. When the father's significant other entered the room, the patient stopped all interaction with the music therapist and looked down at his bed. When the significant other left the room to obtain a syringe, the patient took the music therapist's hands and clapped them together, presumably to begin the music. The music therapist continued the initial song with similar responses from the patient. The patient mimicked animal sounds and behaviors in response to song lyrics. He handed the music therapist a baseball glove and tossed the ball to begin the game of catch. The patient bounced up and down on the bed when the music therapist initiated the game of eating after every five catches. The patient counted aloud with the music therapist and took at least one bite of food after each round. After eating the food, the patient would hold up five fingers, and the music therapist confirmed the number of catches needed before the next bite. Patient did not verbalize in sentences longer than three or four words, and he utilized hand motions and demonstrations to ask and answer most questions. After the patient ate half of his food, the music therapist invited another family member to continue playing the game while the patient finished his dinner. The music therapist scheduled a follow-up session with the family and then exited the room. The music therapist consulted with nursing staff about the patient's noncompliance with eating and shared methods of reinforcement for nursing staff to use to encourage oral self feeds versus bolus feeds.

Goal 1:   Increase compliance with necessary oral feeds
    Objective 1: Patient will consume a sufficient amount of solid foods to prevent the need
            for supplemental nutrition via bolus feeds.
    Objective 2: Patient will initiate self feeds without continual reinforcement.

Goal 2:   Increase opportunities for developmentally appropriate socialization including
    conversation
    Objective 1: Patient will respond to therapist interactions with observable social
            behaviors including, but not limited to, smiles, eye contact, change in
            physical proximity, and vocalizations.
    Objective 2: Patient will verbalize at least one personal need per 30-minute session.

The music therapist will provide the next follow up session 10/21/2004. 20- to 30-minute sessions will occur two times per week.

Treatment Environment and Intervention

Determining the Appropriate Treatment Environment

Patients on a medical/surgical unit are generally more medically stable than patients on intensive care units and specialty units. Some are ambulatory (or mobile via wheelchair or walker) and may be required to leave their rooms for scheduled periods of time during the day to maintain or regain strength and baseline levels of functioning. These patients are appropriate candidates for music therapy group sessions and music-related hospital-wide events (e.g., performances, karaoke, or musicals). Some patients cannot or should not leave their rooms. Reasons could include:

1. Medical bed-rest
2. **Externalized shunt**
3. Fever
4. Mechanical breathing assistance

5. Isolation
   a. Barrier
   b. Respiratory
   c. Transplant
   d. Strict

These patients should be seen in their rooms by the music therapist. The music therapist must follow posted hospital policies when working with patients in isolation, which could include the use of gowns, gloves, shoe covers, and masks. The music therapist must also pay close attention to the types of instruments and props used with an isolation patient. For most types of isolation, ALL materials used with the patient MUST be cleaned with hospital-approved disinfectant prior to being used with another patient. The hospital music therapist may want to have a few inexpensive or homemade instruments that can be left with the patient who is in isolation.

Individual patient sessions can occur at the bedside, in a therapy gym, or in the unit activity room during non-posted times. If a music therapy session is scheduled to occur at a patient's bedside, the music therapist must take several potential situations into consideration prior to conducting the bedside session. While many pediatric hospitals provide private rooms for patients and family members, some pediatric medical/surgical units still have semiprivate rooms (i.e., two or more patients sharing a room and bathroom facilities). As a result, the music therapist must consider the needs of the referred patient's roommate prior to introducing music stimuli into the room environment. If musical stimulation is contraindicated for a referred patient's roommate, the music therapist should arrange for the sessions to be held in another area. If this is not possible (e.g., patient medical bed-rest), then the music therapist should meet with treatment team members to advocate for room reassignment. In the event that neither of these options is available, the music therapist should collaborate with treatment team members to develop an alternative form of intervention.

If musical stimulation is not contraindicated for the referral patient's roommate, the music therapist can proceed with assessment and treatment planning. Upon completion of an initial assessment, the music therapist might consider inviting the patient's roommate to participate in the music therapy session. This decision would be affected by the referred patient's desire to interact with his or her roommate and by the nature of the treatment goals.

Patient Goals: Individual Sessions

Goal areas for medical/surgical patients can vary as greatly as the patients themselves. The pediatric music therapist must be capable of collaborating with the patient's treatment team to address the goals that most directly affect the patient's ability to cope with hospitalization and ultimately prepare for discharge. Table 1 demonstrates sample goal areas and patient objectives for this population. In addition to these areas, the music therapist will often address secondary goals during patient sessions. These may include developing pre-educational skills with young or developmentally delayed patients, strengthening peer and family relationships, and creating opportunities for general socialization and creative expression.

Table 1

Sample Goal Areas and Patient Objectives for Individual Sessions

Patient Goal Areas	Patient Objectives
Alleviate Symptoms of Anxiety Related to: • Hospitalization • New diagnosis • Separation anxiety • Fear of medical providers • Fear of medical procedures	a. Patient will verbalize feelings about anxiety. b. Patient will express feelings through musical improvisation. c. Patient will identify methods for coping with hospital-related anxiety.
Alleviate Symptoms of Depression Related to: • Altered self-image • Fatigue • Loss of functioning • Long term hospital stay • Decreased peer contact	a. Patient will engage in self-selected leisure activities. b. Patient will verbalize feelings about depression. c. Patient will express feelings about altered self-image/loss of functioning through musical improvisation. d. Patient will develop methods for staying connected with peers.

Decrease Perception of Pain:
• Acute pain
  – during procedures
  – following surgery
  – following injury
• Chronic pain
  – following injury
  – due to chronic illness (e.g., Crohn's disease, lupus)
	a. Patient will report decreased levels of pain perception.
	b. Patient will exhibit decreased frequency of observable pain indicators (e.g., physical tension, facial grimaces, crying).
	c. Patient will engage in preferred musical interaction.
	d. Patient will demonstrate one method of coping with chronic pain

Promote Multisensory Stimulation • Auditory • Visual • Tactile • Cognitive • Social	a. Patient will make eye contact with music therapist. b. Patient will turn head in the direction of auditory and visual stimuli. c. Patient will initiate social contact. d. Patient will achieve or maintain therapeutically appropriate rate of respiration.
Promote Relaxation	a. Patient will demonstrate decreased physical tension. b. Patient will achieve deep, even breaths. c. Patient will report decreased levels of pain, anxiety, and depression. d. Patient will fall asleep.
Maintain Functional Movement Skills: • Fine motor skills • Gross motor skills	a. Patient will grasp percussion instruments. b. Patient will tolerate passive range of motion exercises. c. Patient will sustain movements prescribed by physical therapist.

A music therapist working with the medical/surgical population will utilize any music *specific - interventions* therapy intervention that addresses the patient goal areas and elicits the patient objectives. These interventions will include songwriting, vocal/instrumental improvisation, musical games, structured instrument play, lyric discussion/analysis, receptive music listening, music assisted relaxation, and music as alternate engagement. Please refer to the following individual session case study for a demonstration of the use of these interventions.

Medical/Surgical Patient Individual Session Case Study

J. was a 16-year-old male with renal failure and multi-organ dysfunction. When J. was referred to music therapy, he was exhibiting symptoms of extreme depression. He spent his days and nights with his shades drawn and his lights off. If nursing or medical staff needed to turn on lights for a procedure or to check his vital signs, he would cover his face with his blanket. He did not initiate communication with any staff members and would grunt, shrug, or shake his head in response to questions from staff members. J. lost ambulatory functioning due to extended bed rest and was not performing any activities of daily living. The physical therapist and occupational therapist had attempted several sessions with J., but he refused to participate at any level.

The following sessions include significant information about the course of J.'s music therapy treatment. J. was in the hospital for 3 months after the commencement of music therapy sessions, and his sessions occurred three to five times per week for an average of 30 minutes per session.

Introductory/Assessment Session:

After reviewing the patient's chart, meeting with nursing staff, and consulting with the patient's child life specialist, the music therapist (MT-BC) approached J. in his room. The lights were off, and the patient was completely covered by his bedcovers. The music therapist softly introduced herself and offered to play the guitar for J. J. showed no response to the MT-BC. The MT-BC sat down next to his bed and began to play a simple chord progression in a soft finger-picking pattern. J. remained under the covers for the entire 20-minute session. When the MT-BC finished playing, J. said, "Will you come back?" The MT-BC said, "Of course. What kind of music should I play next time?" J. responded, "Country." The MT-BC said goodbye to J. after scheduling a follow-up session.

Session #2: The MT-BC arrived to a darkened room again. J. was under the covers. The MT-BC introduced herself and asked if she could play for J. again. J. said, "Yes." The MT-BC began to play and sing a popular country song. J. removed the covers from his face and watched the MT-BC as she played. He then asked if he could hold the music while the MT-BC played. After playing and singing several songs, J. made a few suggestions for songs during the next session. The MT-BC scheduled a follow-up session after a 30-minute session with J.

Over the next two weeks, J. became increasingly involved in the sessions with the MT-BC. He searched through songbooks to find songs he wanted to hear. He played music on his CD player for the MT-BC. He sang along with the MT-BC when she played his chosen songs. J. still refused to turn on his lights and remained laying in the bed despite requests from the MT-BC to elevate the head of his bed during the sessions.

Music Therapy as Positive Reinforcement:

During a treatment team meeting, J.'s physicians and psychiatrist determined that J. should spend at least 1 hour a day with the lights on in his room. Due to J.'s positive response to music therapy, the team asked the MT-BC to reinforce this behavior by conducting sessions during this time. During the first session after this meeting, the MT-BC greeted J., who was under his bed covers with the lights off. The MT-BC explained that she could conduct sessions only with the lights on. J. said, "Okay, I'll see you later." The music therapist left after scheduling a follow-up session. When the MT-BC returned for the next session, J. asked, "Do I have to turn on the light?" When the MT-BC affirmed this, J. thanked her and said goodbye. After five sessions, J. asked the MT-BC to turn on the lights when she arrived. The MT-BC reinforced this behavior by playing and singing J.'s preferred songs.

Music Therapy as Co-Treatment with Physical Therapy and Occupational Therapy:

The MT-BC received a request from the hospital's physical therapist (PT) to co-treat with J. The PT's requirement for J. was to sit on the edge of his bed, stand with assistance, and pivot to a bedside chair. J. was then supposed to sit in the chair for a predetermined amount of time. When the PT and MT-BC approached J. together, he immediately refused to participate. The MT-BC explained to J. that he would not have to accomplish all of the required tasks immediately. The MT-BC and PT suggested that J. try to sit up in bed as a first step. The MT-BC asked J. to choose a favorite song to sing. As they sang, the PT assisted J. in elevating the head of his bed. J. verbally indicated pain and discomfort, but he did not refuse. Once J. was comfortable, the PT asked if he could try to move to the edge of the bed. J. refused and asked the PT and MT-BC to leave the room. Both asked to return the following day, and J. agreed. During the next co-treatment session, J. sat up in bed but still refused to move to the edge of the bed.

Introduction of Percussion Instruments to Encourage Proper Positioning:

For the next session, the PT and the MT-BC determined that the MT-BC should begin the session prior to the arrival of the PT. The MT-BC introduced small, hand-held percussion instruments to J. J. stated, "I can't play these. I don't know how." The MT-BC demonstrated and described each instrument. She then encouraged J. to choose one that looked or sounded interesting. J. chose a cowbell. The MT-BC suggested to J. that it would be easiest to play the cowbell if he sat up in bed. J. agreed with this request and elevated the head of his bed without assistance. After playing a few of the instruments, the PT arrived. The MT-BC invited J. to choose an instrument for the PT to play. He selected an instrument for the PT, and the two played their instruments as the MT-BC accompanied them on the guitar. The PT asked J. if he would sit on the edge of the bed to play his instruments. J. stated, "I can play them just fine sitting here." The MT-BC asked J. if he would like to strum the guitar. J. was hesitant, but then said he would like to try. The MT-BC asked again if would sit on the edge of the bed so he could properly reach the guitar as the MT-BC fingered the chords, and J. agreed to try. As the PT assisted J., he indicated physical discomfort and verbally protested. The MT-BC and the PT praised J. for his attempts and offered to help him try the next day. J. agreed.

During the next several sessions, the PT and MT-BC reinforced J.'s successive approximations towards his PT goals. J. eventually moved to the edge of the bed to play his instruments. The PT and MT-BC gradually increased the length of time J. was required to sit on the edge of the bed, and then the PT introduced standing with assistance. The same process of successive approximations was required to achieve this goal. The MT-BC continued to introduce new instruments to encourage J. to reach forward and extend his arms after he stood. J. was eventually able to pivot and sit in his bedside chair. This was an uncomfortable position for J. due to his **continuous ambulatory peritoneal dialysis** (CAPD). As a result, the MT-BC began to conduct sessions after the bed-to-chair transfer was complete to provide music as alternate engagement (MAE) during this time of pain and discomfort.

Referential Improvisation:

During the series of sessions conducted in his bedside chair, the MT-BC asked J. if he knew what the word *improvisation* meant. J. responded, "Doesn't it mean to make stuff up?" The MT-BC said, "That's right. Would you like to try to improvise with the percussion instruments?" J.

said, "I don't know how." The MT-BC introduced the process of referential improvisation. She asked J. to choose an event in his life that was special or memorable for him. She asked him to briefly describe this event. J. chose to talk about a trip he had taken with his family to a theme park. The MT-BC encouraged J. to choose one aspect of this trip to represent musically. The MT-BC asked J. to choose an instrument that represented this aspect of his trip. She also encouraged him to choose an instrument for the MT-BC to play. As J. began to play his instrument, the MT-BC followed his musical cues (e.g., tempo, dynamics, style). When J. finished, he asked the MT-BC, "How did I do?" The MT-BC stated, "You just finished your first improvisation!" J. smiled broadly and asked, "Could you tell what I was playing about?" J. had chosen his aspect of the trip but had not let the MT-BC know what it was in advance. The MT-BC asked, "Was your improvisation referring to a roller coaster ride?" J. became visibly excited and exclaimed, "Yes! It was! How did you know?" The MT-BC described aspects of his improvisation that mimicked a roller coaster ride (e.g., slow, deliberate playing with a sudden shift to fast and sharp sounds). This process led to a discussion of the importance of J.'s trip and how it represented his desire for freedom (i.e., discharge from the hospital). The MT-BC discussed J.'s goals for discharge (e.g., ambulation and self-feeding). J. expressed a determination to complete these goals and a strong desire to go home.

J. requested to complete several further improvisations and initiated a game with the MT-BC. This was the first time J. initiated this type of interaction with the MT-BC. He chose a person to reference during his improvisation, and the MT-BC had to guess the object of the referential improvisation. J.'s first reference to a person involved the use of a small xylophone. He played a very light, sweet melody and then began to rapidly strike the highest note on the instrument. He then returned to his original melody. He did this several times and then ended his improvisation and posed the question to the MT-BC, "Who was that?" The MT-BC knew immediately that J. was referring to his mother, but was silent for several seconds before answering his question. J. confirmed this answer with excitement and began to describe his own musical cues. The melody represented how kind and sweet his mother was to him and how much he loved her. The repeated high note represented the times when she had to "tell him what to do." The MT-BC had interacted with J.'s mother several times prior to this session, and the improvisation was an accurate portrayal of J.'s relationship with her. During this session, J. sat in his bedside chair for an hour and a half with no complaints of discomfort or pain.

These improvisations were J.'s first expression of personal feelings about his family and his hospitalization. As a result, the MT-BC suggested that J. participate in songwriting during the next session. J. was skeptical, but he agreed to try.

Songwriting:
The MT-BC chose one of J.'s favorite songs and created a lyric substitution worksheet for him. Each line of lyrics was followed underneath with a blank line. When the MT-BC arrived, J. was sitting in his bedside chair. He stated, "I don't think I can write songs." The MT-BC said, "Let's try it today. If you don't like it, we will try something else." J. agreed to try. The MT-BC played the chosen song for J. to listen to the melody. The MT-BC then asked J. what he would like to write a song about. J. chose to write about his trip to a theme park. The MT-BC facilitated a brainstorming session with J. using a **mind map**. The MT-BC assisted J. with the first line of his song, and then J. began to compose his own lines. The MT-BC left J. to complete his song in privacy. When the MT-BC returned for the follow-up session, J. had completed the entire song and asked the MT-BC to sing it with him. He was visibly energized by this process and requested to sing the song five times. J. was ready to write his next song, so the MT-BC created a new worksheet for him. J. chose to write about his nursing staff. After completing the song, J. sang through it several times with the MT-BC. He then asked the MT-BC to find his nurses so they could hear their song. After J. performed his song, the nurses praised him. J. smiled broadly. The nurses began to dance around the room singing loudly. He said to them, "Okay, we can go on the road together. I will write the songs, and you can be my backup singers."

As J.'s music therapy sessions continued, he began to leave his room and go to the rehabilitation gym for PT sessions. The MT-BC conducted co-treatment sessions when J. first went to the gym for sessions. Together, they created a workout tape of J.'s favorite songs to serve as a timekeeper and motivation for his sessions. Just before J. was discharged from the hospital, he spent the majority of his days sitting up in bed with his lights on. He wrote songs, learned to play the keyboard, and sang for any eager listener.

This series of sessions demonstrates how a music therapist may utilize several forms of music therapy interventions before determining the best intervention for a particular client. For example, when the MT-BC first met J., it would not have been appropriate to begin with songwriting. The MT-BC had to establish a rapport with J. and provide him with opportunities for success in a nonthreatening environment. After 2 months of daily music therapy sessions, J. was still overwhelmed by the prospect of writing a song. His ability to complete the songwriting task empowered him to initiate interaction with his nursing staff and marked a turning point in his physical rehabilitation. The MT-BC chose interventions based on J.'s mood, energy level, and his assessed needs. As J. successfully participated in early interventions, the MT-BC increased the challenge of the tasks. J. continued to participate in music at home by taking piano lessons from his homebound schoolteacher. Despite his continued medical challenges, J. completed high school and is currently taking college courses.

Patient Goals: Group Sessions

For patients who can attend a group session, the music therapist generally has two options. If space and personnel resources allow, the music therapist may be able to conduct groups that are referral-based to address specific treatment goals (e.g., coping with depression, coping with anxiety, increasing range of motion/physical functioning). The acute nature of most hospital settings does not always allow for a referral-based group session. At any given time, there may be only one patient who is experiencing a particular treatment need. As a result, the music therapist may want to conduct a more general, open-referral group session. The music therapist can invite patients and families from several medical/surgical units to participate. An open-referral group can address general goal areas that most pediatric patients experience while addressing general developmental needs. Table 2 provides examples of these goal areas for pediatric medical/surgical group sessions and possible interventions for each goal area. This is not a comprehensive list of patient needs, nor is it an exhaustive list of music therapy group interventions. A sample group session outline, including sample interventions and the rationale for each intervention, is provided in the Appendix of this chapter. In addition, a detailed task analysis of one intervention is included in the Appendix as an example.

Co-Treatment in Medical/Surgical

Coordinated treatment among the patient's entire treatment team is vital for the success of music therapy interventions on the pediatric medical/surgical unit. The chaotic and busy environment of the pediatric general medical/surgical unit may warrant co-treatment sessions

Table 2

Goal Areas and Possible Interventions for Pediatric Medical/Surgical Group Sessions

Patient Goal Areas	Music Therapy Group Interventions	Patient Objectives
Increase Socialization: • Peers • Staff • Family members	Group member introductions: • Opening song • Hot potato • Leadership opportunities: • Drumming • Solo instrumental improvisation within group improvisation • Improvisational dance • Teamwork opportunities: • Name that tune • Group drumming	a. Patient will introduce self and family members to group members. b. Patient will initiate social interaction. c. Patient will verbally and musically respond to staff and group members when appropriate. d. Patient will accept leadership opportunities e. Patient will collaborate with group members to accomplish assigned task.
Educational Opportunities: • Object identification (e.g., preschool skills—colors, numbers) • Instrument instruction	Identification songs: • *Down on Grandpa's Farm* (traditional) • *Old MacDonald* (traditional) • *Look at All the Fruits and Vegetables* (Hannan) Instrumental instruction: • Percussion instruments • Guitar • Keyboard • Recorder	a. Patient will correctly identify object names, characteristics, and purposes verbally and musically. b. Patient will demonstrate ability to produce musical sounds demonstrated by the therapist. c. Patient will demonstrate unique methods of producing musical sounds.
Opportunities for Creative Expression Related to: • Hospitalization • Diagnosis • Relationships • Spirituality • Mood state (e.g., depression, anxiety)	Songwriting: • Lyric substitution • Story songs • Improvised • Call and response • Blues format • Musical Games: • Magic Circle • Name that Tune Vocal and Instrumental Improvisation	a. Patient will contribute lyrical material for songwriting process. b. Patient will sing or accompany song with group members. c. Patient will demonstrate methods for coping with hospital related situations (e.g., anxiety, depression, new diagnosis) d. Patient will exhibit creative thought through verbalizations, musical performance, and physical movement.

Table 2—Continued

Patient Goal Areas	Music Therapy Group Interventions	Patient Objectives
Maintain Functional Movement Skills: ▪ Fine motor skills ▪ Gross motor skills	Dance: ▪ Improvisational ▪ Patient choreographed ▪ Action Songs (traditional): ▪ *Wheels on the Bus* ▪ *Itsy Bitsy Spider* ▪ *Hi, My Name is Joe* ▪ *The Princess Pat*	a. Patient will demonstrate physical movement for group dance. b. Patient will execute or approximate movements related to action songs.
Increase Decision Making	Occurs during all group interventions.	a. Patient will choose instruments, songs, movements, or methods of musical interaction. b. Patient will choose group members to participate in group interactions (e.g., pt may choose who plays the gathering drum next).

to meet the patient's needs in a time-efficient manner. As the medical/surgical patient recovers from acute illness, injury, or surgery, he or she may receive rehabilitative intervention from the PT/OT.

For example, the music therapist can co-treat with the physical therapist (PT) or occupational therapist (OT) to address tasks such as transfer from the bed to the chair, ambulation, strength training, or the redevelopment of activities of daily living (ADLs). These interventions often include physical endurance tasks of specific frequency and duration (e.g., sitting in the bedside chair for 30 minutes, walking to and from the activity room three times per day). The music therapist can assist the medical/surgical patient by scheduling music therapy interventions during these endurance tasks (e.g., the patient may engage in songwriting with the therapist while sitting in the bedside chair, the music therapist can conduct sessions in the activity room to facilitate scheduled ambulation).

The medical/surgical child life specialist (CLS) may also receive specific referrals for individual patients. The Child Life Council describes a child life specialist as one who "use[s] play, recreation, education, self-expression, and theories of child development to promote psychological well-being and optimum development of children, adolescents, and their families" (Child Life Council, n.d.). Many music therapists in the hospital setting are affiliated with the hospital's child life department. Others work closely with child life specialists assigned to inpatient units and outpatient clinics or centers. Child life specialists can assist the medical music therapist by identifying patients who are appropriate candidates for music therapy assessment. CLSs formally or informally assess each patient and family on their units and their collaboration can provide valuable information for the music therapist to triage patient referrals.

For group sessions, the music therapist relies on child life specialists, assistants, and interns to round on their units and invite patients to the group session. In order to ensure a safe patient-to-staff member ratio during the group sessions, these child life staff members often assist the music therapist during the group session. They can provide hand over hand assistance, hold young children, greet patients and families who arrive after the session has begun, and alert nursing staff when IV pumps are occluded or malfunctioning, or when infusions are complete. These staff members can also assist the music therapist in the event of an emergency such as a medical code.

Music therapists can assist nursing staff by addressing goal areas such as medical compliance and painful procedure support. These interventions can be timesaving for the nursing staff by decreasing patient agitation and combativeness. Patient compliance and satisfaction with a prescribed treatment regimen facilitates a decreased number of patient requests for direct nursing intervention. Recovery from conscious sedation requires careful monitoring from a registered nurse. This requires more frequent vital sign checks, possibly once every 15 minutes. A music therapy intervention such as music as alternate engagement during nonsurgical procedures can result in the decreased use of sedative or pain medication. This results in a subsequent decrease in required direct nursing contact.

Co-treatment among hospital personnel is common across units and can incorporate a diverse group of professionals. The intent of co-treatment is to enhance the treatment intervention through diverse modalities and to intensify outcomes for the patient. A comparable section on co-treatment in the PICU is found in Chapter 3 of this monograph and expands on this topic in greater detail.

Outcome Measures and Documentation

The music therapist evaluates the medical/surgical patient's progress by utilizing behavioral observation; monitoring of vital signs; and feedback from the patient, family members, and medical staff. Behavioral observation can include the documentation of frequency and duration of desired behaviors (e.g., eye contact, social interaction, musical behaviors) and observable indications of mood (e.g., facial movements, verbalizations, physical tension, alertness). Feedback may include the patient's verbal assessment of the intervention and family members' verbal and written comments about the patient's responses during and after the session. Medical staff members may formally (documentation in the patient's chart) or informally (verbal comments directly to the music therapist) relay their observations of the lasting effects of music therapy intervention (e.g., positive self comments, increased compliance with medical regimen, improved mood, display of positive and supportive coping mechanisms).

Documentation may be in a written or electronic format depending on the hospital. Some facilities may require a short checklist style of documentation, while others may be narrative. In this author's experience, all outcomes are documented in a narrative note format in the patient's legal medical chart. The progress note format is similar to the assessment note format. A sample progress note is included below, following this format:

Description of Event:
1. Referral date, referral source, referral reason (if available)
2. Basic patient information from chart review, patient/family interview, and medical staff consultation
3. Patient music therapy goals and objectives
4. Description of session environment

Action:
1. Type and duration of music therapy session
2. Brief description of music therapy assessment interventions

Response:
1. Description of patient behaviors, verbalizations, strengths, and needs
2. Description of patient outcomes related to goals and objectives
3. Reevaluation of goals and objectives
4. Plan for subsequent music therapy sessions or discharge from services

---

Sample Music Therapy Progress Note

Pediatric General Medical Surgical Unit

Date: 10/21/2004
Time: 17:55

D: Patient is a 4-year-old male with cystic fibrosis. Patient was admitted due to cystic fibrosis exacerbation. Patient lives with his father and his father's significant other who refers to herself as "mom." Patient was referred to music therapy by his child life specialist on 10/19/2004. Referral reasons include:
1. Increased risk for depression due to barrier and respiratory isolation
2. Treatment regimen noncompliance

Goals and objectives include:

Goal 1:   Increase compliance with necessary oral feeds
   Objective 1: Patient will consume a sufficient amount of solid foods to prevent the need for supplemental nutrition via bolus feeds.
   Objective 2: Patient will initiate self feeds without continual reinforcement.

Goal 2:   Increase opportunities for developmentally appropriate socialization including conversation.
   Objective 1: Patient will respond to therapist interactions with observable social behaviors including but not limited to smiles, eye contact, change in physical proximity, and vocalizations.
   Objective 2: Patient will verbalize at least one personal need per 30-minute session.

Patient was seated on his bed watching television when this writer arrived. Patient's father was present at the bedside.

A: The music therapist introduced a Q-chord and hand-held percussion instruments to the patient. Patient participated in an introductory song and children's folksongs. Patient also participated in songwriting. When the patient's tray was delivered for dinner, the music therapist encouraged him to eat. Patient's father showed him all the food options on his tray, and patient chose his first food to eat. The music therapist sang a closing song and scheduled a follow-up session.

R: Patient exhibited animated facial expressions and high levels of physical energy as evidenced by constant movement and reaching for musical instruments. Patient asked simple questions about the instruments such as, "What is that?" or "Can I play that?" Patient would point to a new instrument before completing a previous task. The patient invited the music therapist to play particular instruments with him. The music therapist initiated a flashcard songwriting process with the patient. Patient independently chose elements of the song from the flashcards (animal, color, action, and place) and was able to identify the pictures and words on each flashcard. Patient participated in the improvised song by choosing an instrument to accompany the music therapist's singing.

Goal 1, Objective 1: Patient consumed a shake in the presence of the writer and had moved close to his food tray prior to the end of the session. This indicates compliance with oral feeds.

Objective 2: Patient required only verbal encouragement from the music therapist and the patient's father to begin eating.

Goal 2, Objective 1: Patient exhibited smiles, laughter, eye contact, and verbalizations throughout the entire 30-minute session in response to the music therapist's interactions.

Objective 2: Patient verbally requested specific instruments five times during the 30-minute session.

Based on therapist observation and subsequent consultation with nursing staff, it was determined that the patient is compliant with oral feeds. Goal 1 has been attained and will no longer be addressed during music therapy sessions. The music therapist will continue to address the patient's need for socialization and stimulation. Follow-up session will occur on 10/26/2004

A patient may be discharged from music therapy services for one of the following reasons. The patient may have achieved the goals and objectives designed by the music therapist. The music therapist should evaluate the patient for other potential goal areas prior to discharging the patient from services. Music therapy services may become contraindicated for a patient. In this case, the music therapist should discontinue services and consult with the treatment team to assure that the patient's needs are met in an appropriate manner. Finally, the patient may be scheduled for hospital discharge. The music therapist should provide closure for the patient when possible and document recommendations for music therapy at home or community-based music involvement. Some hospitals will provide the music therapist with an interdisciplinary discharge summary document. If no document is available, the music therapist should include discharge recommendations in a narrative note format.

Future Areas for Development and Growth

Music therapy interventions and protocols are well documented for certain aspects of pediatric healthcare. Research in specific areas of healthcare such as **neonatology**, cardiology, and hematology/oncology continues to flourish in music therapy and related healthcare journals. After review of the current literature, this author discovered that the pediatric medical/surgical population was not identified as a specific patient population. Music therapists may want to consider whether this general medical/surgical patient population possesses enough of a shared experience to warrant future study, definition, and development of specific music therapy interventions. Since many medical/surgical patients have chronic medical conditions (e.g., cystic fibrosis, asthma, Crohn's disease, and diabetes), researchers might consider investigating the implication of current research conducted for other chronic conditions such as the areas of hematology/oncology and cardiac care.

While many music therapists are providing procedural support for pediatric patients, more studies are needed to document the cost-effectiveness of this intervention and to develop and pilot intervention protocols. Results of continued research in the area of procedural support may also create opportunities for the inclusion of music therapists on pediatric perioperative teams.

For the general medical/surgical patient, guidelines for the development of treatment goals and interventions are frequently documented in the current literature (Standley & Whipple, 2003). To support the development of methods of best practice in music therapy, the clinical determination of frequency and duration of sessions should be investigated. In addition to enhancing the quality of care provided by the music therapist for this patient population, development of such guidelines could help potential employers of music therapists evaluate the cost effectiveness and viability of music therapy as a treatment option for their patients. The issue of frequency and duration of music therapy interventions also encompasses the method of planning for an acute care patient. The development of methods for conducting a complete intervention process within one session could assist music therapists who do not have the opportunity for a formal process of assessment, treatment planning, intervention delivery, evaluation, and discharge planning. Many music therapists in the pediatric hospital setting must complete all five aspects of service delivery within one 20- to 30-minute session.

The pediatric general medical/surgical unit is perhaps one of the most diverse environments within a pediatric healthcare setting. Patients with chronic illnesses walk the halls with patients who are recovering from an acute condition requiring simple pharmacological intervention. Surgical patients attend activities and group sessions with patients whose set of symptoms eludes a diagnosis from the medical team. Teenaged patients, whose hospital admissions number in the hundreds, share rooms with young or newly diagnosed patients experiencing their first admission. These diverse patient experiences create a rich and challenging environment for the pediatric music therapist. These clinicians are faced with the exciting responsibility of continuing to conduct research with this population to enhance the delivery of music therapy interventions to general medical/surgical pediatric patients.

References

American Academy of Pediatrics (AAP), Surgical Advisory Panel. (2002). Guidelines for referral to pediatric surgical specialists. *Pediatrics, 110,* 187–191.

Bare, M. R. (1997). Confronting a life threatening disease: Renal dialysis and transplant programs. In T. S. Kerson, (Ed.), *Social work in health settings: Practice in context* (2nd ed., pp. 269–290). Binghamton, NY: Haworth Press.

Brenn, B. R. (2003). Preoperative evaluation and testing. In P. Mattei (Ed.), *Surgical directives: Pediatric surgery* (pp. 3–12). Philadelphia: Lippincott, Williams & Wilkins.

Chase, S. K. (1995). The social context of critical care clinical judgment. *Heart & Lung, 24*(2), 154–162.

Child Life Council (n.d.). *Child life professionals.* Retrieved October 17, 2008, from www.childlife.org

Clair, A. A. (1996). The effect of singing on alert responses in persons with late stage dementia. *Journal of Music Therapy, 33,* 234–247.

Humes, H. D. (2000). *Kelley's textbook of internal medicine* (4th ed.). Philadelphia: Lippincott, Williams & Wilkins.

Kampschroer, A., & Schumacher, K. (2002, March). *Hands on! Interventions to use with children and adolescents.* Session presented at the Great Lakes Regional Music Therapy Conference, St. Charles, IL.

Robb, S. (2000). The effect of therapeutic music interventions on the behavior of hospitalized children in isolation: Developing a contextual support model of music therapy. *Journal of Music Therapy, 27,* 118–146.

Robb, S. (2003). Coping and chronic illness: Music therapy for children and adolescents with cancer. In S. Robb (Ed.), *Music therapy in pediatric healthcare: Research and evidence-based practice* (pp. 101–136). Silver Spring, MD: American Music Therapy Association.

Schwartz, M. (2003). *The 5-minute pediatric consult.* Philadelphia: Lippincott, Williams & Wilkins.

Standley, J. (1986). Music research in medical/dental treatment: Meta-analysis and clinical applications. *Journal of Music Therapy, 23,* 56–122.

Standley, J. M., & Whipple, J. (2003). Music therapy with pediatric patients: A meta analysis. In S. Robb (Ed.), *Music therapy in pediatric healthcare: Research and evidence-based practice* (pp. 1–18). Silver Spring, MD: American Music Therapy Association.

Wong, D., & Baker, C. (1988). Pain in children: Comparison of assessment scales. *Pediatric Nursing, 14*(1), 9–17.

Wong, D. L., Hockenberry-Eaton, M., Wilson, D., Winkelstein, M. L., & Schwartz, P. (2001). *Wong's essentials of pediatric nursing* (6th ed.). St. Louis, MO: Mosby.

Appendix

Sample Group Session Outline and Rationale
Pediatric General Medical Surgical Unit

OPENING SONG

Rationale:

A clearly defined beginning to a group session focuses the patients on the tasks of the group. An opening or welcoming song is an appropriate method to begin a group and to create a foundation for open communication and shared creative expression. The opening application also allows for an assessment of the group members' level of functioning.

Procedure and Examples:

Example #1:

Lyrics substituted to *Come on Over* performed by Shania Twain

I   IV^7
Come on over. Come on in. Join us today for music therapy group.
I   IV^7 I
Come on over. Come on in. Tell us your name and your favorite game.

Patients sing and clap or play egg shakers while the music therapist sings and plays an accompaniment instrument (e.g., guitar). The music therapist demonstrates the behavior requested in the song lyrics and then chooses the next person to respond to the song lyrics. The music therapist can invite patients to respond in a structured manner, such as in the order in which they are seated in the circle. Or, the music therapist can add a level of socialization and decision making by allowing patients to choose who responds next, regardless of seating. This also gives young patients and patients who are developmentally delayed an opportunity to test their social skills. For example, a patient may decline to introduce himself or herself to the group. The music therapist can validate this choice and encourage the patient to ask another member of the group to respond first. The music therapist can also provide opportunities for successive approximation of response for the patient who does not wish to introduce himself or herself (e.g., the patient could have someone else introduce him or her; the patient could wait until others have completed the task).

INSTRUMENT PLAYING

Rationale:

The use of hand-held instruments involves the patient in the creation of a musical experience. In addition to potentially learning a new skill, patients may develop problem-solving and decision-making skills during this process. Playing instruments requires fine and gross motor skills, and limited opportunities for exercise during hospitalization necessitates the creation of opportunities for patients to maintain physical functioning. Patients who are engaged in instrument play can expend excess energy or become energized by the musical interaction. Patients may be motivated by musical interaction, thereby offsetting the potential effects of symptoms of depression or anxiety.

Procedure and Examples:

The music therapist introduces a variety of percussion instruments to the members of the group. Each patient has the option of choosing an instrument for himself or herself and for members of the family who attend the group. Once each group member has an instrument, the music therapist facilitates structured or improvised instrument play.

Structured Instrument Play:

The therapist chooses a song to encourage the following patient responses (this is determined by the needs of the group):

- Identification of instrument names
- Demonstration of traditional and non-traditional methods of instrument play
- Auditory discrimination
- Sequencing
- Demonstration of leadership skills
- Demonstration of teamwork through musical support

Example #1:

Momma Don't Allow (traditional)

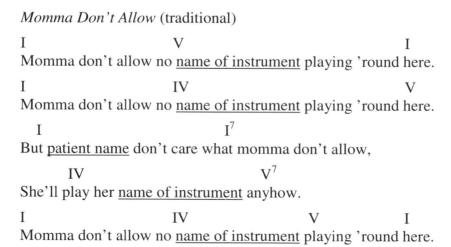

I   V   I
Momma don't allow no <u>name of instrument</u> playing 'round here.

I   IV   V
Momma don't allow no <u>name of instrument</u> playing 'round here.

  I   I^7
But <u>patient name</u> don't care what momma don't allow,

        IV   V^7
She'll play her <u>name of instrument</u> anyhow.

I   IV   V   I
Momma don't allow no <u>name of instrument</u> playing 'round here.

During this song, patients can play quietly while the lyrically identified patient plays a solo over the accompaniment. The music therapist can encourage the patient to choose who goes next (i.e., to promote socialization), can use a predetermined order (e.g., around the circle), or can randomly choose patients to be the soloist (i.e., to promote attention to task). One adaptation can include acknowledging patient behaviors, physical characteristics, and situational information. Using this information to create verses can include patients who do not want to play an instrument or who cannot participate in a traditional manner. Acknowledging common characteristics assists the patient to develop similarity-based connections for social interaction.

Patient Behaviors:

Momma don't allow no <u>dancing</u> 'round here.
Momma don't allow no <u>dancing</u> 'round here.
But <u>patient name</u> don't care what momma don't allow,
She'll <u>dance</u> anyhow.
Momma don't allow no <u>dancing</u> 'round here.

Physical Characteristics:

Momma don't allow no <u>pajama wearing</u> 'round here.
Momma don't allow no <u>pajama wearing</u> 'round here.
But <u>patients who possess this characteristic</u> don't care what momma don't allow,
They'll <u>wear their pajamas</u> anyhow.
Momma don't allow no <u>pajama wearing</u> 'round here.

Situational Information:

Momma don't allow <u>patient's name</u> to be <u>discharged</u> today.
Momma don't allow <u>patient's name</u> to be <u>discharged</u> today.
But <u>patient's name</u> don't care what momma don't allow,
She'll <u>be discharged</u> today anyhow.
Momma don't allow <u>patient's name</u> to be <u>discharged</u> today.

Example #2:

Let's Play Our Instruments (Hannan)

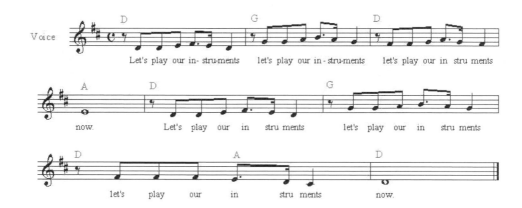

After this introductory verse, the music therapist suggests different ways to play the instruments, including varying positions, contrasting dynamic levels, and contrasting tempi.

> Let's play our instruments,
> Let's play our instruments,
> Let's play our instruments <u>up high</u>.
> Let's play our instruments,
> Let's play our instruments,
> Let's play our instruments (pause to ask the patients, "What is the opposite of up high?") <u>down low</u>.

The music therapist can also encourage patients to demonstrate or verbally introduce a specific method of playing the instrument. Patients can choose who goes next, or the therapist can use a predetermined order.

Improvisational Instrument Play:

The music therapist chooses a basic structure (e.g., blues progression, specific drumming style, or topic for referential improvisation) for the improvisation. The music therapist solicits input from the patients and facilitates the musical interaction by utilizing the chosen structure. The music therapist processes the improvisation with the group members when it is developmentally appropriate to do so. Patients can participate as a group or can be given opportunities for solo improvising. For example, one patient might volunteer to "solo" first. The music therapist may provide a limit to the duration of the solo (e.g., two phrases or two minutes), or the music therapist may encourage the patient to indicate when he has finished his solo. This could include choosing the next patient to play a solo.

Example #1:

Blues in the Key of E flat:

The music therapist plays a simple walking bass line in E flat on the keyboard. Patients are given choices of instruments to play. The music therapist solicits volunteers to "solo" on the keyboard and instructs them to play only the black keys. The music therapist can limit the duration when there are a large number of group members. The music therapist can also allow the patient to "solo" until he or she is ready to stop. This flexibility can allow for:

- Increased demonstration of positive self-esteem
- Socialization with peers
- Development of positive coping skills

MUSICAL GAMES

Rationale:

Pediatric medical professionals recognize that games and other forms of play are a child's "work." Opportunities for play enable children to define themselves and organize their environment according to their own constructs. They also provide opportunities for socialization, appropriate competition, education, and the development of coping strategies.

Procedure and Examples:

Example #1:

Magic Circle (idea adapted from presentation at 2001 Great Lakes Regional Conference, Kampschroer & Schumacher, 2002):

I   IV   V   I
Come into the magic circle where you can be what you want to be.

I   IV   V   I
Come into the magic circle and set yourself free.
Patient's name is in the magic circle where he can be what he wants to be.
Patient's name is in the magic circle. Let's all count to three: 1, 2, 3 magic word!

The music therapist "draws" a large circle on the floor with masking tape. The music therapist explains that a magic circle requires a magic word and encourages the patients to choose a magic word. After practicing the recitation of the magic word, the music therapist explains that when a patient stands in the center of the circle, he or she can act out a person, animal, object, or action. The rest of the group tries to guess the patient's charade. For younger children, the music therapist can add the use of vocalizations. The music therapist sings the verse prior to each child's charade. Once a patient provides a correct guess, the group praises the patient for participating. The patient who provides the correct guess can be the next person in the magic circle, or the music therapist can take volunteers to participate.

For patients who are uncomfortable standing in front of the group or who cannot physically enter the circle due to medical equipment or other limitations, the music therapist can "throw" the magic circle around the patient's chair. The music therapist invites the patients to count to three, say the magic word, and mime the action of picking up and "throwing" the circle. The music therapist can facilitate "deals" between group members during this intervention. For example, if a patient demonstrates behaviors that indicate a desire to participate combined with shyness or reluctance, the music therapist might ask, "If your mom goes into the circle first, would you go next?" or "If the child life specialist goes with you, will you enter the circle?" Some patients have difficulty choosing an object or action to mimic, so staff, volunteers, and family members can assist the patient by making suggestions. This intervention provides opportunities for:

- Socialization
- Positive peer support
- Creative expression
- Decision-making
- Problem solving

Example #2:

Hot Potato:
Hot potato, hot potato, 'round it goes. Where it stops, nobody knows.

The music therapist has patients sit in a circle close enough to pass an object from person to person. The music therapist invites patients to pat their legs and clap their hands in a simple pat, pat, clap, clap pattern. The music therapist then begins to pass a potato shaker (or beanbag) around the circle. Group members complete the chant. The patient who is holding the potato at the end of the chant has a chance to answer one question from the group. Group members learn how to ask appropriate questions, and the person with the potato decides whether or not he or she is going to answer the question. If the patient receives the potato a second time, he or she chooses one member of the group and asks this person a question. The primary focus of this intervention is to develop appropriate methods of social interaction. In addition, this intervention can address:

- Hand/eye coordination
- Turn taking
- Decision making
- Development of a positive self image

SONGWRITING:

Rationale:

Songwriting can address multiple goals simultaneously in a group setting. The experiences of hospitalization create the need for pediatric patients to have an opportunity for creative expression. The music therapist chooses a method of songwriting that is developmentally appropriate for the patients in the group. The music therapist should make this decision based on the majority of the group and adapt the process to include other members. For example, if the group is comprised of eight teenaged patients and two toddlers, the therapist should choose a method that will be engaging for the teenagers (e.g., lyric substitution) and provide opportunities during the process for the toddlers to make choices and participate in the final performance.

Procedure and Examples:

Songwriting in a group setting can be challenging, especially when the group members' ages range from birth through young adult. Since most groups on a pediatric medical/surgical unit are comprised of different members during each session, the music therapist must choose a method of songwriting that will allow group members to complete the song in one session. These methods may include:

- Fill-in-the-blank
- Lyric Substitution
- Story Song
- Original Composition
- Blues

Example #1:

Fill-in-the-blank Songwriting:

To the tune of *Mary Had a Little Lamb* (traditional)

<u>Patient's name</u>'s favorite color is <u>patient's color choice</u>, color is <u>patient's color choice</u>, color is <u>patient's color choice</u>.

<u>Patient's name</u>'s favorite color is <u>patient's color choice</u> and he/she likes it because <u>patient's reason</u>.

This example represents a benign topic and serves as an introduction to the songwriting process. If the group writes more than one song, the patients may introduce topics related to hospitalization, peer relationships, or family situations.

Example #2:

Hospital Blues:

I
We're here at <u>name of hospital</u>. We're here at <u>name of hospital</u>.

                                IV   I
We've got the hospital blues. We've got the hospital blues.

IV   V   I
Sometimes it's bad and sometimes it's good at <u>name of hospital</u>.

The music therapist sings through the song once for the patients. The music therapist asks for a volunteer to fill in something bad about being in the hospital and something good about being in the hospital. The music therapist can pause and vamp on the IV chord while the patient sings or verbalizes the "bad thing" and can then pause and vamp on the V chord while the patient sings or verbalizes the "good thing" about being in the hospital.

MOVEMENT AND DANCE

Rationale:

Movement during hospitalization is important to maintain levels of physical functioning, regain lost functioning, and improve mood by the release of natural endorphins. The following are examples of how to use movement paired with music in a group setting.

Procedure and Examples:

The music therapist must adapt movement interventions to include patients with varying levels of physical mobility. In a group setting, most patients will be seated in chairs, wheelchairs, strollers, or wagons. The music therapist can encourage patients to execute movements from a seated position while extending the opportunity for patients to stand and move through space if desired. This ensures that the basic movements can be performed by all patients while providing an opportunity for additional challenge for higher functioning patients.

Example #1:

Copycat Movement:

The music therapist engages patients in a demonstration of movements and sounds that can be made by the body. The music therapist should encourage the patients to initiate these examples. The music therapist then provides live or recorded musical accompaniment while instructing one patient (volunteer or predetermined order) to initiate a movement for the rest of the group to mimic. The patient can indicate when he or she is ready for another person to lead the group in a new movement.

Example #2:

Dance Choreography

This intervention begins in the same manner as the first example by exploring possible movements and sounds. The music therapist then asks each patient to demonstrate a movement or sound (e.g., clapping, stomping, twisting). The patient also chooses the duration of the movement. The music therapist can encourage patients to choose a number of counts that is divisible by 4. As each patient adds his or her movement to the choreographed dance, the music therapist may choose to periodically practice the sequence of movements with the group. After each patient has made a contribution, the music therapist provides a "dance track" for the performance. The music therapist can use recorded music or a rhythm track from a drum machine or synthesizer. A rhythm track can be set to loop continuously to facilitate varied lengths of dance performance. After performing the choreographed dance, the music therapist may decide to challenge the group by performing the movements in reverse order.

CLOSING SONG:

Rationale:

A closing or goodbye song provides closure for patients in a group session. It signifies a clearly defined end to the group and can summarize the interactions that occurred during the group.

Procedure and Examples:

The music therapist should choose a closing song to support the needs of the patients. A closing song can review group member names, validate accomplishments of the group members, or review commonalities among group members to facilitate socialization outside the group setting.

Example #1:

The music therapist may choose to use an existing or familiar goodbye song. Many children's television shows use goodbye songs to signify the end of the show. These can be adapted to include each group member's name or accomplishments.

Example #2:

Original Composition (A. Hannan):

I   IV
So long <u>patient's name</u>, we're glad you came,

IV   I
You <u>patient action during group</u> so well in group today.

I   IV
So long <u>patient's name</u>, we're glad you came,

IV   V   I
To our group today.

So long <u>Heather</u>, we're glad you came,
You <u>sang</u> so well in group today.
So long <u>Heather</u>, we're glad you came,
To our group today.

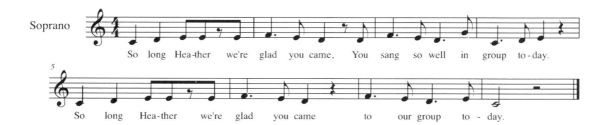

A Detailed Task Analysis of One Intervention

Population/Age Range: preschool – adolescent

Title: Group Story Songwriting

Goals: Facilitate verbal or nonverbal self-expression, improve self-esteem, decrease anxiety, improve choice-making and control, alleviate depression, improve coping with illness and hospitalization

Objective(s):
1. Pts will demonstrate active participation in songwriting to extent capable.
2. Pts will demonstrate verbal or nonverbal self expression depending upon ability.
3. Pts will demonstrate choice-making during songwriting interaction.
4. Pts will validate suggestions made by other group members.
5. Pts will demonstrate improvement in frequency or quality of positive affect.
6. Pts will demonstrate awareness of one positive strategy for coping with illness and hospitalization.

Response Definition:
1. Therapist will assess pts' level of active participation (e.g., frequency/duration of eye contact, level of verbal engagement, level of musical engagement).
2. Therapist will note frequency of pts' verbal or nonverbal communication attempts.
3. Therapist will note frequency of pts' positive self-statements or positive comments about the songwriting process or product.
4. Therapist will note frequency of pts' choice-making.
5. Therapist will observe pts' frequency and quality of positive affect before, during, and after songwriting.
6. Therapist will note pts' ability to verbalize positive skills for coping with illness and hospitalization.

Materials: Accompanying instrument (e.g., keyboard, guitar, Q-chord), hand-held percussion instruments, drawing materials

Procedural Steps:
1. Therapist establishes rapport with the group members through opening song or other developmentally appropriate group music therapy interventions.
2. Therapist offers option of songwriting to the group members.
3. If group members agree to participate, the therapist solicits suggestions for songwriting topics from the group.
4. Therapist facilitates the decision-making process of choosing a topic.

5. Therapist requests a volunteer from the group to provide initial information about the chosen topic.
6. If patients are reluctant to provide information, the therapist may ask questions about the topic or provide choices for the group members (e.g., if the topic is "turtles," the therapist may ask, "What color is the turtle?" or "What is the turtle's name?").
7. Each group member is given an opportunity to add to the "story" about the chosen topic (i.e., the therapist facilitates group member participation at developmentally appropriate levels).
8. Therapist improvises song lyrics based on the patient-expressed story.
9. Therapist uses a call-response song style to involve patients in the performance of the song.
10. Therapist facilitates patient discussion about the song.

Measurement Tools:
1. Patient verbalizations
2. Frequency of musical expression
3. Frequency of choice making
4. Frequency and duration of interaction with peers

Possible Adaptations: The music therapist may record the improvised song and provide printed lyrics or copies of the recorded song to the group members after the session. The music therapist may also invite group members to illustrate the song by decorating lyric sheets or by artistically expressing aspects of the song.

Sample Story Song Process and Lyrics [therapist questions are in italics. Patient responses are in plain text]:

"What would you like to write a song about?"

"Superheroes." "Turtles." "Going home."

"Should we choose one of these topics, or should we write about all three?"

"All three!"

"Okay, is our turtle a superhero?"

"Yes! And he is in the hospital."

"Do superheroes get sick sometimes?"

"Yes, but they don't cry when they get poked."

"Is it okay to cry when you get poked?"

"Yes, and I cry, but superheroes don't cry."

"You're right, it is okay to cry." "Okay, does our turtle have a name?"

"Brandon."

"What color is Brandon?"

"He is blue."

"Okay, so our blue, superhero turtle is in the hospital, and his name is Brandon. What happens to Brandon?" [The therapist might choose to direct this question to a patient who hasn't provided any lyrical input.]

"I don't know."

"Do we know why Brandon is in the hospital?"

"He has diabetes. And he can't eat cookies."

"Oh, diabetes. Okay, so Brandon has diabetes and can't eat cookies. What CAN he do?"

"He can ride on the elevators."

"Where does he go after he rides on the elevators?"

"Outside. To play on the playground."

"What happens on the playground?"

"Somebody falls down and gets hurt."

"Does Brandon get hurt?"

"No, he is a superhero. He helps the person that gets hurt."

"What does he do?"

"He says, 'There, there, it will be okay. I'll give you some medicine.'"

"Why does he give the person medicine?"

"'Cause medicine makes you better!"

"What happens after Brandon helps the person who fell?"

"They go back to the unit together."

"Anything else?"

"No."

"Okay, we have a story for our song. I will sing a line and you can all sing it back to me. After four lines, we repeat them again."

[The therapist can create a melody for a call-and-response song or use a preexisting song. One example is the camp song *The Other Day I Saw a Bear* (traditional).]

This is a song (This is a song)
About a turtle. (About a turtle.)
A superhero turtle (A superhero turtle)
Whose name is Brandon. (Whose name is Brandon.)

This is a song about a turtle. A superhero turtle whose name is Brandon.

[Continue with each verse in the same manner.]
Even though he is a superhero,
Brandon is in the hospital.

'Cause he has diabetes,
And he can't eat cookies.

Even though Brandon
Can't eat cookies,
He can have some fun
Riding on the elevator.

When he gets off the elevator,
He goes to the playground.
And there he sees,
Someone fall and get hurt.

So being a superhero,
He goes to help.
And he says,
"I'll give you some medicine."

When you get medicine,
Sometimes there is a poke.
It's okay to cry,
'Cause the medicine makes you better.

After Brandon helped his friend,
They went back to the unit.
And this is the end
Of our song about a turtle.

This example demonstrates the use of an imaginative story song to validate patients' fears about hospitalization and to address the development of coping strategies.

CHAPTER 5

Hematology, Oncology, and Bone-Marrow Transplant

Claire Ghetti
Joey Walker

General Characteristics and Definition of Population

Historical Perspectives of Pediatric Hematology/Oncology

The diagnosis of childhood **cancer** has evolved from a state of acute disease with probable fatal outcome to a treatable life-threatening illness with a possibility of a cure (Patenaude & Last, 2001). Treatment advances during the past four decades have led to increased disease-free states known as **remissions**, lengthened survival, and, in some cases, apparent cures (National Institutes of Health [NIH], 1993). For example, the average survival after diagnosis of **acute lymphoblastic leukemia** (ALL) in 1940 was less than 3 months (Pearson, 2002). Today, children diagnosed with ALL have approximately an 80% chance of total remission. Likelihood of long-term survival for all childhood malignancies has increased from 20% in the 1960s to 70% in the 1990s (Pearson, 2002). These successful outcomes are largely due to the formation of multi-institutional pediatric oncology groups that develop and assess state-of-the-art treatment protocols across numerous treatment sites (Bertolone, 1997; Corrigan & Feig, 2004; Pearson, 2002). These national initiatives have led to improved surgical outcomes, new **chemotherapy** agents, less toxic **radiation therapy**, and the development of biotherapy approaches to cancer treatment (Bertolone, 1997).

As childhood cancer survival rates have improved, emphasis has shifted from an exclusive focus on life-saving to a more holistic focus on improving quality of life during the treatment phase and beyond. An example of this shift is the emergence of the field of psycho-oncology, which investigates the psychosocial consequences of cancer and its treatment, as well as studies the relationship between particular psychosocial factors and positive adjustment to the illness (Patenaude & Last, 2001). Outcomes of these inquiries help to validate and shape psychosocial clinical intervention. Researchers are also studying the "late effects" of rigorous cancer therapies in adult survivors of childhood cancer. The latent effects of chemotherapy and radiation treatments for childhood cancer on subsequent physical growth, intellectual development, pubertal development, and the aging process are studied in an attempt to eventually decrease the long-term negative medical and social consequences of these treatments (Schwartz, 1999).

The context in which the child experiences diagnosis and treatment has also changed dramatically in recent decades. As childhood cancer in the 1960s was more pervasively a fatal illness, children were often left uninformed of their condition (Patenaude & Last, 2001). An atmosphere of secrecy and denial was maintained to "protect" the child from the truth of his or her condition and prognosis. This left the child isolated from vital sources of emotional support, and often left the child with misunderstandings or hidden suspicions that led to additional anxiety and worry. Today, an environment of open communication is emphasized, with health care workers encouraging families to discuss patient concerns and fears openly. Through open and honest discussion, parents are able to provide support to the child while he or she is experiencing the treatment process. Treatment providers also emphasize a return to normalcy, encouraging patients and families to engage in preferred activities and rituals to the extent possible during the treatment phase. While the patient is at the hospital, this may be achieved through the resources provided by child life, music therapy, therapeutic recreation, creative arts therapy, and/or chaplaincy programming. School reintegration programs help smooth the transition of the child back into school, providing education to teachers and peers and easing a potentially anxiety-producing social transition for the child (Patenaude & Last, 2001). Child life programs also address the greater needs of the family unit by providing developmentally appropriate illness-related education and support for siblings of children with cancer. Multidisciplinary treatment in pediatric oncology settings is strongly recommended by the American Academy of Pediatrics, who urges the involvement of social workers, pediatric psychologists, and child life specialists in patient care (Corrigan & Feig, 2004).

Historical Perspectives of Music Therapy in Pediatric Hematology/Oncology

The clinical use of music therapy within pediatric **hematology** or **oncology** settings was consistently documented in the literature beginning in the 1980s (Brodsky, 1989; Clinton, 1984; Fagen, 1982; Schwankovsky & Guthrie, 1982). These authors described the benefits of music therapy for pediatric cancer patients, focusing on those who were terminally ill or who required placement in isolation. Music therapy was deemed effective for providing social interaction; sensory and developmental stimulation; physical activity; and for reducing loneliness, depression, and confusion associated with terminal illness or prolonged treatment in isolation environments. Music therapy interventions cited in these early references for this population included singing, song selection, songwriting, lyric substitution, improvisation, guided imagery, and playing keyboard and rhythm instruments (Brodsky, 1989; Fagen, 1982). These writings of the 1980s helped form a preliminary rationale for the use of music therapy with this population. Since that time, significant developments in theory, research, and clinical practice have occurred regarding the use of music therapy within pediatric hematology/oncology settings.

More recent clinical works have developed upon preliminary rationales for the use of music therapy with pediatric hematology/oncology patients and have offered recommendations for implementation practices. Clinicians have described the importance of modifying music therapy goals and interventions based on stages of treatment, such as diagnosis, intensive treatment, bone marrow transplantation, and palliative care (Daveson, 2001), or by the phases of the treatment itself, as in the case of bone marrow transplantation (Hadley, 1996; Kennelly, 2001; Robb & Ebberts, 2003a). Current clinical literature continues to emphasize the importance of supporting the specialized needs of pediatric patients undergoing prolonged isolation as a part of cancer treatment (Hadley, 1996; Lane, 1996) and highlights the ability of music therapy intervention to help support the entire family in coping with a patient's life-threatening illness (Lane, 1996; Magill, Coyle, Handzo, & Loscalzo, 1997). Clinicians have also documented in greater detail the therapeutic value of specific music therapy interventions for pediatric hematology/oncology patients. Various forms of songwriting, including improvisation, have been used to encourage expression of feelings, empower patients, improve coping skills, and facilitate adjustment to illness (Hadley, 1996; Kennelly, 2001; Ledger, 2001; Turry & Turry, 1999). Themes that emerge during song selection, song discussion, and songwriting may also serve a diagnostic function in identifying how a patient is adjusting to illness and coping with treatment (Hadley, 1996).

Specific theories that guide research and clinical practice are also emerging within the field of pediatric hematology/oncology music therapy. Robb (2000, 2003a, 2003b) developed a contextual support model of music therapy that emphasizes the use of music therapy methods to improve adaptive coping strategies and facilitate adjustment to illness in children and adolescents with cancer. Live music engagement techniques are implemented to reduce the impact of stress upon the pediatric patient and promote expansion of the child's repertoire of adaptive coping strategies. The music therapist uses music interaction and play experiences to provide structure, autonomy support, and involvement that improve the context within which the child experiences illness and hospitalization (Robb, 2003a).

Research regarding the use of music therapy or therapeutic music in pediatric hematology/oncology is currently limited to a few studies, but these studies have demonstrated positive outcomes. Children undergoing **bone marrow aspiration** demonstrated less distress during the procedure when listening to patient-chosen relaxation music (Pfaff, Smith, & Gowan, 1989), or engaging in either music listening or Lamaze pant-blow breathing (Schur, 1986). Similarly, pediatric patients in the process of bone marrow transplantation (BMT) demonstrated improvement in observed levels of pain when given live music therapy interaction (Robb, 2000) and reported significantly reduced pain and nausea after receiving music therapy and relaxation imagery sessions (Sahler, Hunter, & Liesveld, 2003). When comparing studies that used active versus passive music approaches with pediatric hematology/oncology patients, a larger treatment effect size was noted for live music therapy interaction (Standley & Whipple, 2003). Live, interactive music therapy sessions were also effective for improving mood for pediatric cancer patients who were hospitalized for treatment or were undergoing medical procedures (Barrera, Rykov, & Doyle, 2002). Levels of self-reported anxiety decreased for adolescents undergoing BMT who engaged in songwriting and music video production sessions (Robb & Ebberts, 2003a), and these sessions also led to the identification of personal strengths and positive coping strategies (Robb & Ebberts, 2003b).

The emerging interest in **psychoneuroimmunology** may lend further support to the use of music therapy in pediatric hematology/oncology settings (Kruse, 2003). The ability of music therapy intervention to influence affective functioning and thereby positively influence immune system functioning is beginning to be supported by research efforts. Lane and Olness (1991) found a significant increase in levels of **salivary immunoglobulin A** (sIgA), an indicator of improved immune system function, in hospitalized children who received a single 30-minute music therapy session versus those in a control group who received attention via play activities. Researchers who previously found that music therapy and relaxation imagery benefited adult and pediatric BMT patients (Sahler et al., 2003), are currently investigating the use of music therapy and relaxation imagery to reduce time to **engraftment** as an indicator of enhanced immune reconstitution. Additional research evaluating the effects of music therapy on the immune responses of pediatric hematology/oncology patients is needed. Research efforts are vital for evaluating the effectiveness of intervention strategies and thereby stimulating the development of evidence-based clinical practice.

Common Characteristics of Pediatric Hematology/Oncology Patients

The population of pediatric hematology and oncology patients and those who receive a **stem cell transplant** (also called bone marrow transplant) is a diverse group of children. Many variables affect the specific characteristics of these children, such as age, developmental level, diagnosis, family support, prognosis, the timeline and progress of the condition, as well as treatment and its side effects. One of the characteristics warranting initial consideration is the pediatric patient's specific diagnosis.

Hematology is concerned with the study, diagnosis, and treatment of diseases of the blood, while **oncology** refers to the study, diagnosis, and treatment of cancer (*American Heritage Dictionary*, 2000). Cancer is a group of diseases in which abnormal cells divide without control (NIH, 2001). The disciplines of hematology and oncology are often grouped together in the hospital, and children are identified as hem/onc patients and are treated on the same unit. Some children have diseases of the blood that are cancerous in nature, while others have solely noncancerous blood disorders. Thus, not all hematology patients have cancer—they may have one of the following diseases of the blood:

- **Hemophilia**—blood is not able to clot properly.
- **Sickle cell anemia**—red blood cells sickle and block the small blood vessels of the body

- **Anemia**—red blood cells are reduced from normal levels

(D'Alessandro & Huth, 2002a, 2002b; Miller, McMillan, Chavez, & Giller, 1993)

Leukemia is one of the most common diseases of the blood that is cancerous in nature. A cancer of the **white blood cells**, leukemia occurs when too many immature white blood cells are produced. This can interfere with the making of **red blood cells** (oxygen carriers) as well as **platelets** (blood clotters). White blood cells are the infection fighters and are formed in the bone marrow (the spongy-like tissue in the middle of bones). When there are too many immature abnormal white blood cells, the function of organs, tissues, and spinal fluid may be damaged (Parmet, Lynm, & Glass, 2004). The four types of leukemia occurring in children are:

- **Acute lymphoblastic** (also called lymphocytic) leukemia (**ALL**)
- **Chronic lymphoblastic** (also called lymphocytic) leukemia (**CLL**)
- **Acute myelogenous** (also called myelocytic) leukemia (**AML**)
- **Chronic myelogenous** (also called myelocytic) leukemia (**CML**)

Most children will have the acute forms of ALL or AML in which symptoms progress rapidly and worsen quickly if untreated. CML and CLL present with milder symptoms, progress more slowly, and are the chronic forms of the disorder (D'Alessandro & Kinzer, 2004). In addition to leukemia, other childhood cancers may involve the lymphatic system, bones, and soft tissues, as well as other parts of the body.

Lymphoma is a tumor of the lymph tissue that may originate and establish itself in many different locations. Bone marrow, lymph nodes, spleen, thymus, and vessels that carry fluid and infection-fighting cells may be affected. Lymphoma interferes with the lymphatic system so that production and storage of cells to fight disease and infections is compromised. The two most common lymphomas in children are:

- **Hodgkin's disease**—affects the lymph nodes close to the body's surface, e.g., neck, armpit, groin
- **Non-Hodgkin's lymphoma**—affects lymph nodes located deeper in the body, e.g., bowel, near appendix, or upper chest

Two types of bone cancer found in children are:

- **Osteosarcoma**—develops from cells that form bone; it is a tumor of the bone that usually affects the leg or arm
- **Ewing's sarcoma**—tumor of the bone or soft tissue that forms bone which usually affects the pelvis, trunk, legs

Another type of cancer that affects mostly young children is a soft tissue sarcoma called **rhabdomyosarcoma**. It begins in muscle tissue, occurs anywhere in the body, and most often is found in the head, neck, kidneys, bladder, arms, legs, and trunk. Other types of childhood cancers include:

- **Brain cancer**— consists of solid tumors called **gliomas**
- **Wilms' tumor**—begins in the kidney
- **Neuroblastoma**—consists of solid tumor located in the nerve cells in the abdomen, adrenal glands, or spine
- **Retinoblastoma**—consists of a solid tumor located near the retina in the eye

(Barr et al., 2001; NIH, 2001)

Problems associated with these illnesses are serious and children are hospitalized when they need treatment. In addition, children who have been diagnosed with cancer may be hospitalized for disease management when they have routine illnesses such as fevers, influenza, or chicken pox. Oncology patients are often on a scheduled medical protocol, where they are admitted to the hospital for a few days every third or fourth week for a number of months or years. Some children are able to receive treatment on an outpatient basis after diagnosis and initial admission.

Though chemotherapy and radiation are commonly used as forms of oncology treatment, they also compromise the immune system, leaving children with little defense against contracting disease. These **immunosuppressed** children may be placed in isolation in their rooms or wear masks to cover their nose and mouth in order to prevent contracting an illness. They may stay away from people or crowds until their immune function improves. In addition, children may develop changes in appearance, such as temporary loss of hair and puffiness or swelling of facial tissue due to side effects of treatment.

If children have been or are being treated for cancer and the illness returns (relapse) or is not responding to treatment, they may be candidates for a stem cell transplant. Oncology and stem cell transplant patients all have a **catheter** (or sometimes a port) surgically placed in their body where they receive chemotherapy and other medications. This catheter, called a central line, is an intravenous (IV) tube that travels from under the skin to a large vein in the heart. This IV tube allows blood to be drawn and tested on a regular basis without poking a needle into the child, and delivers transfusions and medications that the child requires (Quinn & Petitgout, 1998). These medications and transfusions as well as liquid nutrition are often hung from a rolling IV pole that contains one or more pumps that infuse the liquid through the line into the child.

Additional general characteristics of hematology/oncology patients include fatigue and loss of appetite. Regression to more familiar behaviors of a younger age or oppositional behavior as a reaction to the stress of hospitalization may occur at any time. The following information concerning more specific characteristics of hematology/oncology patients is grouped together by developmental levels.

Infant and Toddler

Perhaps more than any other age group, hospitalized infants and toddlers need consistency in caregiving. As infants grow, they may display stranger and separation anxiety as part of normal development. They need parental or consistent caregiver contact to establish trust and bonding. Hospitalized infants may develop attachment issues due to the brevity of interactions with multiple caregivers (G. E. Senio, personal communication, August 19, 2004). They may create attention-seeking behaviors if left alone for long periods, and also may fall behind developmentally if not given appropriate stimulation. Babies may be restrained at times in order to keep them from pulling out tubes and other medical equipment. Infants may have an IV line placed in their head, hand, or foot, while toddlers usually have an IV in their hand or foot until a central line is placed. Movement is severely restricted if a toddler has an IV catheter in his or her foot. Toddlers may be fearful of all hospital staff and may regress to more familiar behaviors.

Families and caregivers of hospitalized children may have additional stresses within the environment. Parents or primary caregivers need to develop trust with other hospital caregivers in order to be able to take a break from caring for their child. Some parents feel they cannot leave their child and may have a difficult time realizing the need for their own self-care as well as caring for their child. Other parents may want to be present with their child, but are unable to do so because of obligations at work. Some parents have to be present at their place of employment in order to receive the health insurance they need to pay for their child's medical fees. In addition, quite often the hospitalized infant or toddler has young siblings who are present with a parent in the room for a great deal of time, which may compound levels of stress.

Preschool

Children who are approximately 2 to 5 years old also need a primary caregiver present for comfort. Preschoolers are frequently fearful of all medical staff and procedures and are often unable to verbally express fears, pain, or discomfort. During this time, receptive language skills are much better than expressive ones. Therefore, children may understand more, but instead of being able to verbally communicate, they may act out, become quiet, scream, or regress to former more comfortable behaviors. For example, a child who has begun to talk may choose not to use words in order to communicate, or a child who has been toilet trained may revert to using diapers.

This age group is an active one—normal preschoolers are constantly on the move. Hospitalized children in this age group may have motor difficulties due to medical equipment or illness. Ambulating preschoolers who have an IV pole require consistent supervision to prevent them from inadvertently pulling out the IV line as they move around their rooms or the playroom. The lack of normal routine is also extremely stressful for these children in particular. Older preschool age children may have misconceptions about their illness and the hospital and may believe that they are receiving punishment or may have caused their illness by something they did or did not do. Children may talk much less, or not at all, to medical staff, or communicate by nodding in answer to questions as a way of control. They may respond or whisper their needs to their parents and have their parents or someone they trust talk for them (Barrickman, 1989).

These children also need consistent discipline. Because of the severity of the illness of hematology/oncology patients, sometimes adults want to do everything they can for a child with cancer. Parents may be tired and stressed and may feel bad that the child is sick; nevertheless, the child needs to have consistent limits set by all who care for him or her.

School Age

Children who are 5 to 12 years of age are more capable of understanding their illness and the hospital routine; however, they may still harbor misconceptions. Younger children within this group appear to be able to adjust better to their situation than older patients, who may have greater identification with their peer group. School is also an important part of a normal routine and, despite best efforts, at times children may fall behind in their studies.

Family difficulties may arise due to the time and attention a child with a severe illness may receive—siblings and spouses may feel jealous or excluded. Children who have formerly been more independent may want mom or dad nearby in their room. The forced dependency of the hospital schedule as well as feelings of helplessness may cause difficulty as well (Robb, 2003b). Children are told when and what to eat and drink (or that they are unable to do so), when to sleep, when to take medicine, when to rest, etc. Control may become an issue, and a child may verbalize much less, remaining quiet as a means of control. Children at this age are also more concerned with their appearance and being different because of hair loss, an amputation, or other side effects of illness or medication that sets them apart from their friends.

Adolescents

Lack of peer support and separation from friends are also key concerns of adolescents. They do not want to be excluded from what friends are doing, and being unable to attend major teenage life events due to hospitalization makes them different from their peers. This can lead to anger that may manifest in depression. Adolescents are quite concerned with appearance, and their fragile self-esteem may be compromised if hair is temporarily lost or other drastic changes occur during treatment. They may become more egocentric, have a difficult time planning for the future, and have a tendency to live in the moment.

Typical adolescents want and need more independence as they develop. In contrast, hospitalized adolescents may want family present in their room, or they may want them close in proximity, but in another area of the unit. This need for privacy and self-sufficiency is important even for hospitalized teens, who may feel some insecurity about normal changes in their bodies. Hospitalized adolescents want autonomy and control, but they also have "an incredible need for comfort" (K. J. Whiteside, personal communication, August 26, 2004). Teens may find consolation with a massage, a wig or different head covering, hair and nail styling, or a makeover at the hospital salon. Being able to communicate with friends by email or phone is of particular importance for adolescents. Additionally, there may be hospitalized peers who may have similar diagnoses, but who are in isolation and unable to physically meet others during a teen group or similar situation. Helping adolescents make connections with other hospitalized peers through email or other means can be comforting and reduce the isolation they may feel.

Current Pediatric Hematology/Oncology Treatment Modalities

Though specific treatments, medications, side effects, terminology, and length of hospitalization will develop and change over time, core music therapy goals for pediatric hem/onc patients remain relatively stable. For example, patients will need assistance in coping with hospitalization—whether they are receiving current treatments or new therapies in the future. Music therapists may tend to feel overwhelmed with the amount of significant information associated with specific client populations. However, a basic understanding of the needs and characteristics of clients serves as a foundation upon which the therapist accumulates knowledge from clinical practice in an effort to improve patient outcomes.

The current primary treatments for hematology/oncology patients are surgery, radiation, chemotherapy, **immunotherapy**, and stem cell transplant. Briefly, these treatments may be defined as:

- **Surgery**—removal of tumor, surrounding tissue and nearby lymph nodes; radiation may be used prior to surgery to reduce the tumor before removal
- **Radiation therapies**—localized treatment with high-energy rays to damage or destroy cancer cells in a specific part of the body that has cancer
- **Chemotherapy**—strong drugs that travel through the bloodstream to kill cancer cells throughout the body
- **Immunotherapy**—supplemental administration of biological substances natural to the body that help fight cancer and other diseases
- **Stem cell (or bone marrow) transplants**—blood cells in the diseased or damaged bone marrow are replaced with immature healthy cells (stem cells) that grow into new healthy cells

(NiH, 2001)

Depending on the type of illness, children may receive a combination of these treatments and be hospitalized frequently for long periods of time over many months. In the case of a stem cell transplant, a child will have an extended hospitalization. A variety of diseases such as leukemia, lymphoma, **anemia**, solid tumors, and some genetic disorders may be treated with a stem cell transplant. During a period of time called "conditioning," which takes place before the transplant, a high dose chemotherapy often paired with radiation is administered. The objective of conditioning is to destroy the marrow, immune system, and cancer cells. This, in turn, will create room for the healthy marrow to be transplanted through the central line into the child (Quinn & Petitgout, 1998).

This marrow, which contains stem cells, may be obtained from the child as well as others. Since stem cells may be found in bone marrow as well as circulating blood and in umbilical cord blood, the more accurate term **stem cell transplant** (SCT) is replacing the term *bone marrow transplant* (BMT) (Youngerman-Cole, 2004). An **allogenic transplant** occurs when stem cells are collected, usually from bone marrow in the hip, from another person. An **autologous transplant** happens when the child's own stem cells are withdrawn, treated, and then infused back to the child. A process of separating certain parts of blood cells from the circulating blood of the child is called **pheresis** or **apheresis**. For a stem cell transplant, the stem cells are removed in this procedure that may take many hours over a period of several days. If necessary, the stem cells are treated to remove the malignant cells and then frozen. These stem cells will be returned through a central line to the child after conditioning and will be responsible for producing red blood cells, white blood cells, and platelets during the time called engraftment (Quinn & Petitgout, 1998).

The time frame for engraftment is variable, but it may take approximately 3 to 6 weeks until normal blood cells begin production (Daveson, 2001). During this time as well as the period of conditioning, children will remain in isolation in their room to minimize exposure to bacteria and viruses. Family, visitors, and hospital staff will use careful hand-washing techniques and at times may wear gloves, gowns, masks, and shoe covers when entering a child's room. The child will receive numerous antibiotics, steroids, and blood transfusions to help fight as well as prevent infection. Blood samples are drawn daily to monitor organ function and to determine whether engraftment has taken place (Stewart, 1992).

Some possible physical changes that occur with a stem cell transplant are mouth sores; hair loss; itchy, red, or tender skin; and swelling or puffiness—especially in the face. Fatigue, nausea, diarrhea, weakness, emotional stress, and loss of appetite are common (Barr et al., 2001; Stewart, 1992). Another complication that may develop is called **graft versus host disease** (GVHD). GVHD occurs when the new stem cells (from a donor) attack and attempt to destroy the child's own cells. Affecting the liver, skin, and gastrointestinal tract, GVHD may be mild or severe enough to cause death (Youngerman-Cole, 2004).

In addition to these problems that affect the child physically, a stem cell transplant "is an emotionally and psychologically taxing procedure for both the patient and the family" (Stewart, 1992, p. 6). Families and the children who have previously been diagnosed with a life-threatening illness are now going through this difficult transplant process and are also waiting for answers and outcomes, knowing there is the possibility of graft failure. This is an extremely upsetting and stressful time to be placed in isolation, away from friends, school, home, and familiar situations. Music therapy may be used within the isolation environment to reduce the stress of SCT and improve coping responses. The music therapist can be most effective in providing stress reduction as well as helping with other problem areas for the patient and family when patients are assessed in an efficient, but thorough manner.

engraftment: the process of transplanted stem cells reproducing new cells.

Assessment

Determination of Eligibility for Services

The determination of a hem/onc patient's eligibility for music therapy services will depend on a variety of circumstances: treatment phase, patient adjustment to illness, level of social support for the patient, and patient responses to music. As the period around an initial diagnosis can be extremely stressful for both pediatric patients and families, the criterion of new diagnosis often warrants consideration for music therapy services. In this case, the music therapy interaction may help to identify specific patient fears as well as serve as a means for assessing and improving the patient and family's current coping abilities. As previously stated, the stress of the prolonged isolation required during SCT also gives a patient precedence for music therapy services.

Patients may be prioritized for music therapy services based on formal or informal assessment. A Likert-scale rating system for prioritizing level of patient need may be included on a formal assessment. For example, as a summary to the assessment process, a music therapist may assign each assessed patient a score of 1–3 in domain areas of diagnosis/severity of illness, fear/distress/agitation, family involvement/availability, and social isolation/withdrawal. Such a scoring system helps summarize the immediacy of need within each domain area. When the domains are considered together, it is possible to determine the priority of a patient's need for services relative to other patients who have been assessed. A similar informal prioritization process may be quickly achieved by considering these domain areas when discussing, during nursing or psychosocial rounds or during consultation with child life staff, which patients would be appropriate for music therapy.

Though infrequent, music therapy services may be contraindicated for certain hem/onc patients. Patients undergoing long-term chemotherapy may occasionally experience sensory alterations that may make the experience of music listening unpleasant or painful. Older patients will often be able to convey this verbally to the therapist, but younger or nonverbal patients may not. The music therapist should be sensitive to behavioral responses that might indicate an adverse reaction to auditory stimuli. At times, a supportive verbal interaction may need to substitute for a musical interaction.

Referral Process

Referrals for music therapy may come from a variety of professionals involved in the multidisciplinary care of the pediatric hematology/oncology patient. Physicians; nurses; child life specialists; psychologists/psychiatrists; social workers; recreational therapists; physical, occupational, or speech therapists; chaplains; or other creative arts therapy staff may make a referral for music therapy services. The referral process may differ depending on the facility and, in some settings, music therapy services can be obtained only through a physician's order. Referrals may consist of a completed written form that is directed to the music therapist, a referral note entered in a patient's electronic or paper chart, an emailed or online referral that maintains patient confidentiality, or a verbal referral. A sample Pediatric Hematology/Oncology Music Therapy Referral Form is included in Figure 1. The music therapist may also receive referrals while participating in medical, nursing, or psychosocial rounds. Formal referrals are ideal as they assist the music therapist in prioritizing patients, as well as educate staff as to the availability and scope of practice of music therapy. Referral source, even when the referral is given verbally, should be documented in the assessment form or summary note.

Music Therapy Referral Form
Pediatric Hematology/Oncology

Patient Information:

Patient Name: _____   Rm. # or Unit: _____

Age: _____

Diagnosis: _____

Referring Person:

Name: _____   Department: _____

Extension: _____   Date of referral: _____

Reason for Referral to Music Therapy (check all that apply):
- ❑   new diagnosis
- ❑   pain management
- ❑   anxiety management
- ❑   expressive difficulties (i.e., patient is withdrawn, aggressive, nonverbal)
- ❑   affective difficulties (i.e., patient appears depressed, hopeless)
- ❑   patient requires prolonged isolation
- ❑   developmental or sensory stimulation needed
- ❑   body-image or self-concept issues
- ❑   social support needed
- ❑   family support needed
- ❑   end-of-life care
- ❑   other: _____

Additional Comments:

_____

_____

_____

Figure 1. Music Therapy Referral Form for Pediatric Hematology/Oncology

Assessment Procedure

Assessment of patients in the pediatric hematology/oncology setting relies on information from a variety of sources. Music therapists may employ a combination of methods, including observation of patient and family during both the presence and absence of musical interaction, chart review to assess medical and social history and treatment progress, and patient and/or family interview. Due to variation in patient health status depending on treatment phase and response to treatment, frequent reassessment of patient needs and strengths will be required to assure appropriate goal and intervention planning. Patients undergoing chemotherapy often have depressed immune system function that requires strict infection control protocols. Isolation precautions, allergies, medical equipment precautions, and activity restrictions should be clearly delineated on the music therapy assessment form.

Several areas of assessment are specific to patients being treated for cancer and blood disorders. The patient's diagnosis, time since initial diagnosis, and number of relapses for those who come out of remission, as well as the occurrence of any secondary malignancies, are important initial considerations. A patient coping with a new diagnosis will present very differently than a seasoned patient accustomed to the rigors of chemotherapy and radiation treatments. Additionally, the patient's treatment protocol should be documented, including need for surgery, chemotherapy, radiation, or SCT. The patient's treatment phase may also be noted. For ALL, this might include remission induction, **CNS prophylaxis** (whole brain radiation and/or intrathecal chemotherapy), intensification phase, and maintenance therapy phase (Daveson, 2001). A patient's current chemotherapy or radiation side effects or those experienced in the past, which may impair active participation in music therapy sessions, should be noted and may include oral ulcers, sore throat, nausea, vomiting, diarrhea, constipation, hair loss, and tender skin at the radiation site. All infection control requirements should be noted in the initial assessment to prevent inadvertent violation. Levels of pain and anxiety are usually assessed at regular intervals for patients undergoing hematology and oncology treatments. Current coping strategies and repertoire displayed by the patient and the family are important to document in the assessment. It is useful to note both positive and negative coping tendencies to serve as a baseline against which adaptive strategies developed during the course of music therapy interventions may be compared. The patient's main support networks, as well as their current availability for the child, should be evaluated (Daveson, 2001). The patient's and family's cultural and spiritual background may also have implications for intervention and may be included in the assessment.

Best practice methods would indicate the completion of a formal music therapy assessment document to be included in the chart of each patient who receives services. In inpatient settings, formal assessment is often more practical, as hematology/oncology patients often require frequent and/or lengthy hospitalizations. The format and length of this assessment form may be altered depending upon the logistical needs and document requirements of the setting in question. In addition to the factors mentioned above, music therapy assessments for pediatric hematology/oncology patients evaluate functioning in psychological, cognitive, physical, communicative, and social domains, as well as document the patient's music history, preferences, and responses to music. A sample Pediatric Hematology/Oncology Music Therapy Assessment Form is included in Figure 2.

The approval and initiation process of adding a new discipline's assessment to an electronic or paper charting system is often daunting or prohibitive for the music therapist who is starting a new program. Documenting a narrative summary assessment note, or including an assessment summary in the first session/progress note within the patient's chart may be an acceptable way to circumvent this obstacle. Sometimes in outpatient hematology/oncology treatment, formal assessment and documentation within a patient's chart may not be feasible or possible. In such cases, the music therapist may create short-term assessment techniques and documentation practices that are more workable. For example, a therapist seeing a patient in the clinic may assess the patient based on informal observation during the course of the music therapy session, document a summary in a daily treatment service log, and re-assess the patient more formally upon inpatient admission. If the therapist has access to patient charts in the outpatient setting, a summary session note with the inclusion of a preliminary assessment summary may be charted. A sample Pediatric Hematology/Oncology Music Therapy Assessment Summary Note is found on page 163. Protocols for determining which patients require formal music therapy assessment will vary depending upon facility and departmental standards.

Approach to Patients

The music therapist will vary his or her approach to patients during assessment depending on the patient's age and developmental level, treatment phase and protocol, and current emotional state. Observed or patient-reported levels of pain, anxiety, or discomfort may be used to prioritize goals for immediate interaction. The initial session is often a combination of formal or informal assessment, immediate goal setting, and corresponding intervention. Needs of the moment are addressed first, and the therapist takes note of long-term or secondary goals to be addressed in following sessions. Patient needs and corresponding interventions may vary dramatically from the outpatient setting to inpatient treatment. Therapists seeing patients in outpatient chemo suites (large rooms or solaria where patients receive chemotherapy or blood products) will generally have less privacy in their interactions with patients. This may necessitate more superficial assessment procedures and interaction in order to maintain patient confidentiality.

Typical Treatment Goals and Objectives

The needs of pediatric hem/onc patients and corresponding music therapy treatment goals and objectives for these patients have remained relatively stable over time; however, recent trends such as managed care have affected actual treatment practices. Kruse (2003) found that inpatients may have higher acuity than in the past, meaning they are sicker and have more serious physical and medical needs. In the decades proceeding managed care, patients were hospitalized for less serious problems and for longer periods of time, and they were

Pediatric Hematology/Oncology Music Therapy Assessment (10/2003 C. Ghetti)

Patient Name: _____   Date: _____   Admit Date: _____   Rm #. or Unit: _____

D.O.B. and Age: _____   Gender: M F

Primary Diagnosis: _____

Date of Initial Diagnosis: _____

| Isolation Precautions: |
| Allergies: |
| Medical Equip. Precautions: |

Pt. aware of diagnosis/prognosis? Yes No Not determined

Secondary/admitting Diagnosis: _____

Number and Date of Relapse(s): _____

Secondary Malignancies: _____   Referred by: _____

Referral reason: _____

Treatment protocol (surgery, chemo, radiation, BMT, etc.): _____

Current treatment phase: _____   Past treatments: _____

Current side effects: _____   Past side effects: _____

Physiological:

Pt.'s current level of pain (0-10 Wong/Baker Faces Rating Scale for verbal; FLACC 1-3 for nonverbal): _____

Observed behaviors indicating pain: _____   Pain tolerance level: _____

Medications: _____   Side effects: ❑ excessive sleepiness, sluggishness

_____   ❑ nausea/vomiting ❑ hyperactivity ❑ other: _____

Physical:

Activity status/restrictions: _____

Limits to ROM: _____   Postural restrictions: _____

Sensory impairments: _____

Cognitive:

❑ typically developing   developmental delay: ❑ suspected ❑ reported (specify _____)

Psychosocial/Emotional:

Mood/affect: ❑ Appropriate affect ❑ Flat affect ❑ Incongruent affect Comments: _____

Self-reported current emotional state: _____

Observed behaviors r/t mood: _____

Observed behaviors indicating anxiety: _____

Level of procedural anxiety: ❑ normal for age   ❑ pronounced   ❑ not determined   Comments: _____

Level of separation anxiety: ❑ normal for age   ❑ moderate   ❑ pronounced   ❑ not determined

Patient sources of support (include names if known): _____

Availability of supports: ❑ consistent   ❑ inconsistent   ❑ not determined   Comments: _____

Parental/familial anxiety: ❑ low   ❑ average   ❑ high   Comments: _____

Compliance w/treatment regimen: ❑ good   ❑ fair   ❑ needs improvement   ❑ not determined

Comments: _____

Attitude towards medical procedures/diagnosis/prognosis: _____

Observed coping strategies: _____

Past coping strategies: _____   Familial coping strategies: _____

Level of engagement in Child Life services: ❑ consistent   ❑ minimal   Referred to CL: Yes No (for: _____)

Communication:

Receptive communication limitations: _____

Expressive communication limitations: _____

Musical Behaviors:

Music preferences:_____

Past uses of music: _____

Responses to music: _____

Patient prioritization (1 = low priority, 3 = high priority)

1	2	3	Domain Area:
			Diagnosis/severity of illness
			Fear/distress/agitation of child
			Family involvement and availability
			Social isolation and withdrawal

Recommended for music therapy: ❏ Yes ❏ No (if no, explain _____)

Plan to follow patient: ❏ Inpatient ❏ Outpatient ❏ Both

Recommended goals of MT intervention:

❏ anxiety management (specify: _____)

❏ pain management (specify: _____)

❏ procedural support (specify: _____)

❏ increase expressive communication

❏ identify fears r/t hospitalization/diagnosis

❏ improve mood

❏ increase range of motion (ROM)

  (recommend co-treat w/OT/PT: Yes No)

❏ provide normalization

❏ preparation for medical procedures

❏ facilitate supportive interaction w/family

❏ decrease parental or sibling anxiety

❏ facilitate social interaction with peers

❏ behavior modification (specify: _____)

❏ accomplish developmental tasks

  (specify _____)

❏ other: (specify:_____)

Recommended MT interventions: ❏ individual ❏ with family ❏ other:

❏ music assisted relaxation (MAR) (specify: _____)

❏ alternate engagement during medical procedures (MAE)

❏ instrument playing (specify: _____)

❏ singing (specify: _____)

❏ music permanent product (specify _____)

❏ songwriting

❏ music-facilitated dramatic play

❏ music listening

❏ music with movement

❏ other _____

Summary and Plan:

_____

_____

_____

Name:_____ Title: _____ Date:_____

Figure 2. **Pediatric Hematology/Oncology Music Therapy Assessment Form**

Sample Music Therapy Summary Assessment Note
Pediatric Hematology/Oncology

Date: 6/16/04
Time: 4:00 pm

History and Assessment:

Patient is a 9-year-old male with pre-b cell ALL, first admitted to the PICU on 6/2/04 for fever of unknown origin, subsequently developed respiratory distress. Pt. diagnosed with ALL on 6/7/04 and transferred to inpatient unit for induction chemotherapy, which has been extended by two weeks due to positive bone marrow biopsy on 6/14/04. Pt. was referred to music therapy by Child Life due to pt.'s new diagnosis and staff's observation of poor parental coping. Though parents originally preferred not to disclose pt.'s diagnosis to him, they did discuss the diagnosis once pt. began induction chemotherapy. Writer briefly followed pt. during PICU admission.

Pt. presents as a precocious 4th grader, easily expresses his needs verbally, and immediately engages verbally and musically with therapist. Pt. reports no pain or discomfort at present, though he did experience weakness and bone pain while in the PICU. Pt. displays a wide range of affect, including positive affect, when engaging in instrument playing or singing. Pt. increases speed of verbal communication and motor behavior when anxious, but is able to tolerate medical procedures without pronounced stress behaviors. Pt. uses verbal communication with family for support, and plays with video games to distract himself during procedures. Pt. appears to have strong bond with parents and older brother, and family is appropriately involved in patient's care. Both parents have a tendency to deny their emotions to pt. when they are upset about his illness, and nursing reports that mom appears to be depressed. Though patient engages easily with therapist in individual sessions, he has demonstrated socially-withdrawn behaviors when surrounded by peers during child life programming as evidenced by minimal verbal responses, lack of self-initiating conversation, and avoidance of eye contact with peers.

Pt. has a strong, positive history with music and has enjoyed singing and recorder playing in school. Pt. demonstrates positive affect and active engagement given familiar supportive songs and instrument play. Pt. easily engages in music making and demonstrates a variety of emotional responses to the music-making process.

Summary and Plan:

Pt. with recent diagnosis of ALL experienced anxiety-producing PICU stay before initial diagnosis was made. Pt.'s parents are demonstrating difficulty coping with his diagnosis and have inconsistent communication pattern related to pt.'s illness. Pt. could benefit from increased expressive outlets to explore emotions related to new diagnosis, increased normalization in activities, and improved peer interaction during potentially lengthy hospitalization. Recommend use of active music engagement (e.g., singing familiar songs, songwriting, and instrument playing) during individual sessions, patient-family interactions, and peer interactions to facilitate emotional expression, improve peer support, and facilitate normalization with overall goal of improving pt.'s adjustment to new diagnosis.

Goal 1: To improve patient's adjustment to new diagnosis of life-threatening illness

Objective 1: Given supportive music therapy relationship, pt. will verbalize one fear related to diagnosis/hospitalization by the end of 2 MT sessions.

Objective 2: Given spontaneous music interaction and songwriting, pt. will identify one positive strategy for relieving illness-related anxiety/stress by the end of 2 MT sessions.

Objective 3: Given small group music therapy sessions with peers, pt. will self-initiate musical or verbal interaction with peers 3 times per session across 3 sessions.

generally more active and felt better. The inpatients of today may be acutely ill; therefore, they may have decreased mental and physical energy and are more passive in general (Kruse, 2003). Inpatients may not be able to receive multiple music therapy sessions due to shorter hospital stays. As a result, music therapists may have to adjust intervention for single-session service. Because inpatient single-session service has become more common, music therapists must often assess a patient, set immediate goals, and provide interventions during the context of one session.

The assessment process and planning of goals and objectives may be completed more thoroughly over time for patients who require extended hospitalizations, such as stem cell transplant patients. Reassessment is also important as some of the needs of hematology/oncology and SCT patients may vary daily due to the unpredictability of the hospital, illness, and treatment. After a first admission for chemotherapy within an extended treatment protocol, a music therapist can have a general idea of patient preferences, developmental level, and coping mechanisms, and then plan for long-term goals accordingly. However, a hematology/oncology patient who is undergoing a treatment protocol in which every third week he or she receives chemotherapy while hospitalized for 4 days, may have different immediate needs each admission. These needs of the moment will be addressed during every session and the therapist will adapt intervention as necessary.

After the careful assessment or reassessment of the needs of pediatric hematology/oncology patients, the music therapist identifies goal areas to target that will ultimately help children cope with illness and hospitalization. The most common goals of music therapy intervention with hem/onc patients are:

- Decrease anxiety
- Decrease perception of pain
- Encourage expression of feeling
- Provide opportunity for control and mastery
- Provide normalization
- Improve self-esteem
- Promote communication
- Provide means for family integration

- Provide opportunity for social interaction
- Offer comfort
- Improve mood
- Provide sensory stimulation
- Offer family support
- Encourage use of motor skills
- Prevent developmental delay
- Reinforce academic skills

One of the most important considerations when establishing music therapy goals for hematology/oncology patients is the assessment of the patient's present level of pain. If a patient is in too much pain, there is usually not enough desire or energy to devote to other needs. Therefore, the music therapist (MT-BC) must always be aware of the variability of pain levels and the expectation versus the reality of addressing other goals.

Table 1 lists the music therapy pediatric hematology/oncology goal areas from above and provides sample objectives for each goal. In addition, the table also indicates if the goal is used primarily with individuals or groups, as well as its usage in the outpatient or inpatient setting. For example, goals that are less frequently emphasized in an outpatient context will

Table 1

Pediatric Hematology/Oncology Music Therapy Goals

Pediatric Hematology/Oncology Music Therapy Goals	Inpatient		Outpatient		Sample Music Therapy Objectives
	1:1	Group	1:1	Group	
Decrease anxiety	✓	✓	✓	✓	Pt. will actively participate in music interaction to extent capable Pt. will verbally or nonverbally express fears related to illness or hospitalization Pt. will identify one positive coping skill for managing anxiety
Decrease perception of pain	✓	✓	✓		Pt. will demonstrate decrease in moaning, crying, agitation when experiencing pain Pt. will tolerate medical procedures while demonstrating minimal stress behaviors
Encourage expression of feelings	✓	✓	✓	✓	Pt. will verbally report current emotional state Pt. will demonstrate behavior associated with emotion
Provide opportunity for control and mastery	✓	✓	✓	✓	Pt. will verbally or nonverbally indicate choices Pt. will initiate ideas
Provide normalization	✓	✓	✓	✓	Pt. will participate in an age appropriate musical situation which would normally take place outside of the hospital Pt. will recognize actual music as familiar to home, school
Improve self-esteem	✓	✓	✓	✓	Pt. will successfully complete a task Pt. will attempt new tasks Pt. will verbalize positive self-statements
Promote communication	✓	✓	✓	✓	Pt. will be able to report misconceptions about hospitalization or illness Pt. will discuss concerns with appropriate medical staff Pt. will use verbal or nonverbal means to express wants and needs
Provide means for family integration	✓	✓	✓	✓	Pt. will interact with family while all are participating in a task Pt. will elicit participation from family members

Table 1—Continued

Pediatric Hematology/Oncology Music Therapy Goals	Inpatient		Outpatient		Sample Music Therapy Objectives
	1:1	Group	1:1	Group	
Provide opportunity for social interaction		✓		✓	Pt. will demonstrate sharing and turn taking Pt. will demonstrate support for peers
Offer comfort	✓		✓		Pt. will cuddle closer to caregiver, family member, or MT-BC Pt. will fall asleep
Elevate mood	✓	✓	✓	✓	Pt. will demonstrate increased energy as exhibited by improved alertness and responsiveness Pt. will display more than one emotion Pt. will display positive affect
Provide sensory stimulation	✓				Pt .will demonstrate auditory and/or visual tracking given sensory prompts Pt. will respond with movement of body part
Offer family support	✓	✓			Family will report benefit from time away while child is with MT-BC Pt. will demonstrate behavioral improvement Family will verbalize improved mood Family will report decreased feelings of stress
Encourage use of motor skills	✓	✓	✓	✓	Pt. will reach for or grasp an instrument Pt. will move body or a body part to music Pt. will demonstrate increased range of motion while manipulating instruments
Prevent developmental delay	✓	✓	✓	✓	Pt. will actively participate in age appropriate interventions Pt. will respond verbally or nonverbally at developmentally appropriate level given musical cues
Reinforce academic skills	✓	✓	✓	✓	Pt. will demonstrate knowledge gained through music interaction Pt. will follow directions Pt. will demonstrate developmentally appropriate academic skills given prompts during music interactions

reflect this by the absence of a checkmark in the table. When creating objectives for individual patients, therapists specify criteria that will indicate when the objective has been met. These criteria state the desired frequency or duration of a patient response, and the desired time frame for successful demonstration of that response. For example, when addressing the goal of improving adjustment to new diagnosis, an objective might state that the patient will verbalize one positive coping strategy for managing illness-related stress by the end of the first two MT sessions. The attainment of objectives indicates that progress is being made towards the targeted goal areas.

Goals and objectives for hem/onc patients tend to vary depending upon their current stage of treatment, such as during new diagnosis, intensive treatment, or palliative care (Daveson, 2001). Targeted goal areas will also vary depending upon the needs of each individual as well as the phase of a specific treatment protocol, such as the phases of SCT (Hadley, 1996; Kennelly, 2001; Robb & Ebberts, 2003a). Patients experiencing new diagnosis will often benefit from the use of music therapy to decrease anxiety, promote normalization, increase communication and emotional expression, and provide family support. Patients undergoing intensive treatment will often need reduction in anxiety/pain, outlets for communication and emotional expression, opportunities for family integration, and improved peer support. During the prolonged SCT process, patients may need increased sensory stimulation, chances for choice and control, increased communication/emotional expression, decreased anxiety/pain, developmental stimulation, and opportunities for normalization. Furthermore, the music therapist will emphasize these goals at differing levels depending upon the changing needs of the patient during each phase of the SCT process. Goals for patients undergoing prolonged isolation may include improving sensory stimulation, increasing social support and peer interaction, improving mood, preventing developmental delay, and encouraging the use of motor skills.

Intervention Environments

Inpatient

Although the inpatient hem/onc environment is evolving and incorporating family-centered care in order to better meet the needs of children and their families, it continues to be an unfamiliar, stressful place for children and their families. Overstimulation of the senses may initially occur. The inpatient unit may be noisy with strange monitors and a variety of electronic machines sounding, many personnel conversing, children in distress, loud ventilation systems removing bacteria, and the sounds of many people living together in a confined area. There may be unpleasant odors from other patients or from medications and disinfectants. Food may taste different as chemotherapy side effect, or it may be unfamiliar or not prepared as it is at home. Seeing other children who appear different due to illness or treatment may be frightening or upsetting to children as well as family members. Routine medical equipment, such as IV tubing and poles, can be intimidating. Immunosuppressed children may wear masks, gloves, and hospital gowns to prevent exposure to infection.

Children may be isolated for their own protection in their rooms in order to reduce infection opportunities. Stem cell transplant patients will undergo isolation precautions for an extended amount of time.

This foreign environment contains additional stressors. Medical procedures or tests and the checking of routine vital signs continue day and night. Patients and families have difficulty sleeping due to hospital noise and the intrusion of nursing staff who are giving medications or taking vital signs such as blood pressure, temperature, heart rate, and pain assessment every few hours or more if warranted. Lack of sleep makes it more difficult for patients and parents to cope with stressful situations. Even infants may sense this stress or anxiety in the parent or caregiver.

Conversely, children and their families who have had many treatments at the same hospital on a familiar unit often become comfortable with the routine and the environment. They become acquainted with and are fond of staff members. The playroom, activities, and library become familiar settings, while family members may use the hospital salon to get their nails done, have their hair styled, or get a much needed massage as they continue with the more mundane tasks of life. However, there is still the stress of missing family, school, friends, and the normal situations of everyday life. Children are worried about medical procedures, relapse, side effects of treatment, family situations, and the efficacy of treatment. They may see other patients who have become their friends at the hospital decline in health and die. Other children with the same illness may not respond to treatment, or perhaps no one else with a rare form of cancer is nearby to help support a child in need. In general, the hospital environment can be a chaotic, unpredictable, and frightening experience for the child and family (Robb, 2003b).

Outpatient

The rise of managed care has led to shorter hospitalizations and increased emphasis on outpatient treatment in an effort to control costs. This trend has been echoed by the rise in the number of music therapists working in outpatient oncology settings (Kruse, 2003). Pediatric hematology/oncology is illustrative of this phenomenon, as many of the treatment protocols are successfully administered on an outpatient basis.

Various types of blood infusions as well as certain invasive procedures that are part of standard hematology/oncology treatment are completed within outpatient settings. Procedures such as **spinal taps** and bone marrow aspirations can be completed in the outpatient clinic within private treatment rooms. Occasionally these treatment rooms are equipped with toys, entertainment centers, and activities to assist in the distraction of children from pain during procedures. Infusion areas, also known as "chemo suites," may be larger rooms or solaria where patients receive blood transfusions and intravenous medications. Children undergoing chemotherapy may receive platelet transfusions, while red blood cell transfusions may be given to patients with sickle cell disease, **thalassemia**, or cancer.

Parents are typically allowed to stay with children during the course of the transfusions, which may take several hours. Infusion areas may have televisions, game centers, computers, toys, and access to child life services. Children may sit in large reclining chairs during infusions, or some rooms may be arranged with central activity tables allowing children to play games or engage in structured activities. During transfusions, children are allowed to eat, play video or computer games, or listen to music with headphones.

Children who have experienced a bone marrow transplant may require outpatient treatment in an isolation room, as their immune systems may be compromised. Some clinics have glass-enclosed isolation rooms where children may interact through the use of walkie talkies or room-to-room telephones with nonisolated children receiving treatment. Isolation rooms also provide patients with activities and entertainment outlets.

The music therapist working in an outpatient setting encounters several logistical challenges when implementing sessions. Foremost, sound insulation is often absent in large chemo suites and solaria. Some clinics may serve both adult and pediatric patients, and the therapist must be mindful of meeting the needs of both the pediatric patients served and nearby adult patients. Instruments that have minimal sound production may be necessary to reduce noise levels that might otherwise disturb neighboring patients. In mixed age group infusion areas, pediatric patients may be seated staggered among adult patients with their infusion bags hung above them, which may necessitate providing individual sessions to patients. A music therapist with a substantial outpatient clinic assignment may be able to coordinate group sessions in advance and organize patients' seating to facilitate the group structure. Often, small group sessions may occur spontaneously as a child desires to join in music making with a peer. Siblings who are staying with the patient during lengthy transfusions may keenly benefit from active engagement in music activities. Patients undergoing transfusions will also experience limitations to movement due to infusion equipment. Patients with restrictions to ambulation may find relief in engaging in music activities that focus on moving body parts to the extent possible without disturbing the infusion apparatus.

The goals and interventions used in an outpatient setting will depend upon the patient served as well as upon environmental and logistical factors. The communal environment of the chemo suite tends to prohibit privacy, which may lead to a more superficial interaction during sessions. Adolescents and more reserved pediatric patients may not feel comfortable actively engaging in music production when surrounded by older patients and unknown adults. The music therapist may temper an interaction based on these considerations, opting to work on slightly different goal areas than would be chosen for inpatient sessions. Reducing anxiety, nausea, and providing outlets for creative action will be important goals for young children. Expressing aggravations related to treatment regimen, gaining peer acceptance and support, and building self-esteem will be relevant to preteen and adolescent patients. In addition, adolescent patients may appreciate learning self-management techniques for countering pain and anxiety and improving wellness. The music therapist may implement a variety of interventions to achieve these goals in an outpatient setting, including singing, instrument playing, songwriting, dramatic play, and music-assisted relaxation. Music therapy may be used as procedural support for patients undergoing IV starts, **lumbar punctures**, or bone marrow aspirations in the outpatient clinic. The music therapist may need to interface with nursing to establish a referral procedure to ensure the therapist's advance notification of these procedures.

Individual Sessions

One-to-one music therapy sessions may occur at bedside or in a playroom, teen lounge, treatment room, clinic, waiting room, or other area of the hospital. Parents, family, visitors, or staff may be present all or part of the time, or they may leave for respite. Parents need time to be able to take a shower, go for a walk, or talk with medical staff, for example. Some parents eat their meals in a location other than the child's room if the child is unable to eat or if the child becomes nauseated at the smell of food. This respite time can be coordinated with music therapy. Most parents will want to have an established relationship before they feel comfortable leaving their child with a music therapist. When parents feel assured that their child will be safe and cared for by the MT-BC, they can comfortably take a break knowing that the child will be working toward predetermined goals and generally will be having a positive experience at the same time. Some parents and caregivers may want to remain in the session to take the opportunity to participate with their child in a more normalized situation. Music provides the stimulus for family integration to take place. Siblings, grandparents, and extended family may all participate within the same session, which may create positive family memories for those involved.

Individual sessions are an efficient way to assess and get to know the patient and family. Looking at greeting cards, emails, personal photographs, artwork, books, recordings, games, and toys can help give a well-rounded picture of the patient. From these items we can assess much about a child—music preferences, family support, absence or presence of peer group and friends, developmental level, coping mechanisms, family dynamics, and general preferences.

One-to-one interventions may be scheduled for a specific time and day, or they may need to be more flexibly attempted between times utilized by the medical team, medical procedures, nursing cares, school work, visitors, quiet time, meals, child life activities, and family time, or when the patient is not feeling well. Frequently, the reality for music therapists is a combination of scheduling a planned session while remaining flexible with music therapy programming in the unpredictable environment of the inpatient unit.

Individual sessions can be rewarding due to the intimacy of the situation. Music can be used by a skilled therapist to quickly establish rapport, while also facilitating the identification and expression of feelings on a deeper level. Intense emotions such as fear, anxiety, and anger that may be present can be balanced when appropriate by humor, joy, and relief within the same session. Hospitalization can be a period of intense volatile emotions, and music therapists can validate these feelings and positively involve children and families within nonjudgmental interventions where multiple emotions can be expressed. In addition, specific goals and interventions for each child can be planned and implemented during individual sessions.

Infection Control Precautions

Within the individual session, all objects used by the MT and the child must be cleaned thoroughly as per infection control policies of the facility. Because hematology/oncology patients often are immunosuppressed, extra precautions may be warranted. If objects are likely to be put in the mouth as with older infants, toddlers, and young children, they need to be cleaned in a bleach solution or with a hospital disinfectant cleaner such as Virex, and then washed again with dish soap or through a cycle of an automatic dishwasher. Instruments or objects that are not able to withstand this constant cycle of cleaning are not appropriate for use with young children in the hospital context.

Other objects and all instruments that will not be mouthed will need to be washed or wiped down with approved cleaning agents. Some instruments should not be selected because of their inability to be cleaned (e.g., a painted surface or finish that might be removed) or because dust may be released during play (natural rainsticks, woven basket type shakers). Fuzzy objects such as stuffed animals or puppets are not typically used with this population due to cleaning problems, but if a fuzzy puppet is washed (through an automatic washer) between patients, it can be used in a careful manner. A better choice would be a puppet made of plastic or rubber that can then be wiped or washed between patients. Scarves should be thoroughly washed between patients as well.

A music therapist may need to wear a mask, gloves, and gown in order to protect the child from infection, as well as to prevent spreading infection to other children. This can be a challenge, as extra equipment may raise body temperature and be uncomfortably warm, and playing an instrument such as guitar is more difficult while wearing latex gloves. Depending upon the infection, objects taken into the room may need to remain in the room for use until the infection clears or the child is discharged.

Group Sessions

In a group session, it may be more difficult to assess a child as thoroughly and goals may need to be more generalized. In contrast, there are also advantages to group sessions. A music therapist is able to observe functioning levels while watching for regression or coping difficulties, and is able to assess how each patient relates to his or her peers. In the hospital, most of a child's interactions are with adults, so peer interaction and support within a music therapy session can provide significant normalization.

When pediatric patients are together within the normalizing environment of a music therapy group session, they often relate to their peers in a more natural and developmentally appropriate way. Young children watch each other and may mimic other children's behavior. Older children may be silly and get caught up in the fun as they interact with other children like themselves. Hematology/oncology patients may notice that other children have central lines connected through pumps on IV poles, that peers have lost their hair, or that they have other side effects or types of medical equipment in common. When a group begins with an intervention that encourages cohesiveness, the children may become totally involved and invested in the group and have normal interactions, just as they would away from the hospital. Hematology/oncology patients may fatigue more quickly than normal children, but the desire for playful interaction remains.

Hematology/oncology patients may attend a regular group session for general pediatric patients, or they may have their own groups that are age-appropriate. There may be a preschool group, one for school age patients, and a teen group. Parents and families may attend these groups as well. Groups may be held in a general inpatient playroom or on treatment-specific units. Groups on the restricted access Bone Marrow Transplant (BMT) unit may contain family and children of all ages who are receiving stem cell transplants. Although this wide age range within a group session may be more challenging for a music therapist, it is quite gratifying to assist children and families in their support for one another. Often the families are not acquainted with each other, and music therapy group sessions serve as an initial meeting place that can contribute to the subsequent establishment of supportive relationships among families.

Children on a restricted access BMT unit may have to wear a mask when outside their room or near other children, even though the unit has specialized ventilation systems. This mask often obscures a large portion of the child's face. At times it may be difficult to see a child's expression behind a mask, because it covers the mouth and nose and ties behind the head or hooks behind the ears. Sometimes the mask will make communication more problematic as well. It can be difficult to hear a young child who may talk softly, or to read the lips of all the children in a noisy room full of people. Nevertheless, the music therapist may be more observant of nonverbal communication and utilize assistance from parents, siblings, or grandparents who may be located in closer proximity to the patient.

Because patients who attend music therapy groups may be functioning on a variety of developmental levels, interventions should be planned with several possible adaptations available to address these divergent developmental needs. A wide variety of music, instruments, and objects are selected for a group session in order to offer and maximize choice and to control opportunities for children and their families. Other general inpatient group goals include providing normalization, reducing anxiety, encouraging expression of feeling and communication, providing social interaction and family integration, improving self-esteem, and elevating mood. The use of music to achieve group or individual goals in a cohesive, supportive manner can also be effectively extended to address the needs of other disciplines during co-treatment.

Co-treatment in Hem/Onc

Although physical therapy is not routinely ordered for all hematology/oncology patients, some children have adverse reactions to chemotherapy and may be bedridden for long periods of time. Music therapy may be used during physical therapy to increase endurance, assist with ambulation, or assist with standing or bearing weight. For example, if a physical therapist is attempting to have a young child bear weight, the MT-BC might use instrument holding and playing to structure and motivate this task. Range of motion can be increased by holding instruments in front of a child in such a way that the child must reach out comfortably to play them. Chimes, guitar, or many other interesting instruments may be selected in order to motivate and encourage a child to play. The focus for the child is on reaching for and playing the instrument, not on the fact that he or she is standing up and weight bearing for a period of time. A young child could also stand with help from a gathering drum, playing it or holding on to the edge for support while the MT-BC is making music. Fatiguing repetitions and long durations of physical movements or positions may be sustained when music therapy is used during co-treatment. In addition, active music making on the part of the patient and physical therapist may lead to elevated mood and actual enjoyment of the physical requirements.

Medical staff from a variety of disciplines are usually willing to participate within group or individual sessions when time permits. Often this is not a formal co-treatment, but more of a team effort at supporting a patient and family. When nursing staff are present in a patient's room on a BMT unit, they routinely play instruments or sing when music therapy is offered. Nursing staff also enter to check IVs during a group session in a playroom and are included in the immediate intervention, or teased appropriately by the MT-BC and the patients until they participate or jokingly include or exclude themselves. Physicians, physician assistants, nurses, and child life specialists are often written into the lyrics of a song composed by a patient. The patient may want the staff to hear a performance of the original song, or show the staff the lyrics in which they are included. These staff members are often involved during special occasions within a patient's hospitalization as well, such as music making during transplantation, a birthday or end-of-chemotherapy party, or discharge from the facility.

The music therapist working in a pediatric hematology/oncology setting where child life services exist often interfaces with child life specialists to provide continuity of care. The music therapist can benefit from an alliance with the child life team to receive referrals for music therapy, co-treat during procedural preparation and support, and inform patients of the availability of music therapy.

Family-Centered Care

Diagnosis and treatment of hematology/oncology disorders can be extremely stressful for both the pediatric patient and family. Health care professionals have acknowledged the impact that illness can have on the entire family unit and have collaborated with consumers to advocate for improvements in hospital policies and services to meet the needs of families during hospitalization. This shift towards family-friendly policies, programs, and facility design is known as family-centered care. In the family-centered care environment, families are viewed as integral members of the health care team, are empowered to be actively involved in their children's health care, and are supported as they undertake this role. The family unit is respected as the most stable source of support in a patient's life, and efforts that reduce parental stress can result in improved parental support for patients. Facilitating the availability and consistency of parental support is imperative for the pediatric hematology/oncology patient's healthy adjustment to illness and hospitalization.

Policies and practices that support families in their role of promoting the well-being of their children are seen in pediatric hematology/oncology inpatient and outpatient settings. Parents are offered open visiting hours in many inpatient hem/onc settings. Hospitals typically have accommodations for one parent or parental designee to sleep on a cot or in a sleeper chair at the patient's bedside. Overnight accommodations for a minimal charge may also be arranged at a nearby Ronald McDonald House for families who live more than 50 miles from the hospital. Families may stay at the Ronald McDonald House while a patient is admitted to the hospital or while a patient receives outpatient treatment. Extended family and friends are able to visit children on hematology/oncology units during regular visiting hours, with most units enforcing a two-person limit at bedside. School-age children can visit a sibling who is hospitalized, and these siblings may also engage in child life services. Many pediatric hematology/oncology units offer family services including showering facilities, telephones, Internet access, kitchen facilities, and family lounge. Depending upon the resources of the hospital, families may engage in support groups, sibling support groups, child life services, music therapy programming, individual counseling, chaplaincy services, or hospice services. Classrooms, equipment, tutors, and educators who coordinate schoolwork from a patient's home school may be provided by the hospital. School re-entry programs are available to ease a patient's transition back to school, an event that often provokes a significant amount of anxiety in the patient.

Parents receive education regarding course of illness and treatment procedures to enable them to participate actively in decision making related to their child's care. Parents may also learn developmentally appropriate techniques for supporting their child through invasive procedures. Child life specialists may work with siblings to resolve misconceptions regarding the patient's illness and treatment, to provide suggestions for meaningful engagement with the patient, and to give developmentally appropriate coping support. Music therapists may use their medium to facilitate normalized family–patient interactions (Dun, 1995) and to provide additional support to parents and siblings. End-of-life services, including anticipatory bereavement services, may also be provided for families through social work, chaplaincy, child life, or music therapy programming.

Bereavement Services/Palliative and End-of-Life Care

As hematology and oncology disorders are often life-threatening illnesses, concerns may arise during treatment regarding the possibility of death. Despite recent advances in medical treatments, death still remains a threat for some patients. When a decision has been made to stop aggressive, curative, or healing treatment, a pediatric patient's family may want involvement of palliative music therapy services. The goal of music therapy palliative care is to increase quality of life and reduce pain and suffering during the time prior to the patient's death (Krout, 2000).

The level of open communication about death will vary from family to family depending on cultural and religious traditions, family communication patterns, and parental coping tendencies. Honest communication is generally advised, tailoring specificity of discussion to the developmental level of the child (Leukemia & Lymphoma Society, 2000). Music therapy may help facilitate a child's exploration of themes related to death during musical and dramatic play and may also promote communication and expression of feelings within a cross-generational grouping of family members (Krout, 2000). The music therapist should generally follow the patient's pace when addressing death issues (Fagen, 1982) and should also be mindful of parental preference regarding openness of communication on the possibility of a patient's death. Occasionally, parents may ask the music therapist or child life specialist to assist them in exploring the possibility of death with a patient or sibling for the first time. The therapist may use songs or books (often available through the child life or social work department) that address death issues at developmentally appropriate levels for the patient to facilitate this discussion.

Sedative, familiar, or religious music may be used within music therapy palliative care to provide comfort to families and patients who have reached end-stage illness. The patient is often minimally responsive or unconscious at this time, and intervention may focus primarily on providing familial support. Live sedative music improvisations can provide a calming effect for families, facilitate release of emotions related to anticipatory grieving, and provide a sense of security and support. The music therapist may improvise songs that express support and love for the patient on behalf of family members who are present. The family may request that the therapist play a patient's favorite songs, or they may provide recordings of these songs. Many families rely more heavily on their spirituality or religious views to lend support when death is a possibility for their child. The music therapist may evaluate the importance of spirituality and religious music to a family and incorporate music that reinforces these beliefs when indicated. Not all families will value religion at this time, and the therapist should be careful not to make assumptions related to a family's desire for religious music.

Families who have experienced the death of their child may receive a bereavement packet from the social work department that gives supportive information as well as referrals for formal bereavement services outside of the inpatient setting. Some pediatric units allow for the arrangement of a private room for families to spend a period of hours with their recently deceased. A music therapist may be asked to make music with the family and the recently deceased, to find specific printed lyrics and music for the family, or to provide live music for services or funerals.

Implementation of Interventions

After consideration of the characteristics, needs, assessment tools, goals and objectives, and treatment environments for pediatric hematology/oncology patients, music therapists must design and implement appropriate interventions to facilitate the attainment of identified goals. Interventions must be developmentally appropriate and provide a balance of familiarity and structure, yet offer sufficient flexibility for the provision of the greatest amount of patient choice and control (Barrickman, 1989). In addition, the MT-BC must be able to assess a situation quickly (due to single session service, variability within the environment, or changes in the patient's needs of the moment), and provide an adaptable intervention that is ever changing to meet the needs of each individual patient.

With these considerations in mind, the MT-BC must prepare, organize, create, and administer the most effective music therapy intervention. The following list of music therapy interventions are commonly used with the population of hematology/oncology patients in order to help children cope with pain, fear, anxiety, and stress experienced during hospitalization:

- Music assisted relaxation (MAR)
- Music as alternate engagement during medical procedures (MAE)
- Active music making (including singing and/or instrument playing)
- Music listening
- Songwriting (structured or improvised)
- Music permanent product
- Music-facilitated dramatic play
- Music with movement

Detailed descriptions of the interventions MAR, MAE, songwriting, music permanent product, and music-facilitated dramatic play are included in the Appendix at the end of this monograph. The music therapist will adapt any chosen intervention to better meet the needs of the patient and will alternate between interventions depending upon patient responses or changes in identified goals.

The overall, general goal for the MT-BC working with hematology/oncology patients is the facilitation and improvement of coping skills. Robb (2003b) investigated how music therapists effectively help patients cope, whether in short-term procedural support or for longer extended hospitalizations, within the context of a supportive environment. She developed the Contextual Support Model of Music Therapy based on child development, models of coping, and principles of music therapy. Robb discusses the contextual support elements of structure, autonomy support, and involvement in relation to the selection of music, the session format, and the client–therapist relationship. The following adaptation of Robb's model may assist the music therapist with planning appropriate interventions by considering the following elements within the intervention design. Each of these critical pieces of music therapy intervention design (selection of music, session format, and client–therapist relationship) are discussed in relation to the three elements (structure, autonomy support, and involvement) of Robb's model, first in a summary format and second with detailed examples in narrative form.

The Selection of Music

Source	Structure	Autonomy Support	Involvement
Music can:	▪ Create comfort/security due to familiarity ▪ Energize and motivate action ▪ Provide structure for participation and response ▪ Provide flexible structure for independent and successful experiences	▪ Allow for creative independence through flexible structure ▪ Support participation; success and security gained through participation result in exploration and independent responses	▪ Facilitate rapport through use of familiar music and shared experience of active music making ▪ Make an enjoyable shared experience through use of familiar and developmentally appropriate music

Structure

The music selected for interventions must be familiar and developmentally appropriate for patients. Choosing music that is patient-preferred and familiar for children of any age provides normalization. The MT-BC must have a strong basic repertoire of music memorized for children of all levels of development in order to be most effective and meet the changing needs of patients. Whether the chosen music is pre-existing or improvised, the MT-BC must also provide a pleasing product—musicality is extremely important.

The structural elements of music provide opportunities for children to respond, which then can be modified to encourage independent responses. For example, if children are initially moving a puppet to the directions given in a song, the song may be adapted to what the children are doing with their puppet, or the children may choose what their puppet will do for another verse of the song. By encouraging patients to choose when to start and stop the music, or to designate tempo and dynamic levels, the structure of live music is easily adapted to maximize choice making. Rhythm can stimulate active responses in children, and it can be modified to meet the specific energy, strength, and endurance capabilities of each child.

Infants, toddlers, and preschoolers need familiar music and routines to provide them with security and comfort. Standard fingerplays like "The Eency Weency Spider" and songs such as "Twinkle, Twinkle Little Star" can be soothing and comforting to children. Young children may also know all the words to country songs, rock music, television themes, or other genres that are played in their home environment. For school age children, familiar music is important, but if the music is developmentally on target, novel music can be mixed with the more familiar. Teenagers have their own preferences but may like to have current music within their desired genres provided. If teens have extended hospitalizations, they may not have independent access to the latest top hits, but these may be able to be provided by the MT-BC.

Autonomy Support

Support for participation as well as creative and independent responses can be provided by the structural elements of music. For example, a structured improvisation may be set up in an ABA format. The A section is a certain number of measures of a structured song, the B section is set aside for improvisation, and the A section is then repeated. There are infinite ways to encourage independent responses through musical structure—call and response, the blues, and song parody/piggybacking (creating new lyrics for existing melodies), to name a few. A song such as "Old McDonald Had a Farm" has a structure that is familiar to many young children. At the appropriate time in the song, children can select and make an animal sound, even if it is the creative chosen response of *and on this farm he had a great big Western painted turtle, E-I-E-I-O.* The skilled therapist can take the construction of music, and adapt it to encourage creative and autonomous responses.

Involvement

By selecting familiar and developmentally appropriate music, as well as actively making music within an enjoyable shared experience, the MT-BC is able to establish rapport quickly. This is important in an environment where children are often fearful of all staff. Involving all personnel and family in a shared pleasant experience can reduce the anxiety of everyone concerned. The MT-BC can structure not only a successful, musically pleasing experience that encourages autonomous behavior, but one that also can create a pleasant association with the hospital environment for the child and family.

The Session Format

Source	Structure	Autonomy Support	Involvement
The **session format** needs:	• Clear opening and closing • Repetition to make it predictable and familiar • Appropriate challenges • Successful experiences	• Choices of instruments and materials • Choices for direction of session • Input of patients into final products	• Placement of patient's needs and interests foremost in session • Flexibility to meet patient's varying needs

Structure

Whether in a group or individual session, the format must have a clear opening and closing. Patients and families need to know when a group is ending. For example, a group with an ambiguous end may actually cause stress—patients and families may be polite and wait for a definitive end from a therapist, even though they would prefer to leave the room. With young children, "bookending" or beginning and ending a session with the same familiar music can be comforting as well as giving advance notice that a transition time is near. For example, a session for toddlers could begin and end with the music "The More We Get Together," and "The Barney Song." Older school age and teenage patients do not need a "hello song" and a "goodbye song" typically written by music therapists, but they do need an obvious starting point and a strong conclusion to a session.

Young children often need repetition of music before they actively participate; this repetition provides the structure and predictability that helps children feel secure. However, the MT-BC must observe closely for inattention, boredom, and restlessness when using repetition. When attempting to keep a child actively engaged, this is a helpful rule of thumb: spend one minute per each year of a child's mental age on a specific activity before changing it in some fashion (D. T. McDonald, personal communication, January 25, 1989).

The MT-BC must also structure every intervention to be successful for the child, allowing for challenges along the way in order for the child to gain some mastery over the situation. Sometimes this may take the form of the child showing the MT-BC how to play an instrument the "right way." Other times, the MT-BC may praise a skill demonstrated by a patient and spontaneously create a task that might be slightly more challenging. For example, the MT-BC might challenge a group who did well playing instruments together on a song, saying, "I bet you guys can't begin the song together, play it one time softly and one time loudly, and end together on your own with me holding this egg on my head." The patients would then work together to begin and end at the same time and possibly play loudly enough to knock a plastic shaker egg off the MT-BC's head.

Autonomy Support

The child will have many choices available in a session, including selecting instruments and objects, and choosing the actual direction of the session. For example, the MT-BC may draw cryptic pictures or place random numbers of the planned interventions on a dry erase board. The patient may select one by throwing a ball at the board, choosing verbally or by pointing or looking at the picture or number. It is up to the MT-BC to make smooth transitions between interventions, as patients are choosing the actual direction of the session. Empowering patients in every way possible is always a consideration. If a child is given a choice of three objects or instruments that are exactly alike, the child needs to be able to select the one he or she wants. The MT-BC needs to foster these choices and not hand an object or an instrument to someone just because the instruments all look the same. In this way, each patient will have choices as well as input into the session. If there is a product created by the group, the MT-BC must ensure that each member has an opportunity to contribute in some way and is involved in the final result.

Involvement

The group or individual session will always be tailored to the needs and interests of the patient. Again, the music therapist must demonstrate considerable skill in remaining flexible, even within a planned structure, in order to meet the patient's changing needs. Having a repertoire of memorized, developmentally appropriate live music enables the MT-BC to concentrate on the needs of the patient and adapt quickly without having to concentrate on the production of the music itself. When using prerecorded music, a wide variety must be available in order to accommodate patient preferences.

The Client–Therapist Relationship

Source	Structure	Autonomy Support	Involvement
Client–Therapist Relationship involves:	<ul><li>Observation, adaptation of interventions to promote mastery and success</li><li>Support and empowerment</li><li>Positive reinforcement</li></ul>	<ul><li>Encouragement of independent decisions</li><li>Connection of decisions and outcomes</li></ul>	<ul><li>Unconditional acceptance</li><li>Authenticity</li><li>Genuine interest in children</li><li>Listening and attending</li><li>Respect and support</li></ul>

Structure

In order to be effective and meet changing needs, the MT-BC must have keen observational skills while multi-tasking within the session. Watching for nonverbal cues from patients and families can provide necessary information with regard to the adaptation of interventions. For example, a group is writing a song using the fill-in-the-blank technique. A patient who is quiet with little eye contact may need support from the MT-BC in order to participate. This patient may need the structure of making a choice between two words suggested by the group or MT-BC, instead of an open-ended fill-in-the-blank question. The patient still has a choice to make, but it does not seem like such an overwhelming task. In this way, the MT-BC uses structure to ensure that the patient will have a successful experience. After patients are able to make choices and successfully participate, and these efforts are supported and reinforced, they are more likely to independently respond, control, and master the environment.

Empowering patients is one of the most important ways to offer control in the unpredictable hospital environment. Encouraging the patient to make choices such as where to sit, who will take the next turn, what instrument to choose for a family member to use, how the music should be played, etc., empowers the patient to be self-sufficient instead of feeling helpless. The following situation is an example of working toward mastering the environment with assistance from the MT-BC. A child who has difficulty reading wants to choose some music to make a recording to use in his or her room. As an alternative to the therapist reading a list of music from which the child may choose, the therapist encourages the child to select music by listening at his or her own pace to the songs on an MP3 player. Empowering patients may take more time and effort on the part of the MT-BC, but patients know they have a supportive person who truly cares about them and wants them to succeed through active involvement with their environment.

The art of giving positive reinforcement takes energy, thought, and authenticity. Frequently, blanket phrases such as "good job" and "that was great" are overused. Effective positive reinforcement must be specific, immediate, and genuine. "Way to go, John! You have a great idea for how we can shake our maracas behind our back" is much more specific than saying, "Good job, John." In order for the reinforcement to be effective, it needs to be delivered as soon as possible after the behavior. Sometimes, because of the nature of the session, this is difficult to do verbally. While singing, an MT-BC can smile at someone, nod his or her head, reach over and touch someone on the leg or arm, make knowing eye contact, give a "thumbs up" sign even while playing guitar, laugh appropriately, say a quick "yes" within the lyrics, etc. Nonverbal reinforcement is very effective and can be directed to one person out of sight of other group members. Sometimes children or teens do not want to look like they are overly involved in a group session (this might not be the "cool thing" to do) but they like to get acknowledgment in a quiet way unseen by peers. Since reinforcement originates from the careful observation of patients, it can be given in a natural, genuine manner. The MT-BC sees the behavior and then gives a specific comment or nonverbal gesture, in a straightforward manner, regarding the behavior. Using a high-pitched or condescending tone of voice with children is not recommended. Children know when the therapist is sincerely excited, interested, and genuinely involved with them as individuals.

Autonomy Support

When children are encouraged to make their own decisions and take control when possible, they realize they have choices and can affect outcomes. The MT-BC can help children become aware of these connections as well. For example, patients may be able to select different instruments for themselves as well as for family members to play during the session. In order to facilitate more control for a child, he or she may hold up a "Stop" sign when everyone in the group is actively making music. The group must stop playing, and the child will control all the adults and peers in the room, indicating that everyone may begin again by turning the sign around to the "Go" side. The therapist may also validate patient skills or unique contributions. For example, when a child creates a different way to play an instrument than in the standard manner, the therapist may be able to make a connection: "Because you were creative and were thinking of new ideas, we will be able to use this with other people, and it will be really helpful."

Involvement

The MT-BC who chooses to work with hematology/oncology patients must be able to respect children's ideas and support their independence with unconditional acceptance. Having a genuine interest in children and being authentic is what is necessary—not merely going through the motions. Children need adults to be there with them, not only physically but also by being fully present. Again, this takes more energy than just doing things in an automatic fashion. The MT-BC needs to be comfortable with flexibility and spontaneity, but needs to be organized and well prepared. A strong sense of self and a level of maturity will be helpful when confronting the issues of pain, suffering, and death. When working with hematology/oncology patients, the MT-BC needs compassion rather than pity, as well as the realization that music therapy can improve the quality of life of children with serious illnesses.

Case Examples

Long-term Patient with Wilms' Tumor

D. was 4½ years old when diagnosed with bilateral Wilms' tumor (i.e., affecting both kidneys). The malignancy had already progressed to Stage 4 when it was discovered, thus his prognosis was poor from the beginning of treatment. D. underwent surgery to remove one kidney and the majority of the second before receiving chemotherapy. D.'s family had recently immigrated to the United States from a Spanish-speaking country.

D. first received music therapy sessions during his treatments in the outpatient clinic. Sessions through the first 6 months were sporadic, occurring approximately twice a month. Though very independent, D. often exhibited elevated anxiety during nursing procedures, including chemo flushes and **mediport** removal, and would pull away from nurses or become combative. The music therapist used music interactions to provide alternate engagement while D. received anxiety-provoking nursing care. Though he used minimal expressive communication at this time, D. was immediately drawn to rhythm instruments including the rainstick, finger cymbals, and thunder tube, and took initiative in requesting to play and swap these instruments. As D. developed rapport with the MT-BC, it became apparent that he was actually quite precocious. D. began speaking in English more often and engaged in dramatic play sequences using a combination of instruments and finger puppets to tell stories of conflict and resolution. D. often presented with flat affect, but would become animated during musical play sessions. After 8 months of treatment, D. demonstrated improved expressive communication but increased impulsivity, requiring the music therapist to use methods to reinforce tolerance of limits, turn taking, and boundaries. D. was also impulsive with staff and needed calming and behavioral cues during nursing procedures to remain compliant.

The music therapist began seeing D. more frequently during inpatient hospitalizations for fevers and **neutropenia** starting in the 8th month of treatment. At 5 years old, D. was often left alone in his room, as his mother worked during the day and also had to care for D.'s three other siblings. D. enjoyed making puppets with the child life staff and acting out familial scenes as the MT-BC played music to accompany the dramatic action. D. demonstrated keen awareness of the improvised music and would request exaggerations in musical style to match the mood he desired to create, making requests such as "make it sound even more angry!" D. also used a doll house in the child life room during his dramatic play and began to demonstrate an attraction to the Cinderella story. D. continued giving directives for the musical accompaniment to his stories, speaking the storyline while the MT-BC accompanied and sang refrains that mirrored the action and emerging themes.

D. began displaying manipulative behavior and increased difficulty tolerating limits during his interactions with child life staff around the 12th month of treatment. As the length and frequency of his hospitalizations increased, he lacked consistent parental presence and therefore did not experience consistent reinforcement of behavioral limits. D. would often become angry and upset when denied a toy or supply from the child life room or when denied a favorite snack or candy, and he had increasing difficulty coping with refusals. During music-facilitated dramatic play, D. would act out themes of violence, frequently with male perpetrators acting aggressively towards his character, which was usually female. D. also demonstrated increasing fascination with feminine interests and preferred playing with female dolls. The child life staff supported D.'s expressive play and did not judge or challenge his interest in the opposite gender. The child life specialist also made a referral for continued MT sessions to increase expressive outlets and assess D.'s coping with illness. The MT-BC documented sessions in D.'s chart and described D.'s recurring themes of aggression, control, and opposite gender interests. The MT-BC also provided continuity of social support for times when D. was without familial presence. Over time, D. began to express his anger more directly, first projecting these feelings onto dolls and puppets, then projecting his negative feelings onto the therapist, and finally expressing his frustrations verbally. With support and clarifying questions from the MT-BC, D. began to reveal his underlying anger toward medical staff, toward limit setting, and toward his perceived abandonment by his family. It was around this time that the nursing staff learned that D.'s mother was being physically and mentally abused by her husband. Suddenly, the themes of D.'s dramatic play gained new significance within this familial context. MT sessions were viewed as a safe and supportive way for D. to act out his unresolved feelings related to the conflicts he might have experienced in his home situation as well as the lack of control and security he felt at home and while in the hospital. Social work staff intervened to support D.'s mother, and she was encouraged to spend as much time at the hospital with D. as possible.

D.'s family decided not to inform him of the details of his medical condition or prognosis, which was worsening as a result of extensive pulmonary disease. This decision was made in part because D.'s mother had great difficulty accepting the severity of his condition. During his 13th month of treatment, D. was granted a wish from the Make-a-Wish Foundation and requested a trip to Disney World. D. was very excited by this possibility, and it provided a positive way for D. and his mother to bond and maintain hopefulness. During this time, D. demonstrated increasing precociousness in sessions and was quite adept at expressing himself verbally. He continued to use music-facilitated dramatic play to express angry emotions, create interpersonal conflicts, and provide resolutions. The Cinderella storyline appeared frequently in his play. D. continued to need support as he coped with refusal and limit setting but now more frequently expressed sadness instead of anger when limits were enforced. Occasionally D. would request that the MT-BC read a Cinderella musical storybook, as D. pressed the buttons to create corresponding sounds. In the last music therapy session, D. appeared sad and lamented his current admission. The MT-BC provided supportive listening while gently strumming the guitar to encourage and sustain D.'s verbal expression.

No formal closure was achieved in the music therapy work with D. When it was clear that the current treatment regimen had not successfully ameliorated his condition, he was transferred to a neighboring hospital to begin a clinical research trial. The MT-BC did not see D. again, as he died at this hospital after 2 weeks of unsuccessful treatment.

The case study presented above demonstrates how the relationship formed within the context of music therapy can play a supportive role throughout the course of a pediatric patient's illness and hospitalization. The nature of this relationship and the goals of the accompanying music therapy intervention change during the course of treatment depending upon the patient's immediate needs. Deeper issues, such as a patient experiencing domestic violence in the home setting, will influence a patient's adjustment to illness and hospitalization, but may or may not be overtly revealed and addressed during hospitalization. In the current case, music therapy interactions provided a safe context within which D. was able to act out and attempt to master the mixed feelings he may have experienced as a witness to conflicts at home. This open expression and the music therapist's documentation of the patient's recurrent themes helped alert staff to the potential of problems in the patient's family setting. This case study also raises the question of the appropriate depth of psychosocial intervention for this time-limited setting. Patients may bring long-term problems to their current hospitalization that cannot be adequately addressed during a brief hospitalization or because of the prioritization of immediate needs related to the crisis state of the patient's current health status. The therapist must address these underlying issues to the extent that they may be ethically ameliorated. The role of the music therapist in an inpatient medical setting is generally supportive in nature, allowing for the safe expression of emotions, providing social support, and facilitating the patient's acquisition of positive coping abilities to improve adjustment to illness and hospitalization. The expressive and coping skills that a child learns through music therapy may also be applied to underlying long-term issues, though additional psychosocial intervention may be required to fully address these issues. When long-term issues arise during music therapy, the therapist should involve other members of the health care team, namely social workers, child psychologists, and child life specialists, in the psychosocial care of the patient to assure that both the patient and family receive the supports they require.

Stem Cell Transplant Patient with Acute Lymphoblastic Leukemia (ALL)

B. was diagnosed with ALL when he was 8 years old and, despite being treated with chemotherapy, relapsed 2 years later. B. was then admitted to the hospital and placed in isolation, where he began his conditioning for stem cell transplantation. B. received his stem cell transplant from a matched-unrelated donor. B. and two younger siblings were adopted and all have been diagnosed with ADD or ADHD.

B. received his initial music therapy session on the day of the SCT, and the MT-BC continued offering sessions 3–4 times a week throughout B.'s 7 weeks of hospitalization. Because of logistical problems such as time constraints, a short workday, and commitments to other patients, the MT-BC went in to B.'s room without benefit of chart review. During a brief 5-minute assessment, the MT-BC found that B. liked a wide variety of music and had an electric guitar at home that he did not get played very often. B.'s mother specifically asked that the MT-BC return at a later time when B.'s sisters would arrive and be in his room. The MT-BC's schedule was adapted hurriedly to accommodate the desires of the family. Later that day, B. and his siblings used three open-tuned guitars to play some of B.'s favorite songs. B. did play several songs on the open-tuned guitars with his sisters but was somewhat reluctant to try to barre a pattern of a favorite song using open, 5th, and 7th frets on his guitar. He did barre the actual frets, but demonstrated difficulty learning a simple pattern of these positions with only verbal cues given by the MT-BC. He also displayed a lack of confidence about playing guitar by himself in front of the MT-BC and other staff members, but was quite willing to play together with his sisters. During this session, his family sang while playing guitars and the atmosphere was fun and casual. B. repeatedly asked for different songs and indicated that he wanted to continue with the music through the actual time of the transplant.

During transplant, a CLS brought in a banner and some gifts, photographs were taken, nursing staff played guitars, a social worker sang, the family played some rhythm instruments, and the physician's assistant was present. At this time, the MT-BC played guitar and sang improvised lyrics about what was happening with the transplant, with B. and people in the room, and the positive aspects of what might happen in the future. The structure of the music and adaptations made by the MT-BC allowed everyone to participate in a joyful atmosphere while reducing anxiety associated with the process. Family stated that they had fun and felt like they were contributing to the process instead of feeling helpless and merely sitting and observing the infusion. B. had a lively joking personality, and this time of laughter and silly participation by staff and family demonstrated for B. that there was a fun, supportive, and cohesive atmosphere within the unpredictability of the hospital. At the end of the session, the three guitars were left in the room for B. and his sisters to use for the weekend.

In the following session, both B. and his mother could play the I, IV, V pattern on the guitar, although B. continued to lack confidence when playing the guitar with the therapist present. He was not shy about talking or joking with the MT, however. B. played the guitar but did not seem to be excited about it or want to learn other ways of playing it. He demonstrated some difficulty following verbal multi-step directions, so the MT-BC modified all further instructions throughout his inpatient hospitalization to involve one-step commands with visual as well as verbal cues. During this session the MT-BC learned of B.'s diagnosis of ADHD.

Due to the fact that guitar was not motivating for B. and that B. expressed interest in playing percussion in the school band, the next few sessions consisted of playing drums of differing sizes. B. was motivated to play the drums and was able to improvise and play along with some favorite recordings. He was more interested in spontaneous play and taking control than learning specific percussion techniques. Drums were left with B. in his room, so that his sisters could play them and interact with B. during their weekend visits.

During the next 2 weeks, sessions involved improvisation and active music making with a variety of percussion and other instruments. These instruments were also left with B. and his family for use on weekends. B.'s isolation room was a difficult place for two energetic young siblings to be for a weekend, and they were able to use new and different equipment with B. in many interactions. B. had many opportunities for normalization, control and choice-making, as well as expression of feelings through active, fun, shared experiences with the MT-BC and his family.

During the week, B.'s mom participated in MT sessions at times, and at other times she expressed gratitude for the time she could spend doing other tasks while the MT-BC was involved with B. The MT-BC was able to facilitate improved self-esteem by positively reinforcing B. for his creativity, intelligence, and the way he would look at things a little differently than other patients. B. needed this support, due to the fact that traditional homework and learning were difficult for him because of his attention deficit disorder.

Another way of showing support for B. involved the MT-BC coordinating a visit from a group of child life specialists, recreational therapists, and music therapists, who sang a humorous song called *Pajama Bottomless Blues* and other songs of B.'s choice to B. and his mother. B. and his mother were able to laugh and joke around with six therapists simultaneously, three of whom worked directly with them.

The next week B. had low energy levels and was snuggled in his bed. The active music making was discontinued temporarily and the MT-BC offered B. choices of prerecorded music to compile as a CD that he could design and listen to while in bed. An MP3 player was used to allow B. to choose from hundreds of songs. This was an effective means—because B. had a harder time reading titles of various songs, he could listen to them instead and select the ones he preferred. This format was also successful because of the wide variety of music that was available for B. to select. Instead of choosing from one style on one recording, he could choose from rap, rock, country and music from movie soundtracks in which he was interested. He then was able to control the order of the songs he wanted for a particular recording, and the MT-BC then burned these onto a compact disc personalized specifically for B.

The next week B. slept most of the time and did not feel like doing much of anything. The one day of this week that he felt better and had a little energy was the day that he was then sedated for some routine tests. Instead of spending time with B., the MT-BC used this time to talk with family and check on any unmet needs they might have. Family support was important at this time—the parents felt helpless, and they needed someone to listen and offer encouragement.

The next week B. was still not feeling well, but he did have a little more energy. One thing that was frustrating him, as well as his mother, was that he could not fall asleep at night. The MT-BC suggested some deep breathing and simple imagery techniques and practiced these with B. Calm, relaxing music recordings were also provided. The MT-BC suggested that the breathing and imagery techniques be used with the recordings. This music sedation did help B. relax and get the rest he needed at night, so that he did not sleep as much during the day.

Another session coincided with nursing staff teaching B.'s mother how to change the central line dressing in preparation for her doing this after discharge from the hospital. Changing a dressing for a catheter is a common occurrence for the patient and nursing staff, but for B.'s mom it was new and somewhat overwhelming. The tape from the old dressing was stuck around the line, and even the nurse was having great difficulty removing it. B. was anxious at this time, stating, "Mom, you're going to pull it out!" The MT-BC sang and played calming music on the guitar in the style B. preferred. The nurse, mother, and B. all stated that the music helped them feel less anxious in a tense situation.

B. gradually began feeling more energetic and was interested in live music making again, and there was discussion of possible discharge to the Ronald McDonald House for a period of a few months before finally going home. He was excited and began to go for walks out of the BMT unit. He was interested in new and different percussion instruments such as a large gong, thunder tubes, flexatone, and ocean drum. For a period of approximately 10 days, B. anticipated discharge each day, but inevitably a fever would keep him from leaving. His mother had cleaned out his room in anticipation of discharge, and B. didn't have his normal things to occupy him during this time. The MT-BC provided him with instruments and opportunities for improvisation and play, as this was a stressful, unpredictable time for B. and his mother.

B. was discharged 50 days after his transplant but still came to the hospital for school and for outpatient clinic on weekdays. The MT-BC gathered staff during B.'s outpatient school time to sing a goodbye song written by the MT-BC with ideas gathered from B. B. was pleased and days later his dad stated that the family had still been singing the song.

This case study illustrates the need for flexibility in modifying goals to reflect the changing needs of each patient. These needs tend to vary in a consistent pattern for SCT patients: an initial period of time in which patients feel pretty good; next, a period when they may not feel like participating in anything; and finally, a period of time in which they gradually feel better. The MT-BC must establish rapport quickly in the initial period, in order for interactions to be more effective during the time when patients do not feel well.

Music therapy goals with B. included reducing anxiety, offering choice and control, supporting B. and his family, providing normalization and opportunities for family integration, improving self-esteem, teaching relaxation techniques, encouraging self-expression, and providing music sedation. Addressing these music therapy goals during implementation of adaptable interventions, along with the supportive role of the MT-BC, successfully helped B. and his family improve coping with isolation, illness, and hospitalization as demonstrated through this case study. It is hoped that long-term outcomes can be positively affected through the coping strategies learned and practiced during B.'s SCT.

Outcome Measures

Evaluation of the effectiveness of music therapy interventions to achieve assessed goals and objectives is an essential part of the treatment process. A patient's level of active engagement in music therapy, pain and anxiety levels, and mood may fluctuate depending on treatment phase (Robb & Ebberts, 2003a), treatment side effects, or changes in a patient's prognosis or remission status. As these factors influence a patient's response to intervention, treatment approaches may need to vary from session to session depending upon the current mood and needs of a patient on a particular day. Techniques chosen to evaluate the efficacy of music therapy interventions may also vary depending upon the type of intervention presented and the kind of behaviors being observed.

Intervention outcomes are informally noted periodically during the intervention itself, and the music therapist uses this information regarding patient responses to modify his or her methods in order to improve efficacy. The therapist may monitor patient reactions by observing behavioral, psychosocial, and physiological parameters. Behavioral measures may include frequency and duration of eye contact, attending, visual or auditory tracking, and physical or communicative responsiveness. Changes in the level of observable agitation and combativeness or changes in the intensity of a patient's crying may be appropriate behavioral indices for some patients. Psychosocial variables include affective responses, self-concept, and changes in quality of social interaction. Mood may be measured informally by noting changes in frequency or quality of positive affect. Formal measurement of mood may include patient self-report of current mood state or indication of mood using a visual analog scale, such as the **Wong-Baker FACES Scale** (Barrera et al., 2002) or a **Likert scale** for mood (Lane & Olness, 1991). Patient attitudes related to self-image and overall self-esteem may be evaluated by documenting patient self-statements across sessions. Changes in level of social interaction may include frequency and quality of patient–caregiver interaction, peer interaction, and interaction with staff. Patient and parent questionnaires may also be completed to evaluate the effectiveness of music therapy methods to achieve certain goal areas.

For patients with pain control needs, a visual analog pain scale, most commonly the Wong-Baker FACES Pain Rating Scale as illustrated in Chapter 3, may be used to assess levels of perceived pain. The patient points or verbally expresses which face indicates his or her current level of pain. Each face has a corresponding verbal descriptor and numeral indicating pain intensity. Numeric rating of pain is also common for older pediatric patients, with a scale of 1–10 used most frequently. For children younger than 3 years old or for nonverbal patients, the **FLACC Nonverbal Pain Scale** is more appropriate and provides a pain rating system based on observable behaviors. The therapist might also use a scale based on observable behaviors indicating pain or stress, such as the **Observation Scale of Behavioral Distress** (OSBD). Other methods may provide qualitative information regarding the patient's pain experience, such as the Loewy, MacGregor, Richards, and Rodriguez (1997) Qualitative Color Pain Scale, in which pediatric patients use crayons on line-drawn human figures to color in the areas where they feel pain. In addition to any qualitative pain measures chosen, the music therapist is encouraged to adopt the quantitative pain measurement scale currently used by his or her facility's nursing staff in order to be consistent with treatment team standards.

Occasionally inpatient hematology/oncology patients may have their vital signs continuously monitored. In such cases, a music therapist can evaluate changes in physiological variables such as heart rate, respiratory rate, oxygen saturation levels, and blood pressure by periodically looking at the patient's vital sign monitors. Stable decreases in heart rate and respiratory rate may indicate an improved relaxation response. Conversely, increases in heart rate in response to music may indicate that a patient is stimulated by the auditory stimuli. When music therapy is used as procedural support for hematology/oncology patients undergoing medical procedures, changes in the level of required sedatives or analgesia may serve as a physiological measure of intervention effectiveness.

Outcomes of music therapy intervention should be documented in a way that is consistent with the protocol for other members of the treatment team. Music therapy services may be documented in a patient's chart under the ancillary services or clinical notes section where social workers, child life specialists, physical/occupational/speech therapists, and chaplains enter notes. A music therapist may observe the documentation methods of these related disciplines and create a progress note format that matches the writing style and content of these disciplines to facilitate ease in interdisciplinary communication. The music therapist aims to convey to the treatment team the goals of music therapy intervention; the methods employed; and specific, objective patient responses indicating attainment of or progress towards the stated goals. Progress notes should also contain further recommendations, including continuation of current treatment plan, revision or addition of new goals and objectives, referral for additional services, or recommendation for discharge (Scalenghe & Murphy, 2000). Notes should be of a level of detail similar to other related disciplines and should generally avoid profession-specific jargon. A sample Pediatric Hematology/Oncology Music Therapy Progress Note is presented below.

Sample Music Therapy Progress Note
Pediatric Hematology/Oncology Unit

Date: 10/10/04
Time: 3:00 pm

A. is a 14-year-old male with history of **aplastic anemia** of unknown etiology, upper and lower GI varices with recurrent bleeds, pulmonary HTN, bicuspid AV (s/p VSD repair), hypothyroidism, fused kidneys, and history of multiple UTIs. Pt. is well known to writer from previous inpatient admissions and from weekly outpatient clinic visits.

A. has received music therapy services for social support during platelet transfusions at outpatient clinic approximately 1x/month since 3/20/03 and has been followed most recently during current inpatient admission of 9/20/04 to facilitate improved expressive communication, increase peer support, and assess pt.'s coping with deteriorating medical status. During 30-minute individual and small group music therapy sessions at bedside, pt. has engaged in verbal communication, expressed emotions during music making, and engaged in developmentally appropriate music making with peers. Pt. has demonstrated improved peer social interactions in music sessions and during child life programming as evidenced by increased frequency of interaction, improved verbal communication with peers, and the display of positive affect when with peers. Pt. is able to express aggravations, anger, boredom, and fears related to treatment regimen and hospitalization during individual music and verbal interactions with writer.

Pt. is making progress towards stated goals as demonstrated by increase in frequency of verbal and nonverbal communication during sessions and improvement in the quality of peer interactions. Pt. has not yet addressed his deteriorating health status directly with writer, but writer plans to be available to support this communication when pt. is ready. Recommend continued MT sessions 1x/wk to facilitate ongoing emotional expression related to illness and hospitalization with goal of enabling pt. to positively cope with deteriorating health status.

Due to time constraints, it may not be possible for the music therapist to complete individual charting. The therapist may need to devise a system for charting based on prioritized needs. These may include significant positive therapeutic outcomes, definitive negative or unusual responses, or concerns for follow-up care from other professionals. Depending upon the requirements of the facility, therapists may be asked to chart on all patients, which would necessitate time in the therapist's schedule to complete the task.

Upon discharge, a multidisciplinary form is completed by a nurse and includes the patient's current status and instructions for follow-up care post discharge. Music therapists may include information if follow-up music therapy services are recommended, and they typically include a summary of goals addressed, an overview of progress, and recommendations for future goals.

Qualities of Music Therapists Needed for the Hem/Onc Setting

Though outcomes for pediatric patients have improved given recent treatment advances, death remains a possibility for many patients, and becomes a probability for others. Music therapists who work in hematology/oncology settings serve as witnesses to the physical, mental, and emotional changes a patient endures during treatment for this potentially ravishing group of disorders, as well as to the frequent heartbreak experienced by families. Music therapists are bound to encounter events and interactions that challenge their very beliefs and values and are at-risk for experiencing burnout as a result of this emotionally taxing work. Kennelly (2001) recommends regular professional supervision for music therapists working with cancer patients, so that feelings, thoughts, and issues that arise for the therapist during intense sessions with the patient can be addressed to prevent them from inadvertently affecting the therapeutic process. Music therapists may also engage in staff support groups, individual psychotherapy, individual or group music making, or stress reduction and wellness programs to balance the stress and emotional toil of working with this challenging, but rewarding, population.

The Future of Music Therapy in Pediatric Hematology/Oncology

The development of music therapy programs in pediatric hematology/oncology settings may be realized by grants, endowments, or funds from the hospital budget. Grants may be research or clinical in nature and may require renewal on an annual basis. In one author's experience, music therapy was brought to the outpatient hematology/oncology clinic and to hem/onc patients on the inpatient pediatric unit by a grant awarded to the child life department. The child life coordinator submitted a proposal for music therapy services to a children's foundation and received a 1-year grant to fund a per diem music therapy position servicing the general pediatric inpatient unit, pediatric hematology/oncology clinic, pediatric intensive care unit, and pediatric patients in the burn center. Hematology/oncology patients receive music therapy services by referral on the inpatient pediatric unit at a maximum of three times per week, and the music therapist sees patients in the outpatient clinic once per week. The grant must be renewed on a yearly basis, and funds from the hospital budget have not been available. In the other author's experience, a grant that is renewable annually provides funding for a full-time pediatric inpatient music therapy position. In addition, hospital funds are also used to support another half-time music therapy position in pediatrics.

Preliminary research results support the use of music therapy with pediatric hematology/oncology patients, but significant additional research is needed to validate current clinical practices and identify potential areas for development. In an environment of managed care, music therapists will increasingly be called upon to demonstrate the medical necessity of the work they do. Additional research may help identify which interventions are most effective for particular diagnosis groups and particular phases of treatment. Further substantiating the use of music therapy to improve immune function will have direct implications for oncology patients who are immunosuppressed as a result of intensive treatments. As hematology/oncology patients often require frequent invasive procedures, continued empirical investigation into the effectiveness of music therapy to ease pain and anxiety during such procedures is imperative. Through a combination of research outcomes and clinical practice, music therapists must demonstrate the cost-effectiveness of their methods within the hospital setting in order for this valuable work to remain viable in a health care environment that is focused on cost-cutting. The responsibility lies with music therapy researchers, clinicians, and educators to assure that our services remain available to the patients who need these services the most.

References

American Heritage Dictionary of the English Language (4th ed.). (2000). Boston: Houghton Mifflin.

Barr, R. D., Crockett, M., Dawson, S., Eves, M., Whitton, A., & Wiernikowski, J. (2001). *Childhood cancer: Information for the patient and family* (2nd ed.). Hamilton, Ontario, Canada: BC Decker.

Barrera, M. E., Rykov, M. H., & Doyle, S. L. (2002). The effects of interactive music therapy on hospitalized children with cancer: A pilot study. *Psycho-Oncology, 11,* 379–388.

Barrickman, J. (1989). A developmental approach for preschool hospitalized children. *Music Therapy Perspectives, 7,* 10–17.

Bertolone, K. (1997). Pediatric oncology: Past, present, and new modalities of treatment. *Journal of Intravenous Nursing, 20*(3), 136–140.

Brodsky, W. (1989). Music therapy as an intervention for children with cancer in isolation rooms. *Music Therapy, 8,* 17–34.

Clinton, P. K. (1984). *Music as a nursing intervention for children during painful procedures.* Unpublished master's thesis, The University of Iowa, Iowa City.

Corrigan, J. J., & Feig, S. A. (American Academy of Pediatrics). (2004). Guidelines for pediatric cancer centers. *Pediatrics, 113,* 1833–1835.

D'Alessandro D., & Huth, L. (2002a). *Anemia*. Virtual Children's Hospital: Pediatrics Common Questions, Quick Answers. Retrieved August 22, 2004, from http://www.vh.org/pediatric/patient/pediatrics/cqqa/anemia.html

D'Alessandro D., & Huth, L. (2002b). *Hemophilia*. Virtual Children's Hospital: Pediatrics Common Questions, Quick Answers. Retrieved August 22, 2004, from http://www.vh.org/pediatric/patient/pediatrics/cqqa/hemophilia.html

D'Alessandro D., & Kinzer, S. (2004). *Childhood leukemia*. Virtual Children's Hospital: Common Questions, Quick Answers: Pediatrics. Retrieved October 2, 2004, from http://www.vh.org/pediatric/patient/pediatrics/cqqa/leukemia.html

Daveson, B. A. (2001). Music therapy and childhood cancer: Goals, methods, patient choice and control during diagnosis, intensive treatment, transplant and palliative care. *Music Therapy Perspectives, 19*(2), 114–120.

Dun, B. (1995). A different beat: Music therapy in children's cardiac care. *Music Therapy Perspectives, 13*, 35–39.

Fagen, T. S. (1982). Music therapy in the treatment of anxiety and fear in terminal pediatric patients. *Music Therapy, 2*(1), 13–23.

Hadley, S. J. (1996). A rationale for the use of songs with children undergoing bone marrow transplantation. *The Australian Journal of Music Therapy, 7*, 16–27.

Kennelly, J. (2001). Music therapy in the bone marrow transplant unit: Providing emotional support during adolescence. *Music Therapy Perspectives, 19*, 104–108.

Krout, R. E. (2000). Hospice and palliative music therapy: A continuum of creative caring. In D. S. Smith (Ed.), *Effectiveness of music therapy procedures: Documentation of research and clinical practice* (pp. 323–411). Silver Spring, MD: American Music Therapy Association.

Kruse, J. (2003). Music therapy in United States cancer settings: Recent trends in practice. *Music Therapy Perspectives, 21*, 89–98.

Lane, D. (1996). Music therapy interventions with pediatric oncology patients. In M. A. Froehlich (Ed.), *Music therapy with hospitalized children: A creative arts child life approach* (pp. 109–116). Cherry Hill, NJ: Jeffrey Books.

Lane, D., & Olness, K. (1991). The effect of a single music therapy session on hospitalized children as measured by salivary immunoglobulin A, speech pause time, and a patient opinion Likert scale. *Pediatric Research, 29*(4, part 2), 11A.

Ledger, A. (2001). Song parody for adolescents with cancer. *The Australian Journal of Music Therapy, 12*, 21–28.

Leukemia & Lymphoma Society. (2001). *Emotional aspects of childhood leukemia: A handbook for parents*. New York: Author.

Loewy, J. V., MacGregor, B., Richards, K., & Rodriguez, J. (1997). Music therapy pediatric pain management: Assessing and attending to the sounds of hurt, fear, and anxiety. In J. V. Loewy (Ed.), *Music therapy and pediatric pain* (pp. 45–56). Cherry Hill, NJ: Jeffrey Books.

Magill, L., Coyle, N., Handzo, G., & Loscalzo, M. (1997). Cancer and pain: A creative, multidisciplinary approach in working with patients and families. In J. V. Loewy, (Ed.), *Music therapy and pediatric pain* (pp. 107–114). Cherry Hill, NJ: Jeffrey Books.

Miller, J. A., McMillan, S. K., Chavez, R., & Giller, R. H. (1993). *Sickle cell trait*. Virtual Children's Hospital: Pediatrics. Retrieved August 22, 2004, from http://www.vh.org/pediatric/patient/pediatrics/faq/sicklecell.html

National Institutes of Health (NIH). (1993). *Young people with cancer: A handbook for parents* (No. 93-2378). Bethesda, MD: National Cancer Institute.

National Institutes of Health (NIH). (2001). *Young people with cancer: A handbook for parents* (No. 04-2378). Bethesda, MD: National Cancer Institute.

Parmet, S., Lynm, C., & Glass, R. M. (2004). JAMA patient page. Childhood leukemia. *Journal of the American Medical Association, 291*, 514.

Patenaude, A. F., & Last, B. (2001). Cancer and children: Where are we coming from? Where are we going? *Psycho-Oncology, 10*, 281–283.

Pearson, H. A. (2002). History of pediatric hematology oncology. *Pediatric Research, 52*, 979–992.

Pfaff, V., Smith, K., & Gowan, D. (1989). The effects of music-assisted relaxation on the distress of pediatric cancer patients undergoing bone marrow aspirations. *Children's Health Care, 18*(4), 232–236.

Quinn, G., & Petitgout, J. (1998). *Bone marrow transplant*. Virtual Children's Hospital: Pediatric bone marrow transplant: a guide for families. Retrieved September 28, 2004, from http://www.vh.org/pediatric/patient/pediatrics/bonemarrowtransplant/bmt.html

Robb, S. L. (2000). The effect of therapeutic music interventions on the behavior of hospitalized children in isolation: Developing a contextual support model of music therapy. *Journal of Music Therapy, 37*, 118–147.

Robb, S. L. (2003a). Coping and chronic illness: Music therapy for children and adolescents with cancer. In S. L. Robb (Ed.), *Music therapy in pediatric healthcare: Research and evidence-based practice* (pp. 101–136). Silver Spring, MD: American Music Therapy Association.

Robb, S. L. (2003b). Designing music therapy interventions for hospitalized children and adolescents using a contextual support model of music therapy. *Music Therapy Perspectives, 21*, 27–40.

Robb, S. L., & Ebberts, A. G. (2003a). Songwriting and digital video production interventions for pediatric patients undergoing bone marrow transplantation, part I: An analysis of depression and anxiety levels according to phase of treatment. *Journal of Pediatric Oncology Nursing, 20*(1), 2–15.

Robb, S. L., & Ebberts, A. G. (2003b). Songwriting and digital video production interventions for pediatric patients undergoing bone marrow transplantation, part II: An analysis of patient-generated songs and patient perceptions regarding intervention efficacy. *Journal of Pediatric Oncology Nursing, 20*(1), 16–25.

Sahler, O. J., Hunter, B. C. & Liesveld, J. L. (2003). The effect of using music therapy with relaxation imagery in the management of patients undergoing bone marrow transplantation: A pilot feasibility study. *Alternative Therapies, 9*, 70–74.

Scalenghe, R., & Murphy, K. M. (2000). Music therapy assessment in the managed care environment. *Music Therapy Perspectives, 18*(1), 23–30.

Schur, J. M. (1986). *Alleviating behavioral distress with music or Lamaze pant-blow breathing in children undergoing bone marrow aspirations and lumbar punctures.* Unpublished doctoral dissertation. The University of Texas Health Science Center at Dallas, Dallas, TX.

Schwankovsky, L. M., & Guthrie, P. T. (1982). *Music therapy for handicapped children: Other health impaired.* NAMT Monograph Series. Washington, DC: National Association for Music Therapy.

Schwartz, C. L. (1999). Long-term survivors of childhood cancer: The late effects of therapy. *The Oncologist, 4*, 45–54.

Standley, J. M., & Whipple, J. (2003). Music therapy with pediatric patients: A meta analysis. In S. L. Robb (Ed.), *Music therapy in pediatric healthcare: Research and evidence-based practice* (pp. 1–18). Silver Spring, MD: American Music Therapy Association.

Stewart, S.K. (1992). *The nuts and bolts of bone marrow transplants.* BMT Newsletter. Retrieved September 8, 2004, from http://cpmcnet.columbia.edu/dept/medicine/bonemarrow/bmtinfo.html

Turry, A., & Turry, A. E. (1999). Creative song improvisations with children and adults with cancer. In C. Dileo (Ed.), *Music therapy and medicine: Theoretical and clinical applications* (pp. 167–177). Silver Spring, MD: American Music Therapy Association.

Youngerman-Cole, S. (2004). *Stem cell transplant (bone marrow transplant).* Healthwise Health Guide A–Z. Retrieved September 8, 2004, from http://my.webmd.com/hw/health_guide_atoz/tv7001.asp

CHAPTER 6

Pediatric Burn Recovery: Acute Care, Rehabilitation and Reconstruction[1]

Christine Tuden Neugebauer

Introduction

One would not argue that sustaining a severe burn is one of the most devastating, traumatic, painful, and life-altering injuries one could possibly experience. According to the 2004 National SAFE KIDS Campaign (NSKC), burn injuries are the fourth most common cause of accidental death in both children and adults each year. In 2002, an estimated 92,500 children ages 14 and under were treated for burn-related injuries. Of these injuries, thermal or flame burns were the most prevalent, with scald, chemical, and electrical burns following sequentially (NSKC, 2004).

Although house fires and flame injuries can strike any age group, there are developmental differences when comparing pediatric age groups with causes of burns. Statistical analysis from NSKC (2004) shows that infants and toddlers are most susceptible to bathtub scalds or kitchen-related accidents such as tipping a pot of boiling water from the stove. Unfortunately, child protective services cases related to abuse or lack of supervision are also more common for this age group. Preschool-aged children tend to have flame burn injuries from playing with lighters and matches or from accidents such as falling into barbecue pits or fireplaces. School-aged children, particularly males, have an increased probability of participating in at-risk behaviors such as fire play, playing with gasoline, or lighting fireworks without supervision. Finally, adolescents may sustain a burn-related injury from automobile accidents or from peer-group interactions involving gasoline or drug use. NSKC further reports that electrical burn injuries are more common in males at this age due to higher risk behavior such as climbing or hanging out near utility poles/high voltage equipment. Overall, children

---

[1] This chapter is dedicated to music therapist Mary Toombs Rudenberg for her distinct role in bringing music therapy into the lives and recovery process of children with burn injuries. Her support and encouragement has been most appreciated, and her continued guidance has been invaluable.

are considered a higher risk population for sustaining a burn injury when compared to adults (Pruitt, Mason, & Goodwin, 1990).

Since it opened in March of 1966, Shriners Burns Hospital for Children in Galveston, Texas, has been providing medical care free of charge to children with severe burn injuries. The philanthropic mission of this Shrine hospital includes providing comprehensive treatment during all phases of burn recovery, including acute clinical care, intensive rehabilitation, and reconstructive care. The hospital maintains an affiliation with its neighboring facility, the University of Texas Medical Branch (UTMB), so that it can better carry out its principal objectives of treatment, research, and teaching. The primary healthcare team consists of the following disciplines: general surgery (burns, orthopedics, and plastics); anesthesiology; nursing; respiratory therapy; microbiology; occupational and physical therapy; exercise physiology; nutrition; social work; care coordination; psychology; psychiatry; child life; and music therapy. This chapter will provide an extensive overview of and rationale for the music therapy program as it is currently practiced at the Shriners Burns Hospital–Galveston (SBH-G). While SBH-G is a specialty hospital, music therapists can apply the concepts, methods, and processes illustrated in this chapter to other settings where the burn treatment services may be integrated within the facility (e.g., a specialty unit in a pediatric or general hospital).

Overview of Music Therapy Services

Currently, the music therapy program at SBH-G offers individual, group, and co-treatment services to patients in all stages of recovery on both an inpatient and outpatient basis. In addition to its 30-inpatient-bed facility, SBH-G also has an extensive residential outpatient treatment program where patients requiring intensive rehabilitation or other long-term medical needs come daily for treatments. Of these residential outpatients, some reside in the in-hospital apartments, while others reside in nearby apartments or at local charity housing facilities. The residential outpatients are seen daily for various treatments until they are ready for discharge home. The Shrine organization is both international and philanthropic; therefore, many patients at SBH-G come from countries outside of the United States, such as Mexico. As a result, a significant number of patients are Spanish-speaking only. Cultural considerations and issues are part of the music therapy assessment process and sessions are conducted in the child's primary language when possible. Length of stay is dependent upon many factors including size, location and depth of the burn, medical complications, rehabilitation needs, and access to medical resources available in the community where the child resides.

At this time, recommendations for music therapy services are determined upon verbal referrals from physicians, nurses, psychologists, case coordinators, and occupational and physical therapists. As an active participant of the multidisciplinary team, the music therapist will also identify patients who may benefit from services based upon information received from team rounds and patient-care meetings. Clinical issues that most often warrant music therapy referrals include inability to effectively cope with pain and anxiety (both background and procedure-related), emotional withdrawal, need for neurological or developmental stimulation, reinforcement of active and functional range-of-motion, increasing patient motivation to actively participate in recovery, and decreasing parental stress interfering with positive parent–child interaction. Also, patients aged 6 and under with burns covering over 40% of their total body surface area (TBSA) are automatically referred to participate in a supplemental music and exercise program upon beginning their rehabilitation phase of recovery. An overview of this specific program is discussed later in this chapter.

Referral Criteria for Pediatric Burn Patients

- Inability to effectively cope with pain and anxiety
- Experiencing emotional withdrawal
- Need for neurological or developmental stimulation
- Reinforcement of active and functional range-of-motion
- Increasing patient motivation for active participation in recovery
- Improving positive parent–child interaction

Upon admission, the family plays a vital role throughout the child's recovery process. Thus, family-centered care is an integral component of the treatment philosophy at SBH-G. Family involvement and active participation are highly encouraged with respect and consideration to each family's unique cultural background, coping styles, and family dynamics. The music therapy service also incorporates a family-centered care approach during the treatment process. Due to the fundamental impact of the burn injury on the entire family, an overview of family and caregiver involvement during music therapy services will be discussed at each stage of recovery. There are three phases of recovery from a burn injury: acute, rehabilitation, and reconstructive. This chapter will address the treatment process of music therapy for each phase.

Acute Phase

Sustaining a severe burn injury not only is traumatic but has the potential to be a life-changing experience for both the victim and family. The injury most often occurs suddenly and unexpectedly. Initial survival critically depends upon the emergency management and treatment at the moment of injury. Emergency treatment includes assessment at the scene, wound assessment, and fluid resuscitation (Herndon, 2002). At SBH-G, a newly burned patient is transported to the intensive care unit via air or ground transport after the patient has been treated at an emergency facility and a referral has been arranged for transfer. Although

SBH-G does not have an emergency room, most patients are transferred within the first 24-hours of injury. For patients from outside the United States, transfer from the referring hospital may take longer than 24 hours, depending upon many extraneous factors.

During the acute phase of treatment, the body rapidly adapts to the injury, thus causing many physiological changes. Patients with severe burns are at high risk for experiencing shock and **edema**, which increases their risk for organ or other systematic failures. Inhalation injuries will further increase their risk for respiratory insufficiency and, as a result, **mechanical ventilation** may be required (Herndon, 2002). The first days and weeks following a severe injury are about survival, and the larger the injury, the higher the risk of mortality. However, over the past 10–20 years, outcome studies in burn research as well as improvements in specialized burn care have resulted in the significantly increased chance of survival for patients with large burns (greater than 40% of their total body surface area or TBSA). Nevertheless, recovery from a severe burn is an extensive process that can be emotionally as well as physically traumatic in itself.

The child with severe burns may undergo numerous operative procedures until all the wounds have been covered and healed. Surgical interventions involve **debridement** and **excision** of the dead tissue, wound closure using skin grafting techniques, and sometimes amputations of digits and limbs that have been fully destroyed or have no potential for recovery (Herndon, 2002). Because a vital role of skin is to prevent infections, covering the burn wounds with skin grafts or other temporary skin substitutes while the wounds are healing is critically important. Skin grafts include **autograft** from donor sites (the patient's own unburned/healthy skin), homograft (tissue from cadavers), cultured skin (skin grown in a laboratory from the patient's own cells), and artificial skin substitutes (which provide a temporary covering as donor sites heal). Length of stay on the burn unit will depend on many variables, including the depth, localization, and size of the burn, and can range from a few days to several months (Munster, 1993).

In addition to surgical intervention, many burn patients will attain their nutritional needs via a **nasogastric tube**, since adequate nutritional support is essential to successful recovery. In cases of severe burn injury, the body enters a hypermetabolic state, which causes a significant increase in energy expenditure and accelerated metabolism of protein and other nutrients (Herndon, 2002). Due to the need to monitor nutritional intake and metabolic state, restriction of fluid intake (such as no water by mouth) is necessary. Restricting fluid intake commonly results in increased distress as patients' anxiety escalates when requests for water are denied until they are medically ready. When the child is able to begin eating and drinking, milk or other high-caloric nutritional supplements are given instead of water, since water has no caloric value. This strict fluid intake poses a substantial psychological challenge to patients who will often perseverate in their request for water.

Level of consciousness the first few days to weeks on the burn ICU will vary for each patient. Some children, even with severe burns, are surprisingly alert and interactive early upon their admission, while others may be disoriented, agitated, sedated, or comatose. Some patients will require mechanical ventilation due to smoke inhalation or other respiratory complications. In some cases, a child may sustain neurological damage from an anoxic brain injury caused from a cardiac arrest. In these situations, techniques from the neurological music therapy model, such as musical sensory orientation training, should be applied.

Music Therapy and Pain Modulation

Pain is more than a stimulus-response reaction of our nervous system. It is a highly complex perception with multiple and interrelated dimensions that are uniquely experienced by each individual. According to the International Association for the Study of Pain, pain is defined as "an unpleasant sensory and emotional experience associated with actual or potential tissue damage, or described in terms of such damage" (Merskey & Bogduk, 1994). Pain is also a subjective experience and includes sensory, emotional, and cognitive components, as well as the impact of personality traits on those components (Goubert, Crombez, & Van Damme, 2003; Neugebauer & Neugebauer, 2003).

Several clinical studies in the music therapy field have found music effective in pain reduction (Barrera, Rykov, & Doyle, 2002; Kenny & Faunce, 2004; Krout, 2001). Other clinical studies using music listening alone further support the premise that music, in itself, has **analgesic** properties that can facilitate coping and pain reduction for various medical procedures and conditions (Aragon, Farris, & Byers, 2002; Good, Anderson, Stanton-Hicks, Grass, & Makii, 2002; Phumdoung & Good, 2003; Voss et al., 2004). Further research has shown music listening to reduce the dosage of pain medication or sedation required postoperatively or during invasive procedures (Koch, Kain, Ayoub, & Rosenbaum, 1998; Lee et al., 2002; Lepage, Drolet, Girard, Grenier, & DeGagne, 2001; Nilsson, Rawal, Enqvist, & Unosson, 2003). Even under conditions where one is not consciously aware of hearing the music, such as under general anesthesia, patients who listened to music intra-operatively have been shown to require one third less pain medication as compared to patients not listening to music intra-operatively, and they may be mobilized sooner with less fatigue upon discharge (Lewis, Osborn & Roth, 2004; Nilsson, Rawal, Unestahl, Zetterberg, & Unosson, 2001).

Despite these findings, an understanding as to how music modulates pain perception along the pain **neuraxis** remains a mystery. One possibility may be the impact of music on an area of the brain known as the amygdala. The amygdala is part of the limbic system and plays a key role in emotional-affective aspects of behavior as well as the emotional evaluation of sensory stimuli (Aggleton, 2000). In regards to pain perception, the amygdala has been shown to play a significant function in modulating the emotional-affective component of pain in an excitatory as well as inhibitory way (Neugebauer, Li, Bird, & Han, 2004). Perhaps music's effectiveness in pain relief may involve this specific pain center in the emotional brain (Neugebauer & Neugebauer, 2003). Decreased activation of the **nociceptive** amygdala may inhibit the descending processes involved in facilitating pain perception. Intensely pleasurable music may have the ability to inhibit activation of the amygdala that may give a hint as to music's beneficial effect on pain management (Blood & Zatorre, 2001).

The potential of music's capacity to manipulate this particular brain area is significant when considering the negative emotional state that may result from the ongoing pain experienced after a severe burn injury. Although burn pain is most often classified as nociceptive pain (pain caused by damage to tissue outside the nervous system), it is important to recognize that peripheral neuropathic pain (pain caused by damage to the nervous system) may also exist if the burn has resulted in limb or digit amputation. Phantom limb pain, a type of neuropathic pain, results from damage to the nervous system and may involve a burning or squeezing sensation in the nonexistent extremity (Stoddard et al., 2002). Nociceptive pain caused by a severe burn is persistent and prolonged, which causes the neurons responsible for pain processing to become sensitized. This sensitization of nociceptive and **dorsal** neurons in the peripheral and central nervous systems, respectively, increases responsiveness to noxious stimuli, thus increasing their ability to activate and transmit signals at a lower threshold. **Hyperalgesia** is the term to describe this abnormal pain sensation. The enhanced response and increased excitability of the nociceptive neurons creates a vicious communication cycle between the ascending and descending pain pathways present in the nervous system. Furthermore, the neurohormonal stress response that occurs from severe tissue injury can have adverse effects on immune function as well as the muscular-skeletal system (Stoddard et al., 2002).

The importance of adequate pain management throughout the burn healing process is critical for optimum recovery. Poor pain management may correlate with long-term deleterious psychological effects, thus potentially worsening symptoms associated with posttraumatic stress disorder (PTSD) (Stoddard et al., 2002). The dosage of morphine has been associated with a decreased reduction in development of PTSD over a 6-month period (Saxe et al., 2001). However, pharmacological management of burn pain cannot completely ameliorate pain sensation.

Using music as a supplemental treatment for pain can be an important therapeutic tool in targeting the emotional and cognitive components of pain by inhibiting the descending mechanisms that exacerbate pain perception. Although it is not yet clear how music modulates pain perception, music's ability to manipulate cognitive and affective reactions may influence descending pain pathways associated with attention and mood. Once pain messages are received and processed in the brain areas linked to the pain neuraxis, descending modulating pathways relay messages back to the spinal cord (Price & Bushnell, 2004). Psychological mechanisms such as attention, cognitive appraisal, and affective response are more than just a byproduct of pain intensity. Basic science continues to reveal how psychological processes impact descending pain pathways involved in pain intensity, pain threshold, and pain coping (Bushnell, Villemure & Duncan, 2004; Tracey et al., 2002).

Scientific understanding of the musical processes in the brain is a relatively new field in neuroscience. It has been proposed that both widespread and bilateral networks appear to be involved in music processing, including areas related to pitch, rhythm, timing, memory, and emotion (Peretz & Zatorre, 2005). Developing an understanding of the impact of music therapy on mechanisms involved in pain modulation will begin when researchers identify brain areas of the pain neuraxis that overlap with music processing. Until then, music therapists must extrapolate information related to pain processing and modulation from other fields, such as neuroscience and psychology, as well as from clinical research studies on music and pain.

Studies on Music and Burn Pain

Relatively few quantitative studies exist concerning the effects of music and music therapy on burn pain. Most of the studies concern the use of music in easing pain during debridement and dressing changes, which are both routine treatments that present a significant pain management challenge. A study with adult burn patients compared active music listening with a technique called sensory focusing, which taught patients to focus and monitor changes in their pain sensation. Interestingly, the sensory focusing intervention group reported greater pain relief than the music distraction group, which did not appear to have any beneficial effects (Haythornthwaite, Lawrence, & Fauerbach, 2001). An earlier study using scenic videos with musical accompaniment showed a significant reduction in both pain and anxiety during dressing changes (Miller, Hickman, & Lemasters, 1992). Another study using music-based imagery and musical alternate engagement, facilitated by a music therapist, revealed a significant reduction in pain intensity under the music therapy condition. This study included adults and children over the age of 7 years who sustained an average burn size of 9.96% of their TBSA (Fratianne et al., 2001).

In regards to severe burns, specifically burns greater than 40% TBSA, providing adequate pain management becomes increasingly difficult as coping resources become quickly exhausted. Music therapy research for this challenging population is essential in order to provide the most effective applications of music. In addition to procedural pain management, studies should also explore coping with background pain. Moreover, evaluating the effectiveness of music therapy interventions according to age and developmental level (e.g., infants vs. adolescents) will further enhance the development of best practice methods.

Music Therapy Applications on the Pediatric Burn Intensive Care Unit

In this early stage of injury, the music therapist should first review the child's medical chart with particular attention to the cause of burn, localization of burn wounds, and psychosocial concerns (e.g., whether others were injured or killed in the accident, identifying the current guardian accompanying the child, any other sustained losses in the fire). Next, the music therapist should establish a positive working relationship with the child's parent or guardian and gather information about the child's pre-burn history (family status, growth and development) as well as previous experiences in the hospital setting. As part of the assessment process, it is important to ask questions about the child's coping responses to pain and stress, the child's previous play and recreational activities, as well as the child's musical exposure and interests.

During this initial phase, primary treatment concerns to address through music therapy include fostering skills to cope with trauma, to cope with pain and anxiety, to facilitate

---

Assessment for Pediatric Burn Treatment

- Review medical chart for cause of burn, location of wounds, and psychosocial concerns

- Establish a positive relationship with child's parent(s) or guardian(s)

- Gather information about pre-burn history and previous hospital experiences

- Determine child's coping responses to pain and stress, previous play and recreational activities, and musical interests and experiences

- Assess response to, and coping strategies with, pain

- Determine family coping and interaction style with child

- Re-assess at subsequent phases of treatment

---

positive caregiver interactions with the patient, as well as to reinforce early physical rehabilitation needs (Neugebauer & Neugebauer, 2003). Most music therapy sessions will occur at the child's bedside. Having the parent or guardian present during the initial sessions is highly recommended in order to more easily establish trust with the child. It is natural and expected that parents feel overwhelmed, uncomfortable, and uncertain about how to interact with their newly injured child. The music therapist can model appropriate behavior and provide alternative ways to engage and respond to the child's emotional needs while creating a supportive atmosphere to promote positive parent–child interaction. For many parents, music therapy sessions have provided an opportunity for them to see their child smile and interact normally for the first time since the injury occurred. Actively including family members as part of the healing process can provide them with an increased sense of control and strengthen depleted coping responses.

M. was an 8-year-old boy from Mexico whose parents were also injured and being treated at another hospital located in Mexico. M.'s uncle was the accompanying guardian and was having difficulty adjusting to the increased responsibility of caring for his injured nephew. During the first music therapy session, the uncle initiated a request to borrow the music therapist's guitar. He then began to strum the guitar and sing a traditional song to his nephew. For the first time, M. and his uncle were able to connect with one another as family and strengthen their bond through singing traditional songs of their country. The music provided a normalcy and comfort that had previously been missing. The music therapist supported this interaction by providing hand-over-hand assistance for M. to play the tambourine in accompaniment to the uncle's guitar playing. The uncle was able to borrow a guitar from the music therapy program for the remainder of M.'s admission on the ICU.

Evaluating the child's pain response is integral to developing appropriate treatment interventions. The American Pain Society (Benjamin et al., 1999) purports pain assessment to ascertain pain status, develop treatment strategies, and measure the effectiveness of those strategies. Burn pain can be assessed as either background pain or procedural pain. Background pain refers to the ongoing pain experienced while the child is at rest and not receiving any invasive treatments or procedures. Conversely, procedural pain concerns the pain sensations associated with procedures (wound dressing changes, staple/suture removals, debridement and wound cleaning, physical and occupational therapy sessions) that are often routine treatments necessary in burn care. Background pain is associated with lower pain intensity for a longer duration of time, whereas procedural pain may induce higher pain sensitivity but for a shorter duration of time (Martin-Herz, Thurber, & Patterson, 2000). In conducting pain assessments, it is important to evaluate the patient's pain intensity for both background and procedural pain. Many assessment tools exist to rapidly measure the sensory-discriminative component of pain.

For music therapists, pain assessment should measure more than pain intensity alone. In addition to the patient's self-report of pain, music therapists should monitor physiological responses such as heart rate, respiration rate, and blood pressure, as well as observe overt behaviors including mood, affect, and activity level. Most patients on the intensive care unit will have vital signs, such as heart rate and blood pressure, continuously displayed on the monitors at their bedside. Observing the patient's ability to engage in pleasant and meaningful activities will provide insight as to the coping style and degree of tolerability the child has for background pain. Another important area to monitor is the interaction between the child and caregiver. Studies have shown that the parent's level of anxiety and coping response may positively or negatively impact the child's coping behavior (Daviss et al., 2000; LeDoux, Meyer, Blakeney, & Herndon, 1998). With support and education, parents can play a key role in reducing their child's pain via active involvement and participation during procedures and role modeling effective coping behavior (George & Hancock, 1993).

Despite adequate pharmacological treatment, patients often experience pain on a daily basis, which increases their risk for long-term deleterious effects associated with persistent pain, such as depression (Geisser, Robinson, Keefe, & Weiner, 1994; Neugebauer et al., 2004). In burn recovery, pharmacological management of both background and procedural pain can be supplemented with music therapy to enhance coping. The primary areas to address clinically for background pain are improving positive affect and increasing ability to attend to pleasant and normalized activities. Research has shown a significant connection between negative affect and decreased tolerance for pain (Goubert et al., 2003; Gracely et al., 2004). Moreover, increased attention to pain can increase perception of pain intensity (Levine, Gordon, Smith, & Fields, 1982), whereas distraction from pain can increase pain tolerance and pain threshold (McCaul & Haugtvedt, 1982).

Music therapy techniques on the burn ICU should integrate both emotional and cognitive components to best target the overall coping response of the patient. Neugebauer and Neugebauer (2003) apply the contextual support model of music therapy developed by Robb (2000) to pediatric burn care. Music therapy interventions (such as active music engagement) that incorporate the elements of structure, autonomy, and involvement can enhance the coping process and can be adapted according to the child's developmental level and physical status. Because the burn-injured child experiences daily procedures that are often painful and traumatic in themselves, music therapy sessions may be one of the few times during the day when the child can assert control and safely express thoughts and feelings within a supportive context.

There are several specific cognitive-behavioral techniques that can be applied in situations associated with persistent pain states (Waters, Campbell, Keefe, & Carson, 2004). Pleasant activity scheduling, cognitive restructuring, and distraction are all techniques that can be adapted and integrated into music therapy sessions on the pediatric burn ICU. Pleasant activity scheduling refers to a systematic approach of increasing the frequency and duration of the patient's involvement in activities that are normalizing and pleasant and that elicit positive affective responses. For pediatric burn patients, an initial goal may be to increase the child's ability to actively participate in and attend to music activities from durations of 5 minutes to 15 minutes. Facilitating the child's involvement in pleasant and meaningful activities through music may then become effective coping methods for later treatments.

D. was a 5-year-old girl who sustained third degree burns over 80% of her body. Despite the fact that D. was hanging in traction from all four extremities, she was highly alert and oriented. During early music therapy sessions, D. sang her favorite songs as the therapist accompanied her on the guitar. As sessions progressed, she tolerated longer periods of activity and initiated directing her mother and sometimes her nurse to play percussion instruments to accompany D. as she sang. Later, music therapy was incorporated during her physical therapy sessions as D. began standing and ambulating. The first time she stood, D. swayed her body in rhythm (trying to dance) as the music therapist sang her favorite song while strumming an autoharp.

Music therapy sessions on the acute burn unit should allow much opportunity for choice and control. However, the therapist should also be aware as to not overwhelm the child by providing too many choices. Initially, the music therapist should offer only simple choices, perhaps choosing which storybook song from two options, and observe the child's decision-making process. Gradually increasing the number of options and difficulty level of specific musical interactions can be helpful in restoring the child's previous level of cognitive functioning by facilitating control over their situation.

Assessing the child's physical capabilities to actively participate is also important. Depending upon the location and severity of the injury, a child may be physically limited, thus inhibiting his or her active control over the environment. The ability to sustain attention to pleasant and normalizing activities may be highly limited due to the child's endurance level, degree of alertness, and/or coping response. The music therapist should identify what the patient can do both actively and passively and then gradually build on those strengths.

V. was a 16-year-old girl who sustained an electrical injury that resulted in the amputation of all her extremities. Opportunity for control was significantly limited with exception for the use of her voice. V.'s musical preference included songs sung by the singer Selena. Early music therapy sessions involved V. choosing songs to sing while the therapist accompanied her on guitar. Then, as V.'s recovery progressed, co-treatment with physical therapy was provided as a means to increase her endurance for weight bearing on her stumps using a tilt-table. V. chose songs for the music therapist to sing so she could listen and better tolerate the difficult exercise. Later in her recovery, V. used an adaptive splint made for her left upper extremity so that she could learn to play the melody of her favorite song on the electronic keyboard. Upon receiving her prosthetic arm, the splint was discontinued as V. began using her prosthesis to independently play the keyboard.

In addition to the initial traumatic event, hospitalization with continuous medical treatments can be a harrowing experience for the child. Trauma reactions, ongoing painful procedures, grief, separation from home and loved ones, and aversive hospital stimulation can all lead to symptoms of acute stress disorder (Daviss et al., 2000; Wintgens, Boileau, & Robaey, 1997). These symptoms may include nightmares, intrusive thoughts, flashbacks of the event, altered sleep patterns, flat affect, memory problems, social withdrawal, poor concentration, and exaggerated startle response (Daviss et al., 2000; Robert, Blakeney, Villareal, Rosenberg, & Meyer, 1999). Music can be an ideal tool in offering structure, control, and creative emotional expression to counter the deleterious cognitive and emotional chaos that often occurs after a traumatic event (Neugebauer & Neugebauer, 2003).

Assisting a child during a painful procedure requires an understanding of the child's coping style and, if possible, an understanding of the child's previous experiences with painful events. A child's coping style can range from complete avoidance (e.g., the child wanting to look away completely and dissociate from the removal of dressings) to full participation (e.g., the child wanting to physically assist in removing the dressings) (Martin-Herz et al., 2000). Classical and operant conditioning also play a role as the child's experiences and memories associated with prior medical procedures can either enhance or exacerbate pain tolerance and coping response. In addition, poor coping styles can inhibit effective wound care practices and prolong the treatment process (Thurber, Martin-Herz, & Patterson, 2000).

In using music with patients as a tool for coping with procedural anxiety and pain, Fanurik, Koh, Schmitz, and Brown (1997) provide a working model outlining four phases associated with medical procedures: anticipation phase, preparation phase, procedure phase, and recovery phase. Ideally, coping techniques should be utilized throughout all phases to elicit the most optimum outcome. The time period prior to the procedure is the anticipation phase. During this time, the therapist should establish a positive rapport with the child, learn of the child's expectations and perceptions of the procedure, and determine the coping techniques to include during the procedure. Depending on the developmental age and previous experience with the child, the music therapist may offer the child choices as to which instruments to bring or music to use during the procedure. Directly informing the child as to what he or she can and cannot do during the procedure can decrease feelings of insecurity and further enhance control (Smith, Doctor, & Boulter, 2004). Depending upon the situation, the anticipation phase may occur a day, hours, or minutes prior to the start of the procedure.

The next phase, preparation, involves the period of time immediately before the procedure when the child enters the treatment room, premedication is administered, and other preparations are made. It is generally during this time when the child's level of anxiety and distress begins to increase as the anticipation of the painful event becomes realized. Increased attention to the anticipated and unavoidable painful event may begin activation of pain-related areas of the brain, thus exacerbating pain perception when the noxious stimulus occurs (Bushnell, 2004). Consequently, anticipatory-related fear may increase pain intensity by priming specific regions along the pain neuraxis. Therefore, during this period, music therapists should facilitate the child's involvement in music activities that elicit positive affective responses and enhance the child's control over the situation. If the child needs to be positioned in a particular manner during the procedure, having the child "practice" the coping techniques in that specific position will further facilitate the coping process.

The invasive treatment period is characterized as the procedure phase (Fanurik et al., 1997). In burn care, some procedures, such as a bolster removal, may last only a few minutes. However, other procedures, such as wound debridement and **tubbing**, may take over an hour to complete. Depending upon the coping style and needs of the patient, music may or may not be utilized during this phase. For children demonstrating an avoidance method of coping, music may be used as a distraction technique, focusing attention solely on the musical stimulus. In cases where the child is an active observer or is actively assisting with the procedure, music can be used to positively reinforce the patient and promote a positive reframing of the experience. For example, improvising a song integrating phrases of encouragement during the procedure can give the child increased confidence to effectively cope during the experience. Regardless of the child's coping style, it is critical that the music therapist continuously monitors the child's response to the music and knows when it is appropriate to vary the music stimulus (in cases of habituation) or remove the music stimulus (in cases of overstimulation).

After completion of the procedure, it is important to help the child regain **homeostasis** during the final recovery phase (Fanurik et al., 1997). The music therapist may again engage the child in music activities that promote positive affect. The opportunity to recover from the stressful event may help the child to feel mastery over the situation and to recall coping strategies (Fanurik, et al., 1997). Improvising songs that use phrases emphasizing that the procedure is over and that highlight the child's observed strengths are helpful in establishing safety and reassurance. Parents are often present during procedures, although their roles may be that of observer, participant, or supporter. In burn care, parents often need to learn specific wound care techniques, and, therefore, are sometimes unable to provide adequate emotional support to their child during wound care procedures. The music therapist's presence in assisting the child with coping skills can provide parents some relief in having to manage these multiple roles they often need to assume.

Treatment Goals During the Acute Phase

- Foster coping skills related to the trauma, pain, and anxiety
- Facilitate positive parent(s) or guardian(s) and family interactions
- Promote emotional expression
- Reinforce physical rehabilitation
- Provide for normal, positive, and pleasant experiences
- Provide opportunities for choice and control
- Increase the child's ability to actively participate in and attend to music activities

Rehabilitation Phase

Although occupational and physical therapies are integral treatments during the acute phase, the most physically rigorous therapy begins after the patient's skin is fully covered and the child is discharged from the intensive care unit. Due to the risk of contractures, muscle loss, and tightening of the burn scars, burn rehabilitation is immediate and ongoing. Range of motion exercises, splinting, casting, and scar massage are common techniques used to prevent contractures and prevent orthopedic complications (Serghiou et al., 2002). Active range of motion exercises are also critical interventions for improving function and increasing strength and endurance. During this time, the patient on rehabilitation status has a demanding schedule of daily treatments. Patients continue to have daily tubbing sessions to keep wounds clean, monitor the skin for open areas, and treat/prevent infections. In addition, patients may receive daily physical and occupational therapy sessions; attend school; participate in a wellness/exercise program; receive psychological counseling; and have scheduled clinic appointments to monitor medications, wound healing, nutritional intake, weight, scar tissue, and other medical concerns.

Although parent involvement and education begins from the moment of admission, this change in hospital routine can be an overwhelming and stressful transition for both patient and family. The parent will now have a significant increase in responsibility in caring for the child, which may contribute to increased feelings of emotional distress or insecurity about their abilities to adequately care for their injured child. Parents become responsible not only for learning wound care, but also for administering medications; reinforcing range-of-motion exercises; and applying splints, pressure garments, or other necessary medical equipment. Compliance to medical treatments is critical during this phase and yet can be a common problem. It is also during this phase of recovery when parents and children become more aware of the potential impact this injury could have on their future quality of life. Because the initial crisis has subsided, the opportunity is made available to begin grieving losses and reflect upon the future on both an intellectual and emotional level.

Pain management also continues to be a challenge at this stage, primarily during physical and occupational therapy sessions. Pain is often due to edema or the stretching of grafted skin, which is often tight and dry. Intense itchiness of the newly healed skin is another common treatment issue at this stage and may further hinder the child's coping responses. Inadequate treatment of pain and itch may interfere with patients' motivation to actively participate in their rehabilitation program and may increase their chances to develop psychological symptoms such as depression and anxiety (Meyer, Marvin, Patterson, Thomas, & Blakeney, 2002). Treatment considerations for pain at this stage include pharmacological therapy and behavioral/cognitive therapy techniques. Developmental age of the patient must also be considered, since younger patients are more difficult to differentiate whether complaints are based upon fear and anxiety or pain sensations.

In addition to determining whether patients are accurately receiving their pain medications prior to painful treatments, pain and anxiety assessment should include observational assessment of the patient prior to, during, and after rehabilitation sessions. Robb (2003) mentions the role of attention, attentional bias, and attentional shift as possible mechanisms in helping patients better adapt to stressful events. Because music contains many elements to divide and sustain attention, music therapy intervention during procedures such as OT/PT sessions can certainly enhance coping responses. For younger patients, establishing a routine and incorporating music and play activities during rehabilitation sessions can be a beneficial supplement to their pain management regimen.

J. was a 2-year-old boy who sustained an 80% burn resulting in significant delays in gross motor developmental milestones. J. received music therapy as co-treatment during his physical therapy sessions. A routine was established early in J.'s treatment to facilitate his ability to cope with pain and anxiety and to ease into the transition of physical therapy exercises. After J. was seated on the exercise mat, developmental music activities were implemented during the initial 5–10 minutes. Dependent upon the current treatment goal, the physical therapist positioned J. (e.g., sidelying, standing, or laying prone) while the music therapist integrated active music activities to engage J.'s attention and tolerate the positioning with less distress. Music activities also served as a motivating stimulus for J. to practice gross motor skills such as rolling, sitting up from a prone position, and walking. Each physical therapy session ended with a quiet music/play time for the final 5 minutes. This structure enabled J. to better cope with the strenuous rehabilitation program while offering attention-driven music activities to facilitate attentional shift from a distressing stimulus.

For patients who received music therapy sessions during the acute phase, the therapeutic purpose for music therapy services during this next phase of treatment must be re-evaluated. Depending upon patient needs, the child in this phase may receive group, individual, or co-treatment sessions. Treatment goals most often include reinforcing active exercise and functional range of motion, improving pain and anxiety management associated with rehabilitation exercises, providing a positive outlet to express feelings related to injury/hospitalization to promote adjustment, increasing patient motivation and compliance to participate in the recovery process, providing developmental and neurological stimulation, and enhancing positive parent–child interaction through normalized music and play experiences.

Treatment interventions are varied and may include Neurologic Music Therapy rehabilitation techniques, songwriting and song improvisation, active music engagement, developmental musical play, and music-assisted relaxation (Neugebauer & Neugebauer, 2003). The following case describes the use of music therapy to increase motivation to ambulate during physical therapy sessions.

> E. was a 15-year old male who sustained a 99% TBSA flame burn after attempting suicide via self-immolation (setting oneself on fire). Motivating E. to actively participate in his rehabilitation sessions was a significant challenge, since he suffered from clinical depression. Because music was something that was meaningful to E., the music therapist and physical therapist developed a unique plan with the patient to integrate his interest with his need to ambulate. E. chose a song that was meaningful to him to use in creating his own personalized music video using a digital camera and a movie computer software program. During his physical therapy sessions, E. chose a place in the hospital where he wanted to film a segment for his music video. In order for E. to film his scenes, he needed to walk to the filming location. Although E.'s mood continued to fluctuate on a day-to-day basis, his level of cooperation to participate in his rehabilitation sessions improved significantly.

Metabolism, Exercise, and Music

A serious concern in sustaining a severe burn is the body's prolonged hypermetabolic response, which has been shown to peak at one-year post injury (with a metabolic rate of 180% of normal) and then decrease over an extended period of time (Blakeney, McCauley, & Herndon, 2002). The consequences of this rapid metabolic change includes severe loss of muscle mass and weakness in bone density, causing patients to be at risk for osteoporosis, muscle weakness, and lowered endurance. In children, this hypermetabolic state makes it challenging for patients to maintain their caloric needs and nutritional intake, thus interfering with their overall growth and physical development. During the past several years, extensive research in this area has shown significant improvements in muscle strength and cardiovascular fitness in those patients who participated in an intensive supplemental exercise program, as compared to those who did not participate and received conventional rehabilitation approaches (Cucuzzo, Ferrando, & Herndon, 2001; Thomas, Suman, Chinkes, & Herndon, 2003). For children over 7 years old who have sustained severe burns, specifically burns covering greater than 40% of the total body surface area, research has shown that participation in intensive rehabilitation programs incorporating strength, resistance, and endurance training has significantly improved functional outcomes and may decrease the number of surgical interventions required later in recovery (Celis, Suman, Huang, Yen, & Herndon, 2003; Cucuzzo et al., 2001; Suman, Mlcak, & Herndon, 2002; Suman, Spies, Celis, Mlcak, & Herndon, 2001).

Due to these observed clinical benefits, a wellness center, under the direction of an exercise physiologist, was implemented at SBH-G to provide strength and endurance training in addition to standard occupational and physical therapy practices. This center offers standard endurance and strength training equipment, like treadmills and free weights, with each patient receiving an individualized exercise program according to their abilities and needs. Recently, SBH-G has made it standard clinical practice that all children with burns greater than 40% TBSA participate in a comprehensive and intensive continued-care wellness program integrating rehabilitation, wound care, endurance and resistance training, as well as psychological support.

For children under the age of 7 years, the wellness center equipment and traditional exercise protocol is not age-appropriate. As a result, for those children aged 6 and under, music therapy has become an integral component of this intensive continued-care rehabilitation program. Music therapy groups, focusing on active exercise, functional movement, and endurance activities, are offered several times each week for those children requiring extensive rehabilitation. Their participation in this "Music & Movement" program begins shortly after discharge from the intensive care unit. Patient goals are established with the family during an interdisciplinary complex-needs team meeting prior to the child starting the program.

Music and Physical Rehabilitation

The evidence base for the use of music in rehabilitation can be found in both the basic and clinical science literature. The strong interconnection between the auditory and motor systems in the brain results in the ability of rhythmic and auditory cues to prime motor programming and synchronize movement (Molinari, Leggio, De Martin, Cerasa, & Thaut, 2003; Popescu, Otsuka, & Ioannides, 2004; Thaut, 2003). Studies further validate the therapeutic benefits of using rhythm and music to improve gait parameters and muscular control in both adults and children (Bernatzky, Bernatzky, Hesse, Staffen, & Ladurner, 2004; Thaut, 1985; Thaut, Miltner, Lang, Hurt, & Hoemberg, 1999).

In the exercise literature, music listening has been found to significantly increase endurance times in both muscular and cardiovascular-related tasks (Crust, 2004; De Bourdeaudhuij et al., 2002). Music has been shown to enhance positive mood during exercise, which may lead to increased participation in exercise programming (Hayakawa, Miki, Takada, & Tanaka, 2000; Murrock, 2002). Further, due to its strong attention-capturing attributes, music listening during exercise can lower the threshold of perceived exertion (Potteiger, Schroeder, & Goff, 2000; Szabo, Small, & Leigh, 1999). In young children, a study by Brown, Sherrill and Gench (1981) revealed significant positive changes in perceptual-motor performance for children who participated in a combined music/physical education program as compared to those who participated in physical education only. Hurt-Thaut and Johnson (2003) give explanation for the therapeutic benefits of music therapy in working with special-needs children, stating that "the possibilities are limitless for creatively challenging children to reach, balance, stretch, and utilize their upper and lower extremities in functional movements" (p. 91) with various instruments and musical cues.

Music with Young Children

For young children, active participation and compliance with rehabilitation treatment can pose a great challenge due to their inability to fully comprehend the importance of rehabilitation, potential behavior problems, and anxiety related to hospitalization. Music serves as an ideal tool for use in pediatrics. Providing an exercise program via group sessions provides opportunities for younger children to practice necessary social skills, such as cooperation. Children may also become increasingly motivated to actively participate when observing their peers doing the same activities. For pediatric burn patients, developmental problems may be a realistic concern, and clinicians should consider integrating developmentally stimulating activities during the recovery process (Gorga et al., 1999). Music has been shown to enhance both cognitive and social skills in various pediatric populations. Researchers found that educational programs for children were more effective in sustaining attention and increasing active participation when music was an integral component of the program (Register, 2004; Robb, 2003). Developing comprehensive rehabilitation programs that simultaneously integrate both physical and developmental components may reveal more successful outcomes in overall quality of life than programs that do not (Dijkers, 1997).

Music and Movement Group Program

Children who are 2–6 years of age can participate together during music therapy sessions offering specialized and developmentally appropriate activities involving movement to music and movement to create music. The format for this music and movement group should follow a specific structure in order to provide a positive and supportive environment. An opening greeting song incorporates a movement warm-up exercise of the upper extremities using shakers and integrating developmental concepts such as high and low and fast and slow. The core group activities include endurance-related musical games (e.g., egg-shaker relay races, obstacle courses), active playing of instruments (using upper and lower extremities), modifications of folk dances, and other developmentally appropriate targeted movements (e.g., throwing and catching), all of which incorporate some component of music.

At this time, Neurologic Music Therapy (NMT) offers the most evidence-based approach for the application of music in rehabilitation; therefore, two NMT techniques serve as the primary interventions for this program: Patterned-Sensory Enhancement (PSE) and Therapeutic Instrumental Music Performance (TIMP). PSE is defined as "a technique which uses the rhythmic, melodic, harmonic and dynamic-acoustical elements of music to provide temporal, spatial, and force cues for movements which reflect functional exercises and activities of daily living" (Hurt-Thaut & Johnson, 2003, p. 90). TIMP is defined as "the playing of musical instruments in order to exercise and stimulate functional movement patterns" (Hurt-Thaut & Johnson, 2003, p. 90). Live music is most often used, since the musical elements can be more easily manipulated and adapted to the specific motor goals targeted. However, recorded music with a strong and up-beat rhythmic pulse is used in some cases as a primer for movement as well as a motivating stimulus. Application of NMT sensorimotor techniques to pediatric burn care is beginning to develop more distinctly, particularly given the remarkable challenge of rehabilitating children with severe burns.

Parents and caregivers are also active participants during these groups, in order to provide supervised assistance to each child and to help the parents develop skills to encourage their child to be as independent as possible. Although helping a child with physical challenges develop increased independence is correlated with improved psychosocial development, many parents of children with **chronic illness** have a tendency to overprotect their child (Patterson, 1991). The music therapist, as well as other parents in the group, can serve as a role model for the parents of new patients starting the program who may be overwhelmed and uncertain about how to parent a child with such physical limitations. Active involvement of parents can also decrease feelings of distress and can facilitate their own psychological adjustment. As they begin to observe their child engaging in normalized play with other children and making improvements in functional independence, parents' own coping responses are strengthened (Daviss et al., 2000; LeDoux et al., 1998).

Preliminary evidence has shown that children who participate in the group music and movement program are less likely to lose passive range of motion and are more likely to improve active range of motion as compared to children who receive standard care (Neugebauer, Serghiou, Suman, & Herndon, 2005). Furthermore, Neugebauer, Serghiou, and Marvin (2005) conducted a survey that showed that parents who participated in the group music and exercise program had a high degree of satisfaction with the overall design, implementation, and results of the group program. The same study also revealed that compliance rate in attending the groups on a consistent basis was over 90%. In conjunction with these preliminary data, additional benefits of this group music and movement program are beginning to unfold. Clinical research for this specific program is in progress with the intention of learning more about outcomes related to range-of-motion, physiological measures of heart rate and caloric expenditure, developmental impact, parenting stress, and the emotional/behavioral adjustment of the burned-injured child.

For patients under the age of 2 or for children who are unable to participate in the group exercise program for other reasons, an individualized music therapy program is offered based upon the child's developmental level of functioning. Developmental assessment tools can be helpful in designing a treatment program targeting the child's areas of deficit (Gorga et al., 1999). The music therapist should also work closely with the treatment team, particularly the occupational and physical therapists, when designing a rehabilitation-focused music therapy treatment program. At SBH-G, a patient "needs" checklist, completed by the rehabilitation therapists, is used to outline the fine and gross motor skills that can be reinforced during music therapy sessions. This form serves as a helpful tool in establishing patient goals and in developing positive working relationships with the rehabilitation team.

Rehabilitation for children with severe burn-injuries is intensely challenging. At SBH-G, using music to facilitate physical rehabilitation goals is a significant component of the music therapy program during this phase of recovery, since positive functional outcomes are strongly correlated with overall adjustment and quality of life (Blakeney, Fauerbach, Meyer, & Thomas, 2002). As clinical research continues in this area, specific protocols can be further developed in order to provide the most effective application of music in pediatric burn rehabilitation.

Treatment Goals During the Rehabilitation Phase

- Reinforcing active exercise and functional range of motion
- Managing pain and anxiety related to rehabilitation exercises
- Promoting adjustment to injury and hospitalization
- Encouraging a positive outlet for the expression of feelings
- Increasing patient motivation and compliance in recovery
- Providing developmental and neurological stimulation
- Enhancing positive caregiver–child interaction
- Providing normalized experiences through music and play

Reconstructive Phase

Even after the wounds are healed and rehabilitation goals have been met, the recovery process continues long after the child has been discharged home. Active and passive range-of-motion exercises must be continued on a regular basis as the newly healed skin matures. Often, pressure garments need to be worn over the affected areas for 1 to 2 years in order to decrease the risk of **hypertrophic** (raised) scarring, smooth the skin, and produce flatter and softer burn scars during the maturation process. If the child has sustained burns to the face, a facemask may be required in order to preserve facial features (Serghiou et al., 2002). Wearing pressure garments and other medical equipment such as splints and mouth spreaders can be physically as well as psychologically challenging for the patients, since they need to be worn nearly 24 hours per day, to be removed only during bathing. Facemasks can also be removed while the child is eating. In pediatrics, many pressure garment companies offer a variety of colors (including pink and blue) in addition to neutral colors in an effort to increase the rate of compliance in wearing this prescribed medical equipment.

For many children, the need for surgery may continue well into adulthood as their bodies continue to grow and develop. These rapid changes in growth often lead to scar contractures resulting in a significant decrease in range-of-motion to the affected joints (Herndon, 2002). As a result, children with severe burns require long-term follow-up care in order to monitor their need for reconstructive or plastic surgical intervention. Surgeries requiring the release of scar contractures are common when burns affect the neck, arms, **axillas**, or other major joint areas. In addition to burn contracture releases, some patients may require plastic surgery for cosmetic or aesthetic reasons. In cases where burns have affected the head or face, plastic surgery may include facial scar revision, nose or ear reconstruction, or correction of burn **alopecia** (hair loss) through tissue expansion (expanding the healthy/unburned skin in order to replace it over an affected skin area) (Herndon, 2002). Plastic and reconstructive surgical procedures are scheduled operations and may be performed on a day surgery unit or may require an inpatient hospitalization. Some children may need multiple surgeries over an extended period of time as part of a step-by-step process for correction of deformities. At SBH-G, children are followed for reconstructive surgical care until the age of 18 years, at which time they begin their transition into adulthood. In some special cases where a significant need for extensive surgery exists, patients may be followed until the age of 21.

In addition to medical needs, psychological and social concerns continue to be monitored during this phase of treatment. According to Blakeney, Fauerbach et al. (2002), "quality of life is arguably the most important outcome to individuals who are seriously ill or injured" (p. 791). Children with severe burns are certainly at risk for long-term problems such as depression, posttraumatic stress disorder, body image dissatisfaction, and difficulties associated with social and occupational functioning. As patients undergo each phase of plastic surgical reconstruction, adjustment to their altering appearance may be an ongoing process.

Because many children with large burns require continuous surgeries and hospitalizations throughout their lives, psychological issues may be similar to children who are chronically ill. Having repeated and extended hospitalizations can cause feelings of helplessness, disrupt family life, cause behavioral regression, and exacerbate emotional distress. Furthermore, repeated hospitalizations can impact the normal growth and development process for children of all ages and may cause short-term or long-term problems depending upon the age of the child and time spent in the hospital. Developmental delays have been found to be more prominent than physical or functional limitations in children with severe burns (Gorga et al., 1999).

Music therapy services are made available during the child's reconstructive phase to address issues related to repeated hospitalizations, body image and self-concept, and developmental growth. In some instances, patients who received music therapy services during the acute and rehabilitation phases are followed to provide continuity of care and to monitor development and social-psychological adjustment. Depending upon length of stay, some patients in this phase may be seen only once during their inpatient stay as a way of maintaining healthy coping skills. In cases where the child has a history of anticipatory anxiety related to surgery, the music therapist may be referred to work with the child prior to surgery to facilitate coping with preoperative anxiety. Music-assisted relaxation techniques have been found to be effective in relieving anticipatory anxiety for pediatric burn patients undergoing reconstructive surgical procedures (Robb, Nichols, Rutan, Bishop, & Parker, 1995). The following example illustrates another music therapy approach to alleviate fear associated with awaiting surgery.

G. was a 10-year-old girl awaiting surgery for tissue expander placement for burn alopecia. Because she was the third scheduled operative case, she was unable to eat or drink and had much time to think about her upcoming operation. During the music therapy session, G. wrote lyrics to a familiar tune that reflected her thoughts and feelings related to having surgery. The first verse and chorus reflected her fears related to the surgical procedure. The music therapist then used a positive reframing approach to encourage G. to reflect upon the positive outcome that having this operation would have on her overall quality of life. The words are below:

Verse 1
Here comes Reyna, she's my nurse and she's crazy
But she's important because she takes care of me
She gives me things like medicine and IV's
So I don't feel pain in my body

Chorus
Just hangin' out, hangin' out
Waiting for surgery
Stuck in my room, but playin' music
Which makes me feel happy and good
But I-------- still don't want surgery
I--------- still don't want surgery

Verse 2
I have a doctor who will do my surgery
He's gonna give me a tissue expander
It's on my head so I can have hair everywhere
I can braid it, put clips in it, and have a ponytail

As the music therapist provided musical accompaniment on the guitar, G. sang her song to other staff that came to listen. Shortly after the performance, G. went off to surgery appearing more confident and relaxed.

Songwriting and song improvisation are also useful methods for children post surgery. Using the contextual support model of music therapy (Robb, 2000), music activities focusing on structure, autonomy, and involvement can be effective in assisting the patient during this period of decreased mobility. Musical improvisation can allow children a safe opportunity to independently practice problem-solving skills and can be an effective means to decrease negative thoughts.

During one song improvisation session, C., a 9-year-old boy, began singing about his "getting a shot" as part of his pre-surgical preparation. Using an improvisational approach (Froehlich, 1996), the music therapist encouraged C. to further process this experience by singing, "What do you think the shot would think if the shot could talk?" While improvising on a small electronic keyboard, C. rhythmically sang this response, "The shot would say, don't be scared C., I will just use my head and poke into your skin and then it would be all done."

A more structured songwriting approach can be a supportive tool for patients restricted to bedrest after surgery. In burn care, neck contracture releases are common surgical interventions that may require the child to lay supine with the neck positioned in extension for 5–7 days postoperatively. Such restricted mobility can be emotionally and psychologically difficult and can wear upon even the healthiest coping skills. The following song was written and later audio-recorded by a 12-year-old girl who had to remain in bed after surgery with her neck in extension for 7 days. In addition to writing her own lyrics, the music therapist assisted the patient in creating an original harmonic and melodic structure (see the Appendix of this chapter for actual music).

> *Being in the hospital is boring*
> *Being on your back all day and all night is no fun*
> *I can't turn on my side*
> *I gotta stare at the ceiling*
> *I gotta wear [prism] glasses to see the TV*
>
> *Being in the hospital is no fun*
> *I take lots of medicine when my leg hurts*
> *I had to have surgery*
> *I really miss walking*
> *I also miss looking out the window*
>
> *I would much rather go to the park*
> *Where I would play on the swings all day*
> *Swimming is one of my favorite things*
> *It's a lot of hard work to make a burn better*
> *I just want to go to school and see my friends*

The above song was later recorded with the patient. An instrumental interlude between the second and third verses allowed the patient to improvise on the glockenspiel as the music therapist musically supported the patient on the guitar. The songwriting process took a few days, which offered her an ongoing project to actively engage in while on bedrest.

Songwriting is an excellent tool for burn-injured children to express, understand, and validate their thoughts and feelings related to their injury. After songs are completed, asking the child's permission to share the song with other children in the hospital offers an opportunity to share thoughts and feelings expressed in the song. Most patients grant this request. Sharing original patient songs in this way can introduce the songwriting process to other patients, while also providing an opportunity for patients to hear that other children have had similar thoughts, feelings, and challenges.

While some patients remain on inpatient status or go home after surgery, others may be discharged as "residential" outpatients, where they remain at a nearby housing facility. These patients come daily for postsurgical care until they are ready for discharge home. Music therapy referrals for this patient population are often due to the following therapeutic reasons: reinforcement of active range-of-motion or functional movement postsurgery; pain and anxiety management for medical procedures, such as bolster, pin, suture, or staple removal; developmental stimulation to improve or maintain developmental milestones; and facilitating positive emotional adjustment through self-expression, social interaction, or mastery over the environment.

For procedural support, the music therapist is often referred by the nurse 15–20 minutes prior to the procedure and then works with the patient before, during, and after the procedure. Techniques generally incorporate active music engagement or passive music listening and vary according to the developmental age of the patient, type and duration of the procedure, prior experience in music therapy, and the physical positioning required for the procedure (some patients may have restricted mobility depending upon the location of the procedure). The importance of offering the patient an outlet for control is highlighted in the following case example.

D. was a 7-year-old patient from Guatemala who had over 20 staples to be removed from her scalp after tissue expander placement. Her previous experience in music therapy included attending some music therapy groups as well as receiving an individual session prior to surgery to assist with anticipatory anxiety. During the procedure, D. was given a "director" role and chose to play the bell chimes and tambourine. The music therapist followed D.'s musical style, dynamics, and tempo. Each time D. suddenly stopped playing, the music therapist also stopped playing, which often elicited a smile or laugh. She then tried to "trick" the music therapist as to when she would start and stop the music. D. and the music therapist continued this musical exchange as the nurse removed all the staples from D's scalp, with minimal to no signs of distress observed.

The above case illustrates the importance of music therapists to address both the emotional and cognitive components of pain perception. A more detailed description of the role of music in pain management can be found in Neugebauer and Neugebauer (2003). For burn patients, the risk of developing anxiety and depressive disorders may be increased due to their persistent and continuous exposure to painful stimuli and anxiety-provoking procedures (Blakeney, Fauerbach, et al., 2002; Neugebauer & Neugebauer, 2003). Simultaneously addressing the multidimensional components of pain is critical in pain management and needs to be further explored both clinically and in basic science research.

Rehabilitation goals for patients in this phase of recovery will most likely be localized to the area that was surgically released and may be short-term as compared to the previous rehabilitation phase of recovery. As described in the previous section, Therapeutic Instrumental Music Performance (TIMP) (Hurt-Thaut & Johnson, 2003) is the most commonly used technique at this stage to encourage active range-of-motion or to regain functional independence. For example, patients with surgical releases of web contractures between fingers, or patients who underwent hand reconstruction, may be referred to music therapy to enhance their fine motor dexterity using piano or guitar instruction. Particularly for adolescents, learning to play the guitar or keyboard can be a motivational means to exercise the fingers. Sometimes patients are referred to music therapy in order to expand functional use of their upper extremity prosthetics.

> P. was a 17-year-old male from Central America who had sustained an electrical injury 2 years earlier, which resulted in the amputation of both upper extremities. P. was admitted for reevaluation of prosthetic needs and received new bilateral prosthetic arms during the admission. P. was highly motivated to learn the electric guitar as part of his therapy, as well as for his own personal enjoyment. Music therapy sessions focused on developing an adapted method for P. to have the most successful fine motor control to both strum and play notes on the guitar. The guitar was positioned flat on a low table in front of him. An Everly Brothers brand "Star" guitar pick was used because the hole in the middle of the pick allowed P. to place the pick into one hook of his prosthesis. P. independently discovered that he could successfully use his left prosthesis to press down on the string between the frets. In addition, P. was shown how to use a guitar slide for an alternative style of playing.

Although the primary goal for P. was to improve functional use of his bilateral upper arm prosthetics, a secondary therapeutic benefit was the enrichment of P.'s quality of life, as he learned a skill that provided meaning and fostered self-confidence. Although patients in this stage of the recovery may have long surpassed the initial crisis phase, the search for understanding and meaning can be an ongoing process. The music therapist's role may be to maximize the recovery of physical skills while also fostering the patient's path to self-acceptance through emotional support, encouragement, and success-oriented accomplishments. Music therapy sessions can provide structured music experiences that allow the burn survivor to express thoughts and feelings within a safe and supportive environment. The following case describes how music therapy offered a creative outlet for a teenage girl to express her gratitude to the hospital staff, while also offering her an opportunity to reflect upon her journey from injury through recovery.

> K. was a 14-year-old girl from Ecuador who was injured a few years earlier in an accident that caused a severe flame burn injury. She was undergoing a long-term reconstructive surgical procedure that required her to remain nearby the hospital for several weeks. During this time, K. initiated the idea to "give back" to the hospital by performing a vocal concert for all patients and staff. K. carefully selected her repertoire, which consisted of five songs that had significant meaning to her life. After weeks of practicing and preparing for the program, K. performed a live vocal concert in the hospital auditorium. The music therapist and music therapy intern provided the instrumental accompaniments to each song. Fliers advertising her performance were displayed in the hospital, and a reception followed the concert. Of special note during the performance was her singing a song in dedication to her mother who had died in the same accident that injured K. Over 50 people attended, including patients and staff. The concert was truly an inspiration to all who listened.

In addition to individual sessions, group music therapy sessions can offer another opportunity for emotional support as well as social interaction. When possible, targeting specific age groups is most beneficial, particularly for adolescents who are in a stage of development where peer interaction is vital to their growth and adjustment process. Therapy groups can facilitate adjustment for adolescents who suffer chronic medical conditions. Integrating developmental tasks such as identity development, positive peer interaction, and promotion of autonomy into the group process can reduce stress and promote skills that are integral to this stage of development. Therapy groups may also help in treatment adherence, as teenagers positively identify with others in their peer group going through similar treatments (Creswell, Christie, & Boylan, 2001). The desire for conformity is one of the significant variables in compliance with medical treatment for adolescents (Shaw, 2001).

Songwriting and music video production can be effective tools in promoting emotional well-being for adolescents (Robb, 1996). In working with adolescent groups, rapport-building exercises through music, such as with egg shaker passes or group drumming, can be an efficient way to quickly develop group cohesion. Once trust is established, writing a song together about their injury and hospitalization experiences can develop positive coping responses through the sharing of insights and expansion of universality. Since adolescents are considered neither children nor adults, they often have unique issues as compared to other pediatric patients. For example, adolescents on the plastic surgery unit are generally scheduled as the final operative cases, since younger patients tend to have more difficulty coping with anticipatory anxiety. Songwriting sessions often reflect themes specific to adolescents (e.g., lack of privacy), as expressed in the lyrics to the following blues song written during an adolescent music therapy group:

> *Sittin' in the hospital got nothing to do*
> *Can't eat a crumb 'cause they won't give us no food*
> *Oh I'm hungry, Oh I'm hungry*
> *I see the kids next door and they're eatin' off the floor*
> *Oh, I'm hungry*
>
> *Being stuck inside with nowhere to go*
> *Flippin' through the channels to find a good show*
> *Oh I'm bored, Oh I'm bored*
> *There's nothin' on TV so I'll stare at my IV*
> *Oh I'm bored*
>
> *Being woken up in the middle of the night*
> *Nurse comes in starts turnin' on the light*
> *Oh my Lord, I'm mad*
> *And what about the pain, remember the pain...*
> *Oh yeah, that HURTS!*

Group music therapy has been a significant component of the program at SBH-G. In addition to specialty age groups, an open group is offered each week to all patients and families regardless of age, primary language, or stage of recovery. This large group has ranged in size from 6 to 20 patients, and family members, including parents and siblings, are also encouraged to attend and actively participate. The primary treatment goals for these groups are to practice developmental tasks, develop problem-solving skills, and foster support among the patients and families (Tuden et al., 2000). Upon readmission to the hospital, many patients express interest and enthusiasm in participating in the group music therapy sessions. The groups also serve as a practical means to monitor progress or reassess patients who require recurrent hospitalizations. Each group session includes music-based activities that integrate cognitive, motor, and social skills. A specific documentation form is used for this group as an objective tool to track patient progress and monitor developmental changes with each readmission. See the Appendix of this chapter for the Group Music Therapy Treatment Record.

As demonstrated, music therapy can be a fundamental supplement to the treatment team in addressing the unique physical and psychosocial needs of the burn patient during this continued stage of recovery. The therapist should reassess the patient upon each admission in order to track overall adjustment and development. Assessment should include tracking developmental gains or deficits, as well as reviewing concerns related to family functioning, social adjustment, and quality of life. Parents and caregivers need to be an integral part of the treatment process from the onset of injury and throughout each phase of treatment. Quality of family support is one of the most influential factors in the adjustment process for pediatric burn survivors (Blakeney, Portman, & Rutan, 1990; Landolt, Grubenmann, & Meuili, 2002). The music therapist can facilitate and enhance familial support throughout the recovery process by encouraging active family involvement during sessions and keeping parents well informed as to the goals and treatment process for their child.

Treatment Goals During the Reconstructive Phase

- Encourage positive body image and self-concept
- Facilitate coping with preoperative anxiety
- Support quality of life issues
- Provide stimulation for developmental growth
- Facilitate expression and validation of feelings, and positive emotional adjustment
- Provide procedural support
- Reinforce postsurgery active range-of-motion and/or functional movement
- Promote social interaction and mastery over environment
- Facilitate pain management
- Foster support among patients and families

Conclusion

Having the opportunity to work with a child recovering from a severe burn injury is both challenging and rewarding. Working with these young survivors is an amazing opportunity for any music therapist. Through the modality of music, it becomes a privilege to support and encourage these children as they encounter various challenges, triumphs, and setbacks. However, it is important to recognize that burnout is a risk for any clinician working in a trauma setting. The music therapist has an ethical responsibility to take care of oneself and be alert to the signs and symptoms leading to burnout. Exercising regularly, eating well-balanced meals, and having healthy interpersonal relationships outside of the work environment are all necessary to maintain and strengthen the therapist's ability to deal with profound suffering on a daily basis.

Although a specialized population, pediatric burn care necessitates the music therapist to develop a versatile skill base to handle the multiple physical and psychosocial concerns experienced in this setting. Having a solid understanding of models of medical music therapy as well as training in a variety of music therapy approaches and techniques will enhance the skill base for this challenging clinical population. Training in Neurologic Music Therapy is highly recommended in order to understand the evidence-base and application of the rehabilitation techniques. One should also study the underlying mechanisms and components of pain processing in order to provide the most appropriate clinical application of music therapy. Knowledge of psychosocial theories related to trauma, grief and loss, child development, family systems, and counseling approaches will also be helpful in order to provide a higher standard of care. Keeping informed through the current research literature related to medical models of music therapy, music and neuroscience, general pediatrics, burn care, and pain is also a recommended practice.

Pediatric burn care is a dynamic clinical field where music therapy has much to contribute. Through continued research, music therapists will develop standardized protocols that are integrated throughout the entire burn recovery process. Clinical research in pediatric music therapy is promising. Integrating knowledge gained from basic science and clinical research in music therapy will generate the most evidence-based practice and effective treatment applications.

References

Aggleton, J. P. (2000). *The amygdala: A functional analysis* (2nd ed.). Oxford, England: University Press.

Aragon, D., Farris, C., & Byers, J. F. (2002). The effects of harp music in vascular and thoracic surgical patients. *Alternative Therapies in Health and Medicine, 8*(5), 52–60.

Barrera, M. E., Rykov, M. H., & Doyle, S. L. (2002). The effects of interactive music therapy on hospitalized children with cancer: A pilot study. *Psychooncology, 11*(5), 379–388.

Benjamin, L. J., Dampier, C. D., Jacox, A., Odesina, V., Phoenix, D., Shapiro, B. S., et al. (1999). *Guideline for the management of acute and chronic pain in sickle cell disease.* Glenview, IL: American Pain Society.

Bernatzky, G., Bernatzky, P., Hesse, H. P., Staffen, W., & Ladurner, G. (2004). Stimulating music increases motor coordination in patients afflicted with Morbus Parkinson. *Neuroscience Letters, 6,* 4–8.

Blakeney, P. E., Fauerbach, J. A., Meyer, W. J., III, & Thomas, C. R. (2002). Psychosocial recovery and reintegration of patients with burn injuries. In D. H. Herndon (Ed.), *Total burn care* (2nd ed.) (pp. 783–797). London: Harcourt.

Blakeney, P. E., McCauley, R. L., & Herndon, D. N. (2002). Prolonged hypermetabolic response over time, the use of anabolic agents and exercise, and longitudinal evaluation of the burned child. In D. H. Herndon (Ed.), *Total burn care* (2nd ed., pp. 611–619). London: Harcourt.

Blakeney, P. E., Portman, S., & Rutan, R. (1990). Familial values as factors influencing long-term psychological adjustment of children after severe burn injury. *Journal of Burn Care & Rehabilitation, 11*(5), 472–475.

Blood, A. J., & Zatorre, R. J. (2001). Intensely pleasurable responses to music correlate with activity in brain regions implicated in reward and emotion. *Proceedings of the National Academy of Sciences of the United States of America, 98,* 11818–11823.

Brown, J., Sherill, C., & Gench, B. (1981). Effects of an integrated physical education/music program in changing early childhood perceptual-motor performance. *Perceptual & Motor Skills, 53*(1), 151–154.

Bushnell, M. C. (2004). Pain modulation by attention and distraction. In D. D. Price & M. C. Bushnell (Eds.), *Psychological methods of pain control: Basic science and clinical perspectives* (pp. 99–116). Seattle, WA: IASP Press.

Bushnell, M. C., Villemure, C., & Duncan, G. H. (2004). Psychophysical and neurophysiological studies of pain modulation by attention. In D. D. Price & M. C. Bushnell (Eds.), *Psychological methods of pain control: Basic science and clinical perspectives* (pp. 99–116). Seattle, WA: IASP Press.

Celis, M. M., Suman, O. E., Huang, T. T., Yen, P., & Herndon, D. N. (2003). Effect of a supervised exercise and physiotherapy program on surgical interventions in children with thermal injury. *Journal of Burn Care & Rehabilitation, 24*(1), 57–61.

Creswell, C., Christie, D., & Boylan, J. (2001). Ill or adolescent? Developing group work on an adolescent medicine unit. *Clinical Child Psychology & Psychiatry, 6*(3), 351–362.

Crust, L. (2004). Carryover effects of music in an isometric muscular endurance task. *Perceptual & Motor Skills, 98*(3), 985–991.

Cucuzzo, N. A., Ferrando, A., & Herndon, D. N. (2001). The effects of exercise programming vs. traditional outpatient therapy in the rehabilitation of severely burned children. *Journal of Burn Care & Rehabilition, 22*(3), 214–220.

Daviss, W. B., Mooney, D., Racusin, R., Ford, J. D., Fleischer, A., & McHugo, G. J. (2000). Predicting posttraumatic stress after hospitalization for pediatric injury. *Journal of the Academy of Child and Adolescent Psychiatry, 39*(5), 576–583.

De Bourdeaudhuij, I., Crombez, G., Deforche, B., Vinaimont, F., Debode, P, & Bouckaert, J. (2002). Effects of distraction on treadmill running time in severely obese children and adolescents. *International Journal of Obesity and Related Metabolic Disorders, 26*(8), 1023–1029.

Dijkers, M. (1997). Measuring quality of life. In M. J. Fuhrer (Ed.), *Assessing medical rehabilitation practices: The promise of outcomes research* (pp. 153–179). Baltimore: Paul H. Brookes.

Fanurik, D., Koh, J., Schmitz, M., & Brown, R. (1997). Pharmacobehavioral intervention: Integrating pharmacologic and behavioral techniques for pediatric medical procedures. *Children's Health Care, 26*(1), 31–46.

Fratianne, R. B., Prensner, J. D., Huston, M. J., Super, D. M., Yowler, C. J., & Standley, J. M. (2001). The effect of music-based imagery and musical alternate engagement on the burn debridement process. *Journal of Burn Care & Rehabilitation, 22*(1), 47–53.

Froehlich, M. (1996). *Music therapy with hospitalized children: A creative arts child life approach.* Cherry Hill, NJ: Jeffrey Books.

Geisser, M., Robinson, M., Keefe, F., & Weiner, M. (1994). Catastrophising, depression, and the sensory, affective and evaluative aspects of chronic pain. *Pain, 59,* 79–83.

George, A., & Hancock, J. (1993). Reducing pediatric pain with parent participation. *Journal of Burn Care & Rehabilitation, 14*(1), 104–107.

Good, M., Anderson, G. C., Stanton-Hicks, M., Grass, J. A., & Makii, M. (2002). Relaxation and music reduce pain after gynecologic surgery. *Pain Management Nursing, 3*(2), 61–70.

Gorga, D., Johnson, J., Bentley, A., Silverberg, R., Glassman, M., Madden, M., et al. (1999). The physical, functional, and developmental outcome of pediatric burn survivors from 1 to 12 months post injury. *Journal of Burn Care & Rehabilitation, 20*(2), 171–178.

Goubert, L., Crombez, G., & Van Damme, S. (2003). The role of neuroticism, pain catastrophizing and pain-related fear in vigilance to pain: A structural equations approach. *Pain, 107,* 234–241.

Gracely, R. H., Geisser, M. E., Giesecke, T., Grant, M. A., Petzke, F., Williams, D. A., & Clauw, D. J. (2004). Pain catastrophizing and neural responses to pain among persons with fibromyalgia. *Brain, 127,* 835–843.

Hayakawa, Y., Miki, H., Takada, K., & Tanaka, K. (2000). Effects of music on mood during bench stepping exercise. *Perceptual & Motor Skills, 90*(1), 307–314.

Haythornthwaite, J. A., Lawrence, J. W., & Fauerbach, J. A. (2001). Brief cognitive interventions for burn pain. *Annals of Behavioral Medicine, 23*(1), 42–49.

Herndon, D. N. (Ed.). (2002). *Total burn care* (2nd ed.). London: Harcourt.

Hurt-Thaut, C., & Johnson, S. (2003). Neurologic music therapy with children: Scientific foundations and clinical application. In S. L. Robb (Ed.), *Music therapy in pediatric healthcare: Research and evidenced-based practice* (pp. 81–100). Silver Spring, MD: American Music Therapy Association.

Kenny, D. T., & Faunce, G. (2004). The impact of group singing on mood, coping, and perceived pain in chronic pain patients attending a multidisciplinary pain clinic. *Journal of Music Therapy, 41*(3), 241–258.

Koch, M. E., Kain, Z. N., Ayoub, C., & Rosenbaum, S. H. (1998). The sedative and analgesic sparing effect of music. *Anesthesiology, 89,* 300–306.

Krout, R. E. (2001). The effects of single-session music therapy interventions on the observed and self-reported levels of pain control, physical comfort, and relaxation of hospice patients. *American Journal of Hospice and Palliative Care, 18*(6), 383–390.

Landolt, M., Grubenmann, S., & Meuili, M. (2002). Family impact greatest: Predictors of quality of life and psychological adjustment in pediatric burn survivors. *Journal of Trauma, 53*(6), 1146–1151.

LeDoux, J., Meyer, W. J., III, Blakeney, P. E., & Herndon, D. N. (1998). Relationship between parental emotional states, family environment and the behavioral adjustment of pediatric burn survivors. *Burns, 24,* 425–432.

Lee, D. W. H., Chan, K., Poon, C., Ko, C., Chan, K., Sin, K., et al. (2002). Relaxation music decreases the dose of patient-controlled sedation during colonoscopy: A prospective randomized controlled trial. *Gastrointestinal Endoscopy, 55*(1), 33–36.

Lepage, C., Drolet, P., Girard, M., Grenier, Y., & DeGagne, R. (2001). Music decreases sedative requirements during spinal anesthesia. *Anesthesia & Analgesia, 93,* 912–916.

Levine, J. D., Gordon, N. C., Smith, R., & Fields, H. L. (1982). Post-operative pain: Effect of extent of injury and attention. *Brain Research, 234,* 500–504.

Lewis, A. K., Osborn, I. P., & Roth, R. (2004). The effect of hemispheric synchronization on intraoperative analgesia. *Anesthesia & Analgesia, 98,* 533–536.

Martin-Herz, B. H., Thurber, C. A., & Patterson, D. R. (2000). Psychological principles of burn wound pain in children. II: Treatment applications. *Journal of Burn Care & Rehabilitation, 21*(5), 458–472.

McCaul, K. D., & Haugtvedt, C. (1982). Attention, distraction, and cold-pressor pain. *Journal of Personality & Social Psychology, 43,* 154–162.

Merskey, H., & Bogduk, N. (1994). *Classification of chronic pain: Descriptions of chronic pain syndromes and definition of pain terms* (2nd ed.). Seattle: IASP Press.

Meyer, W. J., Marvin, J. A., Patterson, D. R., Thomas, C. R., & Blakeney, P. E. (2002). Management of pain and other discomforts in burned patients. In D. H. Herndon (Ed.), *Total burn care* (2nd ed., pp. 747–765). London: Harcourt.

Miller, A. C., Hickman, L. C., & Lemasters, G. K. (1992). A distraction technique for control of burn pain. *Journal of Burn Care & Rehabilitation, 13*(5), 576–580.

Molinari, M., Leggio, M. G., De Martin, M., Cerasa, A., & Thaut, M. (2003). Neurobiology of rhythmic motor entrainment. *Annals of the New York Academy of Sciences, 999*, 313–321.

Munster, A. M. (1993). *Severe burns: A family guide to medical and emotional recovery*, Baltimore: Johns Hopkins University Press.

Murrock, C. J. (2002). The effects of music on the rate of perceived exertion and general mood among coronary artery bypass graft patients enrolled in cardiac rehabilitation phase II. *Rehabilitation Nursing, 27*(6), 227–231.

National SAFE KIDS Campaign (NFKC). (2004). *Burn injury fact sheet*. Washington, DC: Author.

Neugebauer, C. T., & Neugebauer, V. (2003). Music therapy in pediatric burn care. In S. L. Robb (Ed.), *Music therapy in pediatric healthcare: Research and evidenced-based practice* (pp. 31–48). Silver Spring, MD: American Music Therapy Association.

Neugebauer, C. T., Serghiou, M., & Marvin, J. (2005). A comprehensive 8–12 week group music and movement program for severely burned children [Abstract]. *Journal of Burn Care & Rehabilitation, 26*(Suppl. 2), S85.

Neugebauer, C. T., Serghiou, M., Suman, O. E., & Herndon, D. N. (2005). Effects of a 12-week therapeutic music and movement-based exercise and rehabilitation program on range of motion in burned children [Abstract]. *Journal of Burn Care & Rehabilitation, 26*(Suppl. 2), S53.

Neugebauer, V., Li, W., Bird, G. C., & Han, J. S. (2004). The amygdala and persistent pain. *Neuroscientist, 10*(3), 221–234.

Nilsson, U., Rawal, N., Enqvist, B., & Unosson, M. (2003). Analgesia following music and therapeutic suggestions in the PACU in ambulatory surgery: A randomized controlled trial. *Acta Anaesthesiologica Scandinavica, 47*, 278–283.

Nilsson, U., Rawal, N., Unestahl, E., Zetterberg, C., & Unosson, M. (2001). Improved recovery after music and therapeutic suggestions during general anaesthesia: A double-blind randomized controlled trial. *Acta Anaesthesiologica Scandinavica, 45*, 812–817.

Patterson, J. M. (1991). Family resilience to the challenge of a child's disability. *Pediatric Annals, 20*(9), 491–499.

Peretz, I., & Zatorre, R. J. (2005). Brain organization for music processing. *Annual Review of Psychology, 56*, 4.1–4.26.

Phumdoung, S., & Good, M. (2003). Music reduces sensation and distress of labor pain. *Pain Management Nursing, 4*(2), 54–61.

Popescu, M., Otsuka, A., & Ioannides, A. A. (2004). Dynamics of brain activity in motor and frontal cortical areas during music listening: A magnetoencephalographic study. *Neuroimage, 21*(4), 1622–1638.

Potteiger, J. A., Schroeder, J. M., & Goff, K. L. (2000). Influence of music on ratings of perceived exertions during 20 minutes of moderate intensity exercise. *Perceptual & Motor Skills, 91*(3, Pt. 1), 848–854.

Price, D. D., & Bushnell, M. C. (Eds.). (2004). *Psychological methods of pain control: Basic science and clinical perspectives.* Seattle, WA: IASP Press.

Pruitt, B. A., Mason, A. D., & Goodwin, C. W. (1990). Epidemiology of burn injury and demography of burn care facilities. In D. S. Gann (Ed.), *Problems in general surgery* (pp. 235–251). Philadelphia: J. B. Lippincott.

Register, D. (2004). The effects of live music groups versus an educational children's television program on the emergent literacy of young children. *Journal of Music Therapy, 41*(1), 2–27.

Robb, S. L. (1996). Techniques in song writing: Restoring emotional and physical well being in adolescents who have been traumatically injured. *Music Therapy Perspectives, 14*(1), 30–37.

Robb, S. L. (2000). The effect of therapeutic music interventions on the behavior of hospitalized children in isolation: Developing a contextual support model of music therapy. *Journal of Music Therapy, 37*(2), 118–146.

Robb, S. L. (2003). Coping and chronic illness: Music therapy for children and adults with cancer. In S. L. Robb (Ed.), *Music therapy in pediatric healthcare: Research and evidenced-based practice* (pp. 101–136). Silver Spring, MD: American Music Therapy Association.

Robb, S. L., Nichols, R. J., Rutan, R. L., Bishop, B. L., & Parker, J. C. (1995). The effects of music-assisted relaxation on preoperative anxiety. *Journal of Music Therapy, 32,* 2–21.

Robert, R., Blakeney, P. E., Villareal, C., Rosenberg, L., & Meyer, W. J. (1999). Imipramine treatment in pediatric burn patients with symptoms of acute stress disorder: A pilot study. *Journal of the American Academy of Child & Adolescent Psychiatry, 38*(7), 873–882.

Saxe, G., Stoddard, F., Courtney, D., Cunningham, K., Chawla, N., Sheridan, R., King, D., & King, L. (2001). Relationship between acute morphine and the course of PTSD in children with burns. *Journal of the American Academy of Child & Adolescent Psychiatry, 40*(8), 915–921.

Serghiou, M. A., Evans, E. B., Ott, S., Calhoun, J. H., Morgan, D., & Hannon, L. (2002). Comprehensive rehabilitation of the burned patient. In D. H. Herndon (Ed.), *Total burn care* (2nd ed., pp. 563–592). London: Harcourt.

Shaw, R. J. (2001). Treatment adherence in adolescents: Development and psychopathology. *Clinical Child Psychology and Psychiatry 6*(1), 137–154.

Smith, M., Doctor, M., & Boulter, T. (2004). Unique considerations in caring for a pediatric burn patient: A developmental approach. *Critical Care Nursing Clinics of North America, 16,* 99–108.

Stoddard, F. J., Sheridan, R. L., Saxe, G. N., King, B. S., King, B. H., Chedekel, D. S., Schnitzer, J. J., & Martyn, A. J. (2002). Treatment of pain in acutely burned children. *Journal of Burn Care & Rehabilitation, 23*(2), 135–156.

Suman, O. E., Mlcak, R. P., & Herndon, D. N. (2002). Effect of exercise training on pulmonary function in children with thermal injury. *Journal of Burn Care & Rehabilitation, 23*(4), 288–293.

Suman, O. E., Spies, R. J., Celis, M. M., Mlcak, R. P., & Herndon, D. N. (2001). Effects of a 12-wk resistance exercise program on skeletal muscle strength in children with burn injuries. *Applied Physiology, 91*(3), 1168–1175.

Szabo, A., Small, A., & Leigh, M. (1999). The effects of slow- and fast-rhythm classical music on progressive cycling to voluntary physical exhaustion. *Journal of Sports Medicine & Physical Fitness, 39*(3), 220–225.

Thaut, M. H. (1985). The use of auditory rhythm and rhythmic speech to aid temporal muscular control in children with gross motor dysfunction. *Journal of Music Therapy, 22*(3), 108–128.

Thaut, M. H. (2003). Neural basis of rhythmic timing networks in the human brain. *Annals of the New York Academy of Sciences, 999*, 364–373.

Thaut, M. H., Miltner, R., Lange, H. W., Hurt C. P., & Hoemberg, V. (1999). Velocity modulation and rhythmic synchronization of gait in Huntington's disease. *Movement Disorders, 14*(5), 808–819.

Thomas, S., Suman, O. E., Chinkes, D. L., & Herndon, D. N. (2003). Effect of exercise on bone formation in burned children [Abstract]. *Journal of Burn Care & Rehabilitation, 24*(Suppl. 2), S76.

Thurber, C. A., Martin-Herz, S. P., & Patterson, D. R. (2000). Psychological principles of burn wound pain in children. I: Theoretical framework. *Journal of Burn Care & Rehabilitation, 21*(4), 376–387.

Tracey, I., Ploghaus, A., Gati, J. S., Clare, S., Smith, S., Menon, R. S., & Matthews, P. M. (2002). Imaging attentional modulation of pain in the periaqueductal gray in humans. *The Journal of Neuroscience, 22*(7), 2748–2752.

Tuden, C., Amrhein, C., Rosenberg, L., Sanford, A., Cucuzzo, N., & Herndon, D. N. (2000). "Thank you for the music": Group music therapy for pediatric burn patients and their families [Abstract]. *Journal of Burn Care & Rehabilitation, 21*(Suppl. 1), S176.

Voss, J. A., Good, M., Yates, B., Baun, M. M., Thompson, A, & Hertsog, M. (2004). Sedative music reduces anxiety and pain during chair rest after open-heart surgery. *Pain, 112*, 197–203.

Waters, S. J., Campbell, L. C., Keefe, F. J., & Carson, J. W. (2004). The essence of cognitive-behavioral pain management. In R. H. Dworkin & W. S. Breitbart (Eds.), *Psychosocial aspects of pain: A handbook for healthcare providers* (pp. 261–283). Seattle, WA: IASP Press.

Wintgens, A., Boileau, B., & Robaey, P. (1997). Posttraumatic stress symptoms and medical procedures in children. *Canadian Journal of Psychiatry, 42*, 611–616.

Appendix

L's Song

music therapy

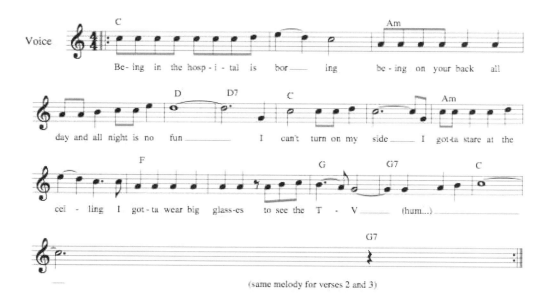

Voice

Be- ing in the hosp - i - tal is bor —— ing   be - ing on your back   all

day and all night is no   fun ____   I   can't   turn on my   side ____ I got-ta stare at the

cei - ling I got - ta wear big glass-es   to see the T - V ____ (hum...) _____

(same melody for verses 2 and 3)

Group Music Therapy Treatment Record

Group Music Therapy Treatment Record

Group Treatment Plan: Goals will address development in social skills, cognitive & problem-solving skills, functional motor skills, and enhancement of positive caregiver-child interaction.
Treatment Techniques: Active Music Engagement, Developmental Musical Play, Therapeutic Instrumental Music Performance, Music-Facilitated Movement

Patient: **MRN #:**   **Date:**

Participation/Motivation Level: Participated in   out of 5 group activities

☐ Refused to participate ☐ Slightly involved ☐ Moderately involved ☐ Highly Involved
☐ Passive observer ☐ Partially active ☐ Extrinsically motivated ☐ Intrinsically motivated

Level of Physical Assistance:
☐ Independent ☐ Minimal ☐ Moderate ☐ Dependent ☐ Adaptive Device Required

Comments: _____

Ability to Adapt to Physical Challenges:
☐ Independently adapts when necessary ☐ Occasionally requires assistance ☐ Always requires assistance ☐ N/A

Comments: _____

Level of Caregiver/Parent Involvement:
☐ Actively participated with child ☐ Assisted child when necessary ☐ Active observer ☐ Passive observer ☐ Not present

Comments: _____

C = Consistently; **O** = Occasionally; **R** = Rarely; **N** = Never; **DA** = Developmentally Appropriate

Social Skills:	C	O	R	N	DA	Comments
Waits turn						
Responds to verbal guidance/cueing						
Cooperates with other children (e.g. sharing)						
Engages in reciprocal play/interaction						
Aware of safety						
Demonstrates impulse control						
Asserts independence						
Smiles/laughs in response to play						
Initiates musical/non-musical interactions						
Assists with group (e.g., collecting instruments)						
Cognitive Skills:						
Follows directions for activities						
Focuses & sustains attention during activities						
Follows visual gestures/movements						
Plays simple rhythmic patterns/beats						
Follows auditory cues (fast/slow; loud/soft)						

Affective Reactions: _____

Plan: ☐ Patient will continue to be encouraged to attend group music therapy sessions during this admission
☐ Patient discharged; Attended   # of groups during this admission
☐ Other: _____

Therapist Signature: _____   **Date:**

MUSIC THERAPY
Shriners Hospitals   Shriners Burns Hospital-Galveston
for children   Treatment Record   **MRN #**
Form Rev. 7/08

GROUP MUSIC THERAPY TREATMENT RECORD

Activity	Skill Area(s) Targeted	GM = Goal met PM = Partially met NM = Not met
Opening Greeting Song	Cooperation Skills: Sustaining attention	
Developmental Musical Play	Following Directions: Basic cognitive skills (e.g. counting, discriminating auditory or visual cues).	
Active Music Engagement & Therapeutic Instrumental Music Performance	Functional Fine Motor Skills: Problem solving skills, discriminating auditory cues of music.	
Music Facilitated Movement	Active Gross Motor Skills: Cooperation skills, promote body awareness/ awareness of safety.	
Closing Goodbye Song	Following auditory cues of music, sustaining attention, functional fine motor skills.	

Therapist Signature: _____ Date:

MUSIC THERAPY
Shriners Hospitals   Shriners Burns Hospital-Galveston
for children   Treatment Record   MRN #
Form Rev. 7/08

Section III:

Resources

GLOSSARY OF TERMS

Acute lymphoblastic (lymphocytic) leukemia (ALL) – a form of leukemia with sudden onset and rapid progression; involves large numbers of immature white blood cells in the blood and bone marrow, specifically those that will become lymphocytes; most common form of cancer in children

Acute myelogenous (myelocytic) leukemia (AML) – a form of leukemia with rapid progression; involves large numbers of immature white blood cells in the blood and bone marrow, specifically those that will become granulocytes or monocytes

Adjunctive – treatment used in conjunction with the primary treatment; purpose is to assist the primary treatment

Allogenic transplant – diseased or damaged bone marrow is replaced by healthy bone marrow from a donor who is not an identical twin of the patient

Alopecia – unusual hair loss; side effect of most chemotherapy treatments

Analgesic – a drug that reduces pain without the loss of consciousness

Anemia – a reduction of red blood cells or hemoglobin from normal levels

Anoxia – absence or near absence of oxygen

Aplastic anemia – lower counts of all three types of blood cells: red blood cells, white blood cells, and platelets

Arterial line (A-line) – catheter inserted into an artery to measure blood pressure or draw blood

Autograft – see **Autologous transplant**

Autologous transplant – diseased or damaged bone marrow is replaced by healthy bone marrow from the patient's own body

Axilla – the cavity at the junction of the arm and body ("armpit")

Bone marrow aspiration – removal of a small amount of bone marrow fluid through a needle inserted into the bone, usually at the hip; used for diagnosis and obtaining bone marrow for transplants

Bone marrow transplant – see **Stem cell transplant**

Cancer – group of diseases in which abnormal cells divide without control and may spread throughout the body

Cardiac monitor (EKG) – measures the electrical activity of the heart in order to monitor heart condition; displays heart rate and rhythm

Cardiologist – a physician who specializes in heart disease

Catheter – a thin, flexible tube used to inject substances such as drugs, fluids, blood products, or nutrients into the body

Central venous pressure (CVP) – the venous pressure of the right atrium of the heart obtained by inserting a catheter into the median cubital vein and advancing it to the right atrium through the superior vena cava

Certified Child Life Specialist (CCLS) – nationally certified professionals who help pediatric patients cope with hospitalization and positively adjust to illness

Chemistry panel – a group of tests performed on a blood sample to evaluate a patient's general health status or the status of a particular organ

Chemotherapy – strong drugs that travel through the bloodstream to kill cancer cells throughout the body; may be administered by intravenous, intramuscular, or oral means

Chemotherapy suite – infusion area where cancer patients receive medications and chemotherapy treatments; often designed to increase patient comfort by providing comfortable chairs, televisions, and other services

Chest tube – tubes inserted through the skin into the space around the lungs to drain fluid or air

Chronic illness – an illness lasting three months or more

Chronic lymphoblastic (lymphocytic) leukemia (CLL) – a form of cancer in which abnormal lymphocytes enlarge the lymph nodes and cause a shortage of red blood cells and platelets

Chronic myelogenous (myelocytic) leukemia (CML) – a form of cancer in which the body produces too many white blood cells

CNS prophylaxis – chemotherapy or radiation therapy used to kill cancer cells in the central nervous system (CNS)

Complete blood count (CBC) – a measurement of various components of blood, including white blood cell count, automated white cell differential, red cell count, hemoglobin, hematocrit, mean cell volume, mean cell hemoglobin, mean cell hemoglobin concentration, red cell distribution width, and platelet count

Computerized axial tomography (CAT or CT) scan – produces images of structures of the body from multiple x-ray images; product is much clearer than a normal x-ray scan

Continuous ambulatory peritoneal dialysis (CAPD) – a method of removing waste from the body when the kidneys are unable to do so; dialysis solution remains in the abdomen until drained; does not require a machine

Debridement – the removal of dead or foreign tissue

Diagnostic test – a test that detects a disease or tracks recovery progress of a disease

Dorsal – the back or posterior of a structure

Edema – the swelling of soft tissues that results from a buildup of fluid

Endocrinologist – a doctor who specializes in disorders of the endocrine system

Endotracheal intubation – the process of placing an endotracheal tube through the nose or mouth into the trachea to maintain an open airway and permit mechanical ventilation and removal of secretions

Engraftment – occurs when donated stem cells reach the patient's bone marrow and begin to produce new blood cells; usually occurs 15–30 days following the transplant

Enteral feeding – providing nutrients and fluids by means of the gastrointestinal tract, such as through a feeding tube

Ewing's sarcoma – a tumor of the bone or the soft tissue that forms the bone; usually affects larger bones such as in the pelvis, trunk, or legs

Excision – surgical removal

Externalized shunt – temporary device used to drain excess cerebrospinal fluid from the ventricles of the brain, thereby reducing pressure in the skull; attached to a drainage container outside the body

Extrauterine – outside the uterus

FLACC Nonverbal Pain Scale – used to asses pain in children or nonverbal patients by rating observable behaviors in five categories: Face, Legs, Activity, Cry, Consolability

Foley catheter – a tube placed into the bladder to drain urine

Gastroenterology – the study, diagnosis, and treatment of diseases of the digestive system

Gastroschisis – a congenital abdominal wall defect where intestines and other organs may develop outside the abdomen

Glioma – a brain tumor originating in a glial cell; frequently resistant to treatment

Graft-versus-host disease – the rejection of transplanted bone marrow by the body's own cells

Hematology – the study, diagnosis, and treatment of diseases of the blood and bone marrow

Hemodynamic monitoring – monitoring the circulation of the blood, such as by measuring blood pressure

Hemophilia – an inherited disorder in which blood is unable to clot properly

Hodgkin's disease – cancer originating in the lymphocytes; affects lymph nodes close to body's surface

Homeostasis – a balanced state that is maintained by the continuous adjustment of biochemical and physiological components of a body or system

Hyperalgesia – increased sensitivity to pain

Hypertrophy – the abnormal or excessive growth of an organ

ICU psychosis – a state in which patients in an intensive care unit may experience impaired intellectual functioning, such as disorientation, confusion, combativeness, paranoia, agitation, or hallucination, resulting from the combination of sleep deprivation and sensory deprivation

Immunosuppression – suppression of the immune system; can be caused by disease or can be deliberately caused by drugs in order to prevent the rejection of a transplant

Immunotherapy – supplemental administration of biological substances natural to the body that help fight cancer and other diseases

Intensivist – a physician who specializes in critical care, usually in an intensive care unit

Intraoperative – during surgery

Intravenous (IV) nutrition – feeding through a vein; see also **parenteral feeding**

Intravenous catheter (IV) – tube placed in several different locations, including veins in the arm, neck, leg or groin, or the scalp in small infants; delivers medications, glucose, or other electrolyte solutions

Intubated – placing of a plastic tube into the trachea (airway) to provide a means of mechanical ventilation to give an individual oxygen

Laparoscopy – incision of the abdominal wall in order to insert tubes, probes, or instruments used to view structures in the abdomen or pelvis

Leukemia – abnormal growth and development of the blood cells

Likert scale – rating scale measuring the strength of agreement with a clear statement; often administered in the form of a questionnaire used to gauge attitudes or reactions

Lumbar puncture – see **spinal tap**

Lupus – chronic inflammation that occurs when unusual antibodies in the blood attack the body's own tissue

Lymphoma – a tumor of the lymphoid tissue, which includes the lymph nodes, tonsils, spleen, adenoids, and thymus

Magnetic resonance imaging (MRI) – a magnetized body scan that is capable of detecting small changes in structure

Mechanical ventilation – provides mechanical assistance for patients who cannot breathe independently; requires intubation

MediPort – a brand of central venous line; implanted under the skin in place of a PICC line to deliver medications to the bloodstream; removal is a simple outpatient procedure

Methicillin-resistant Staphylococcus aureus (MRSA) – a type of staph bacteria resistant to antibiotics; often occurs when the entrance site of a catheter becomes infected

Mind map – a nonlinear visual diagram that contains a central idea with related ideas and words clustered around the center

Multisensory stimulation – stimulation occurring simultaneously in two or more modes, including auditory, tactile, vestibular, or visual

Nasogastric tube (NG) – a tube placed through the nose to the stomach to administer medications or nutrients or to remove fluids or small solids

Neonatology – the science of providing medical care for newborns

Nephrology – relating to the care of the kidneys

Neuraxis – axis of the central nervous system, including the spinal cord, rhombencephalon, mesencephalon, and diencephalon

Neuroblastoma – consists of a solid tumor located in the nerve cells in the abdomen, adrenal glands, or spine; affects infants and children

Neurosurgeon – a physician who specializes in surgery of the brain and nervous system

Neutropenia – state of compromised immune system due to reduction of neutrophils (a type of white blood cell) in the body

Nociceptive – caused by, or in response to pain

Non-Hodgkin's lymphoma – cancer originating in the lymphocytes; affects lymph nodes located deep in body

Observation Scale of Behavioral Distress (OSBD) – a scale with a set of twelve operational definitions used to gauge the behavioral distress of patients, especially children, during painful medical procedures

Omphalocele – a congenital malformation in which amounts of the abdominal contents protrude through the base of the umbilical cord

Oncology – the study, diagnosis, and treatment of cancer

Orthopedist – a doctor specializing in injuries and disorders of the musculoskeletal system

Osteosarcoma – cancer of the bone; half of the cases in children originate in the bones around the knee

Parenteral feeding – providing nutrients and fluids directly to the bloodstream by intravenous methods

Pathologist – a doctor who studies cells and tissues to identify disease

Perioperative – refers to the three phases of surgery: preoperative (before), intraoperative (during), and postoperative (after)

Peripherally inserted central catheter (PICC) line – an intravenous catheter designed for long-term use, often to provide chemotherapy or total parenteral nutrition

Pheresis (apheresis) – the process of filtering blood to remove a certain component, after which the remainder of the blood is returned to the patient

Platelets – particles found in blood involved in the clotting process

Psychoneuroimmunology (PNI) – the study of the interrelationships between psychological, behavioral, neural, endocrinal, and immune processes

Pulse oximeter – a device used to monitor the concentration of oxygen in blood

Radiation therapy – localized treatment with high-energy rays to damage or destroy cancer cells and stop them from growing and dividing

Red blood cells – blood cells that contain hemoglobin, which allows them to carry oxygen and carbon dioxide

Remission – a temporary or permanent disappearance of the signs and symptoms of cancer

Retinoblastoma – a malignant tumor located near the retina in the eye; affects children, usually under the age of five

Rhabdomyosarcoma – a malignant muscular tumor affecting mostly children

Salivary immunoglobulin A (sIgA) – an immunoglobulin present in saliva that is linked with immune response in the upper respiratory system

Sickle cell anemia – a condition in which abnormal hemoglobin causes distorted red blood cells prone to rupture, thereby causing anemia; the irregular cells may also block small blood vessels

Spinal tap (lumbar puncture) – procedure in which spinal fluid is removed from the spinal canal, usually for diagnostic purposes

Stem cell (or bone marrow) transplant – cells in diseased or damaged bone marrow are replaced with immature healthy cells (stem cells) which grow into new cells

Suctioning – removal of mucous and fluid from the nose, mouth, or endotracheal tube

Surgeon – a physician who treats disease or injury by operation or manual methods

Thalassemia – a group of inherited blood disorders that interfere with the body's normal production of hemoglobin

Total parenteral nutrition (TPN) – intravenous feeding that provides all fluids and nutrients necessary for the patient's health

Tubbing – daily bathing of a patient's burns in order to prevent infection and remove dead skin

Ultrasound – a procedure that uses high-frequency sound waves to produce an image of structures of the body

Vascular access device (VAD) – a catheter placed inside a major blood vessel to provide a long-term method of drawing blood or providing nutrients or drugs

Venipuncture – a method of drawing blood from the body by the puncture of a vein

White blood cells – a class of cells that help the body fight infections

Wilms' tumor – a cancer of the kidney caused by the lack or inactivity of a tumor suppressor gene; occurs during childhood

Wong-Baker FACES Pain Rating Scale – a visual analog scale often used with children; the patient chooses which illustrated face matches his or her current pain level

COMPREHENSIVE BIBLIOGRAPHY

Pediatrics

Newborn Intensive Care

Arnon, S., Shapsa, A., Forman, L., Regev, R., Bauer, S., Litmanovitz, I., et al. (2006). Live music is beneficial to preterm infants in the neonatal intensive care unit environment. *Birth, 33*, 131–136.

Blumenfeld, H., & Eisenfeld, L. (2006). Does a mother singing to her premature baby affect feeding in the neonatal intensive care unit? *Clinical Pediatrics, 45*, 65–70.

Caine, J. (1991). The effects of music on the selected stress behaviors, weight, caloric and formula intake, and length of hospital stay of premature and low birth weight neonates in a newborn intensive care unit. *Journal of Music Therapy, 28*, 180–192.

Calabro, J., Wolfe, R., & Shoemark, H. (2003). The effects of recorded sedative music on the physiology and behaviour of premature infants with a respiratory disorder. *Australian Journal of Music Therapy, 14*, 3–19.

Cassidy, J. W., & Ditty, K. M. (1998). Presentation of aural stimuli to newborns and premature infants: An audiological perspective. *Journal of Music Therapy, 32*(4), 208–227.

Cassidy, J. W., & Standley, J. M. (1995). The effect of music listening on physiological responses of premature infants in the NICU. *Journal of Music Therapy, 32*(4), 208–227.

Cevasco, A. M., & Grant, R. E. (2005). Effects of the Pacifier Activated Lullaby on weight gain of premature infants. *Journal of Music Therapy, 42*(2), 123–139.

Chou, L. L., Wang, R. H., Chen, S. J., & Pai, L. (2003). Effects of music therapy on oxygen saturation in premature infants receiving endotracheal suctioning. *Journal of Nursing Research, 11*, 209–216.

Collins, S. K., & Kuck, K. (1991). Music therapy in the neonatal intensive care unit. *Neonatal Network, 9*(6), 23–26.

Dureau, S. J. (2005). The effect of gender on one-day-old infants' behavior and heart rate responses to music decibel level. *Journal of Music Therapy, 42*, 168–184.

Graven, S. N. (2000). Sound and the developing infant in the NICU: Conclusions and recommendations for care. *Journal of Perinatology, 20*, S88–93.

Hanson-Abromeit, D. (2003). The Newborn Individualized Developmental Care and Assessment Program (NIDCAP) as a model for clinical music therapy interventions with premature infants. *Music Therapy Perspectives, 21*(2), 60–68.

Kemper, K., Martin, K., Block, S. M., Shoaf, R., & Woods, C. (2004). Attitudes and expectations about music therapy for premature infants among staff in a neonatal intensive care unit. *Alternative Therapies in Health and Medicine, 10*, 50–54.

Lorch, C. A., Lorch, V., Diefendorf, A. O., & Earl, P. W. (1994). Effect of stimulative and sedative music on systolic blood pressure, heart rate, and respiratory rate in premature infants. *Journal of Music Therapy, 31*(2), 105–118.

Shoemark, H. (1999). Singing as the foundation for multi-modal stimulation. In R. Pratt & D. Grocke (Eds.), *MusicMedicine 3: MusicMedicine and music therapy: Expanding horizons* (pp. 140–152). Victoria, Australia: The University of Melbourne.

Shoemark, H. (2000). The use of music therapy in treating infants with complex bowel conditions. In J. V. Loewy (Ed.), *Music therapy in the neonatal intensive care unit* (pp. 101–109). New York: Satchnote Press.

Shoemark, H. (2004). Family-centred music therapy for infants with complex medical and surgical needs. In M. Nocker (Ed.), *Music therapy for premature and newborn infants* (pp. 141–157). Gilsum, NH: Barcelona.

Shoemark, H. (2006). Infant-directed singing as a vehicle for regulation rehearsal in the medically fragile full-term infant. *Australian Journal of Music Therapy, 17*, 54–63.

Shoemark, H. (2008). Mapping progress within an individual music therapy session with full-term hospitalized infants. *Music Therapy Perspectives, 26*(1), 38–45.

Shoemark, H., & Dearn, T. (2008). Keeping parents at the centre of family centred music therapy with hospitalized infants. *Australian Journal of Music Therapy, 19*, 3–24.

Standley, J. M. (1998). The effect of music and multimodal stimulation on responses of premature infants in neonatal intensive care. *Pediatric Nursing, 24*, 532–538.

Standley, J. M. (2000). The effect of contingent music to increase non-nutritive sucking of premature infants. *Pediatric Nursing, 26*, 493–499.

Standley, J. M. (2001). Music therapy for the neonate. *Newborn and Infant Nursing Reviews, 1*(4), 211–216.

Standley, J. M. (2001). Music therapy for premature infants in neonatal intensive care: Physiological and developmental benefits. *Early Childhood Connections, 7*(2), 18–25.

Standley, J. M. (2002). A meta-analysis of the efficacy of music therapy for premature infants. *Journal of Pediatric Nursing, 17*, 107–113.

Standley, J. M. (2003). The effect of music-reinforced nonnutritive sucking on feeding rate of premature infants. *Journal of Pediatric Nursing, 18*, 169–173.

Standley, J. M. (2003). *Music therapy with premature infants: Research and developmental interventions*. Silver Spring, MD: American Music Therapy Association.

Standley, J. M., & Moore, R. S. (1995). Therapeutic effects of music and mother's voice on premature infants. *Pediatric Nursing, 21*, 509–512, 574.

Stewart, K., & Schneider, S. (2003). The effects of music therapy on the sound environment in the NICU: A pilot study. In J. V. Loewy (Ed.), *Music therapy in the neonatal intensive care unit* (pp. 85–101). New York: Satchnote Press.

Whipple, J. (2000). The effect of parent training in music and multimodal stimulation on parent-neonate interactions in the neonatal intensive care unit. *Journal of Music Therapy, 37*, 250–268.

Whipple, J. (2005). Music and multimodal stimulation as developmental intervention in neonatal intensive care. *Music Therapy Perspectives, 23*, 100–105.

Whitwell, G. E. (1999). The importance of prenatal sound and music. *Journal of Prenatal and Perinatal Psychology and Health, 13*, 255–262.

Pediatric Intensive Care

Dun, B. (1995). A different beat: Music therapy in children's cardiac care. *Music Therapy Perspectives, 13*, 35–39.

Edwards, J. (1999). Anxiety management in pediatric music therapy. In C. Dileo (Ed.), *Music therapy and medicine: Theoretical and clinical approaches* (pp. 69–76). Silver Spring, MD: American Music Therapy Association.

Ghetti, C. (2007). A personal reflection: Tactile music therapy at night for patients on ECMO in the pediatric intensive care setting. *Dimensions of Critical Care Nursing, 26*, 173.

Johnston, K., & Rohaly-Davis, J. (1996). An introduction to music therapy: Helping the oncology patient in the ICU. *Critical Care Nursing Quarterly, 18*(4), 54–60.

Kennelly, J., & Edwards, J. (1997). Providing music therapy for the unconscious child in the paediatric intensive care unit. *Australian Journal of Music Therapy, 8*, 18–29.

Malone, A. B. (1996). The effects of live music on the distress of pediatric patients receiving intravenous starts, venipunctures, injections, and heel sticks. *Journal of Music Therapy, 23*, 19–33.

Stouffer, J. W., & Shirk, B. (2003). Critical care: Clinical applications of music for children on mechanical ventilation. In S. Robb (Ed.), *Music therapy in pediatric healthcare: Research and evidence-based practice* (pp. 49–80). Silver Spring, MD: American Music Therapy Association.

Updike, P. (1990). Music therapy results for ICU patients. *Dimensions of Critical Care Nursing, 9*(1), 39–45.

Walworth, D. D. (2003). Procedural support: Music therapy assisted CT, EKG, EEG, X-Ray, IV, ventilator, and emergency services. In S. L. Robb (Ed.), *Music therapy in pediatric healthcare: Research and evidence-based practice* (pp. 137–146). Silver Spring, MD: American Music Therapy Association.

General Medical/Surgical

Aitken, J. C., Wilson, S., Coury, D., & Moursi, A. M. (2002). The effect of music distraction on pain, anxiety, and behavior in pediatric dental patients. *Pediatric Dentistry, 24*, 114–118.

Aldridge, K. (1993). The use of music to relieve pre-operational anxiety in children attending day surgery. *The Australian Journal of Music Therapy, 4*, 19–35.

Barrickman, J. (1989). A developmental music therapy approach for preschool hospitalized children. *Music Therapy Perspectives, 7*, 10–16.

Caprilli, S., Anastasi, F., Grotto, R. P., Abeti, M. S., & Messeri, A. (2007). Interactive music as a treatment for pain and stress in children during venipuncture: A randomized prospective study. *Journal of Developmental and Behavioral Pediatrics, 28*, 399–403.

Chetta, H. D. (1981). The effect of music and desensitization on preoperative anxiety in children. *Journal of Music Therapy, 18*, 74–87.

Colwell, C. M., Davis, K., & Schroeder, L. K. (2005). The effect of composition (art or music) on the self-concept of hospitalized children. *Journal of Music Therapy, 42*, 49–63.

Edwards, J. (1999). Music therapy with children hospitalised for severe injury or illness. *British Journal of Music Therapy, 13*, 21–27.

Edwards, J. (2005). A reflection on the music therapist's role in developing a program in a children's hospital. *Music Therapy Perspectives, 23*, 36–44.

Froehlich, M. A. (1984). A comparison of the effect of music therapy and medical play therapy on the verbalization behavior of pediatric patients. *Journal of Music Therapy, 21*, 2–15.

Han, P. (1998). The use of music in managing pain for hospitalised children. *Australian Journal of Music Therapy, 9*, 44–56.

Hatem, T. P., Lira, P. I., & Mattos, S. S. (2006). The therapeutic effects of music in children following cardiac surgery. *Jornal de Pediatria, 82*, 186–192.

Hendon, C., & Bohon, L. M. (2008). Hospitalized children's mood differences during play and music therapy. *Child Care, Health, & Development, 34*(2), 141–144.

Jacobowitz, R. M. (1992). Music therapy in the short-term pediatric setting: Practical guidelines for the limited time frame. *Music Therapy, 11*, 45–64.

Joyce, B., Keck, J., & Gerkensmeyer, J. (2001). Evaluation of pain management interventions for neonatal circumcision pain. *Journal of Pediatric Health Care, 15*, 105–114.

Kain, Z. N., Caldwell-Andrews, A. A., Krivutza, D. M., Weinberg, M. E., Gaal, D., Wang, S. M., et al. (2004). Interactive music therapy as a treatment for preoperative anxiety in children: A randomized controlled trial. *Anesthesia and Analgesia, 98*, 1260–1266.

Kennelly, J. (2000). The specialist role of the music therapist in developmental programs for hospitalized children. *Journal of Pediatric Health Care, 14*, 56–59.

Klein, S. A., & Winkelstein, M. L. (1996). Enhancing pediatric health care with music. *Journal of Pediatric Health Care, 10*, 74–81.

Mathur, A., Duda, L., & Kamat, D. M. (2008). Knowledge and use of music therapy among pediatric practitioners in Michigan. *Clinical Pediatrics, 47*, 155–159.

McDonnell, L. (1984). Music therapy with trauma patients and their families on a pediatric service. *Music Therapy, 4*, 55–63.

Noguchi, L. K. (2006). The effect of music versus nonmusic on behavioral signs of distress and self-report of pain in pediatric injection patients. *Journal of Music Therapy, 43*, 16–38.

Robb, S. L. (2003). Designing music therapy interventions for hospitalized children and adolescents using a contextual support model of music therapy. *Music Therapy Perspectives, 21*, 27–40.

Stouffer, J. W., Shirk, B. J., & Polomano, R. C. (2007). Practice guidelines for music interventions with hospitalized pediatric patients. *Journal of Pediatric Nursing, 22*, 448–456.

Walworth, D. (2005). Procedural-support music therapy in the healthcare setting: A cost-effectiveness analysis. *Journal of Pediatric Nursing, 20*(4), 276–284.

Whipple, J. (2003). Surgery buddies: A music therapy program for pediatric surgical patients. *Music Therapy Perspectives, 21*, 77–83.

Whitehead-Pleaux, A. M., Zebrowski, N., Baryza, M. J., & Sheridan, R. L. (2007). Exploring the effects of music therapy on pediatric pain: Phase 1. *Journal of Music Therapy, 44*, 217–241.

Hematology/Oncology/Bone Marrow Transplant

Aasgaard, T. (1999). Music therapy as milieu in the hospice and paediatric oncology ward. In D. Aldridge (Ed.), *Music therapy in palliative care*. London: Jessica Kingsley.

Aasgaard, T. (2000). 'A suspiciously cheerful lady': A study of a song's life in the paediatric oncology ward, and beyond. *British Journal of Music Therapy, 14*, 70–81.

Aasgaard, T. (2001). An ecology of love: Aspects of music therapy in the pediatric oncology environment. *Journal of Palliative Care, 17*, 177–181.

Abad, V. (2003). A time of turmoil: Music therapy interventions for adolescents in a paediatric oncology ward. *Australian Journal of Music Therapy, 14*, 20–36.

Barrera, M., Kykov, M., & Doyle, S. (2002). The effects of interactive music therapy on hospitalized children with cancer: A pilot study. *Psycho-Oncology, 11*, 379–388.

Brodsky, W. (1989). Music therapy as an intervention for children with cancer in isolation rooms. *Music Therapy, 8*, 17–34.

Daveson, B. A. (2001). Music therapy and childhood cancer: Goals, methods, patient choice and control during diagnosis, intensive treatment, transplant, and palliative care. *Music Therapy Perspectives, 19*, 114–120.

Hadley, S. (1996). A rationale for the use of song with children undergoing bone marrow transplantation. *Australian Journal of Music Therapy, 7*, 16–27.

Kemper, K. J., Hamilton, C. A., McLean, T. W., & Lovato, J. (2008). Impact of music on pediatric oncology outpatients. *Pediatric Research, 64*(1), 105–109.

Kennelly, J. (2001). Music therapy in the bone marrow transplant unit: Providing emotional support during adolescence. *Music Therapy Perspectives, 19*, 104–108.

Ledger, A. (2001). Song parody for adolescents with cancer. *Australian Journal of Music Therapy, 12*, 21–28.

O'Callaghan, C., Sexton, M., & Wheeler, G. (2007). Music therapy as a non-pharmacological anxiolytic for paediatric radiotherapy patients. *Australasian Radiology, 51*, 159–162.

O'Neill, N., & Pavlicevic, M. (2003). What am I doing here? Exploring a role for music therapy with children undergoing bone marrow transplantation at Great Ormond Street Hospital, London. *British Journal of Music Therapy, 17*, 8–16.

Pfaff, V., Smith, K., & Gowan, D. (1989). The effects of music-assisted relaxation on the distress of pediatric cancer patients undergoing bone marrow aspirations. *Children's Health Care, 18*(4), 232–236.

Robb, S. L. (2000). The effect of therapeutic music interventions on the behavior of hospitalized children in isolation: Developing a contextual support model of music therapy. *Journal of Music Therapy, 37*, 118–146.

Robb, S. L. (2003). Coping and chronic illness: Music therapy for children and adolescents with cancer. In S. L. Robb (Ed.), *Music therapy in pediatric healthcare: Research and evidence-based practice* (pp. 101–136). Silver Spring, MD: American Music Therapy Association.

Robb, S. L. (2003). Designing music therapy interventions for hospitalized children and adolescents using a contextual support model of music therapy. *Music Therapy Perspectives, 21*, 27–40.

Robb, S. L., Clair, A. A., Watanabe, M., Monahan, P. O, Azzouz, F., Stouffer, J. W., Ebberts, A., Darsie, E., Whitmer, C., Walker, J., Nelson, K., Hanson-Abromeit, D., Lane, D., & Hannan, A. (2008). Randomized controlled trial of the active music engagement (AME) intervention on children with cancer. *Psycho-Oncology, 17*(7), 699–708.

Robb, S. L., & Ebberts, A. G. (2003). Songwriting and digital video production interventions for pediatric patients undergoing bone marrow transplantation, part I: An analysis of depression and anxiety levels according to phase of treatment. *Journal of Pediatric Oncology Nursing, 20*, 2–15.

Robb, S. L., & Ebberts, A. G. (2003). Songwriting and digital video production interventions for pediatric patients undergoing bone marrow transplantation, part II: An analysis of patient-generated songs and patient perceptions regarding intervention efficacy. *Journal of Pediatric Oncology Nursing, 20*, 16–25.

Standley, J. M., & Hanser, S. B. (1995). Music therapy research and applications in pediatric oncology treatment. *Journal of Pediatric Oncology Nursing, 12*, 3–10.

Burn

Barker, L. (1991). The use of music and relaxation techniques to reduce pain of burn patients during daily debridement. In C. Maranto (Ed.), *Applications of music in medicine*. Silver Spring, MD: National Association for Music Therapy.

Bishop, B., Christenberry, A., Robb, S., & Rudenberg, M. T. (1996). Music therapy and child life interventions with pediatric burn patients. In M. Froehlich (Ed.), *Music therapy with hospitalized children: A creative arts child life approach.* Cherry Hill, NJ: Jeffrey Books.

Christenberry, R. B. (1979). The use of music therapy with burn patients. *Journal of Music Therapy, 16*, 136–148.

Daveson, B. A. (1999). A model of response: Coping mechanisms and music therapy techniques during debridement. *Music Therapy Perspectives, 17*, 92–98.

Edwards, J. (1994). The use of music therapy to assist children who have severe burns. *Australian Journal of Music Therapy, 5*, 3–6.

Edwards, J. (1995). "You are singing beautifully": Music therapy and the debridement bath. *The Arts in Psychotherapy, 22*, 53–55.

Edwards, J. (1998). Music therapy for children with severe burn injury. *Music Therapy Perspectives, 16*(1), 21–26.

Rudenberg, M., & Royka, A. (1989). Promoting psychosocial adjustment in pediatric burn patients through music therapy and child life therapy. *Music Therapy Perspectives, 7*, 40–43.

Sahler, O. J., Hunter, B. C. & Liesveld, J. L. (2003). The effect of using music therapy with relaxation imagery in the management of patients undergoing bone marrow transplantation: A pilot feasibility study. *Alternative Therapies, 9*, 70–74.

Turry, A., & Turry, A. E. (1999). Creative song improvisations with children and adults with cancer. In C. Dileo (Ed.), *Music therapy and medicine: Theoretical and clinical applications* (pp. 167–177). Silver Spring, MD: American Music Therapy Association.

Whitehead-Pleaux, A. M., Baryza, M. J., & Sheridan, R. L. (2006). The effects of music therapy on pediatric patients' pain and anxiety during donor site dressing change. *Journal of Music Therapy, 43*, 136–153.

Palliative Care

Daveson, B. A., & Kennelly, J. (2000). Music therapy in palliative care for hospitalized children and adolescents. *Journal of Palliative Care, 16*, 35–38.

Fagen, T. S. (1982). Music therapy in the treatment of anxiety and fear in terminal pediatric patients. *Music Therapy, 2*, 13–23.

Hilliard, R. E. (2001). The effects of music therapy-based bereavement groups on mood and behavior of grieving children. *Journal of Music Therapy, 38*, 291–306.

Hilliard, R. E. (2003). Music therapy in pediatric palliative care: A complementary approach. *Journal of Palliative Care, 19*, 127–132.

Hilliard, R. E. (2006). Music therapy in pediatric oncology: A review of the literature. *Journal of the Society for Integrative Oncology, 4*, 75–79.

Hilliard, R. E. (2007). The effects of Orff-based music therapy and social work sessions on grieving children. *Journal of Music Therapy, 44*, 123–138.

Sheridan, J., & McFerran, K. (2004). Exploring the value of opportunities for choice and control in music therapy within a paediatric hospice setting. *Australian Journal of Music Therapy, 15*, 18–32.

Population/Age Range: Infants–adolescents (relaxation method will vary depending upon developmental level)

Title: *Music-Assisted Relaxation* (MAR)

Estimated Time for Implementation: 10–30 minutes

Goals: To facilitate relaxation, to decrease perception of pain, to promote sedation, to improve compliance during procedures

Objective(s):
1. Pt. will demonstrate stability or reduction in HR and RR.
2. Pt. will demonstrate increase in deep inhalations.
3. Pt. will demonstrate decrease in physical tension.
4. Pt. will report less pain.
5. Pt. will fall asleep.
6. Pt. will tolerate painful procedures with minimal stress behaviors.

Response Definition:
1. Therapist will record baseline heart rate (HR) and/or respiratory rate (RR) and will observe/record changes during session.
2. Therapist will observe depth of breathing (shallow frequent breaths vs. deep, slow inhalations).
3. Therapist will note changes to observable signs of tension (clenched fists, wincing, contracted arms or legs).
4. Therapist will record pt.'s reported level of pain (use Wong-Baker FACES scale).
5. Therapist will observe behavior state and vital sign indications of sleep (maintenance of decrease in HR and/or RR).
6. Therapist will note pt.'s compliance with procedural requirements (e.g., holding affected limb still for blood draw or IV start).

Materials: Quiet portable accompanying instrument (usually guitar, could be folk harp or keyboard); optional: sound effects percussion (ocean drum, rainstick)

Procedural Steps:
1. Introduce self to pt.; assess developmental level, current mood state, and level of reported pain or anxiety.
2. Assess baseline measures of HR, RR, behavior state, observable physical tension, and pain (if applicable).
3. Decide upon relaxation method based on assessment of pt.'s developmental level, pain level, anxiety level, and procedural requirements (e.g., sedative music listening, music-facilitated deep breathing, music and guided imagery, active or passive progressive muscle relaxation).
4. Begin sedative music accompaniment approximating tempo of breathing (depending on MT-BC's assessment of pt., therapist may choose to begin with voice alone first, then add gentle accompaniment).
5. Assess pt.'s tolerance of auditory stimuli by observing responses to music and add voice (or accompaniment) quietly if stimuli are well-tolerated.
6. Gradually slow tempo if pt. is currently agitated.
7. Begin cues for chosen relaxation method (e.g., cues for breathing in and out or visualization to assist with deep inhalations, cues for imagery, or prompts to tighten and release muscle groups for active progressive muscle relaxation or imagery for muscle groups if using passive progressive muscle relaxation).
8. Assess changes in vital signs and observable behaviors.
9. If vital signs or observable behaviors are moving towards preferred direction for sedation, continue with current relaxation method.
10. If there is no change in vital signs or observable behaviors, either discontinue verbal prompts, repeat current cues, or change to alternate relaxation method.
11. If vital signs or observable behaviors change in negative direction, reduce complexity of auditory stimuli, wait for stabilization of vital signs or behaviors, then either repeat current relaxation method or try an alternate method.
12. When concluding relaxation method, phase out if pt. appears to be asleep or help pt. gradually transition back to being aware of surroundings.

Measurement Tools:
1. Heart rate (HR) and/or respiratory rate (RR)
2. Changes in breathing pattern
3. Observable signs of tension
4. Pain level as measured on Wong-Baker FACES analog scale
5. behavior state
6. Patient verbalizations
7. Amount of pain or sedation medication required for procedure
8. Pt. level of compliance with procedure

Possible Adaptations:
The relaxation method chosen within the MAR technique will vary depending on patient's developmental, pain, and anxiety levels, as well as upon the ultimate goal of intervention (e.g., relaxation, procedural compliance, sleep). The technique also requires adaptation or adjustment throughout, depending upon patient responses.

Population/Age Range: Toddler–preteen

Title: *Music as Alternate Engagement during Medical Procedures* (MAE)

Estimated Time for Implementation: 10–30 minutes

Goals: Alternatively engage attention during procedure, decrease perception of pain, decrease anxiety, improve choice-making and control, improve compliance with procedures

Objective(s):
1. Pt. will redirect attention to the music interaction.
2. Pt. will demonstrate active participation in music interaction to extent capable.
3. Pt. will demonstrate decrease in crying/agitation.
4. Pt. will demonstrate choice-making during music interaction.
5. Pt. will tolerate painful procedures with minimal stress behaviors.

Response Definition:
1. Therapist will assess pt.'s level of active participation (e.g., frequency/duration of eye contact, level of physical engagement, level of verbal engagement, frequency of choices made).
2. Therapist will observe behaviors indicating agitation/anxiety at session onset and during MAE (e.g., wailing cry, flailing arms, attempting to hit staff).
3. Therapist will note frequency of pt.'s choice-making during procedure.
4. After the procedure, therapist will record pt.'s reported level of pain during the procedure (use Wong-Baker FACES scale).
5. Therapist will document pt.'s affective response to procedure (with pt.'s evaluation of the experience if developmentally appropriate).
6. Therapist will note pt.'s compliance with procedural requirements (e.g., holding affected limb still for blood draw or IV start).

Materials: Novel and attractive instruments such as rainbow rainstick, thunder tube, and colored shaker eggs; accompanying instrument that allows pt. participation (e.g., strumming on guitar); optional: puppets or toy props for songs (must be immediately washable or owned by the pt.)

Procedural Steps:
1. Assess nature of pt.'s upcoming procedure, obtain consent for MT procedural support from physician/nurse if necessary.
2. Introduce self to pt.; assess developmental level, current mood state, and level of reported pain or anxiety.
3. Decide upon MAE method based on assessment of pt.'s developmental level, pain level, anxiety level, and procedural requirements (e.g., music listening or song singing with choice-making; instrument exploration; action songs with cued movements, sounds or instruments).

4. Briefly assess music preferences through pt. or parent interview, if appropriate.

5. Incorporating pt.'s musical preferences, start with interactions requiring visual engagement (e.g., demonstrate rainbow rainstick or other visually-oriented instrument, encourage eye contact).

6. Progress to increasing levels of active engagement to extent permissible by procedure (e.g., holding and playing shaker egg when cued by song; turning rainstick); if physical engagement is restricted due to procedural requirements, focus on increasing pt.'s active vocal responses (e.g., choosing songs and singing along, filling in sounds or counts for songs).

7. Discontinue or decrease level of active engagement required if pt. requests to stop music during procedure.

8. Validate pt.'s negative feelings during procedure and allow pt. to occasionally attend to procedure if pt. desires, then gradually guide back to music interaction.

9. If pt. resists engaging in music and desires only to attend to procedure, support with sedative music and consider switching to MAR approach.

10. Provide sedative/comforting music incorporating pt.'s preferences once procedure is completed to calm and sooth pt.

Measurement Tools:

1. Frequency and duration of eye contact
2. Observable signs of agitation
3. Behavior state
4. Frequency of choice making
5. Pain level as measured on Wong-Baker FACES analog scale
6. Pt. verbalizations
7. Amount of pain or sedation medication required for procedure
8. Pt. level of compliance with procedure

Possible Adaptations: Use of either MAE or MAR during medical procedures should be based upon patient assessment in the moment. With experience, the music therapist will learn how to assess when MAE would be more effective than MAR for a particular patient and vice versa.

Population/Age Range: Infants–adolescents

Title: *Multisensory Stimulation*

Estimated Time for Implementation: 10–30 minutes

Goals: To facilitate developmentally appropriate auditory, visual, vestibular, and tactile stimulation, to improve active cognition, to provide opportunities for socialization, to decrease agitation, to maintain current levels of physical functioning

Objective(s):
1. Pt. will demonstrate auditory and/or visual tracking given auditory or visual stimuli.
2. Pt. will initiate physical movement.
3. Pt. will exhibit social behaviors (e.g., eye contact, smiles, reaching for instruments).
4. Pt. will exhibit decreased signs of agitation (e.g., non-purposeful limb movements, grimaces, crying).

Response Definition:
1. Therapist will record baseline pt. vital signs (heart rate, rate of respiration, pulse, pain level) and will observe/record changes during session.
2. Therapist will observe pt. behaviors at session onset and during multisensory stimulation (e.g., alertness, purposeful and non-purposeful physical movements, signs of agitation).
3. Therapist will note frequency of social behaviors.
4. Therapist will document pt.'s affective response to stimuli (with pt.'s evaluation of the experience if developmentally appropriate).

Materials: Accompaniment instrument (guitar or Q chord could allow for pt. participation), small percussion instruments of varying materials and textures (for auditory and tactile discrimination), hand drums

Procedural Steps:
1. Introduce self to pt.; assess developmental level, current mood state and level of reported pain or anxiety.
2. Assess music preferences through pt. or parent interview, if appropriate.
3. Determine pt.'s potential level of involvement (passive or active).
4. Provide opportunities for choice-making if developmentally appropriate (e.g., songs, instruments, staff/family involvement).
5. If pt.'s participation will be passive:
   a. Initiate musical stimulation such as therapist-accompanied singing while assessing pt. response to stimuli.
   b. If there are signs of agitation, decrease complexity of auditory stimuli (e.g., singing only or accompaniment only) until pt. returns to baseline behaviors.
   c. If pt. tolerates the auditory stimuli, add tactile stimuli when appropriate (e.g., soft touch (can be provided by family member), hand-over-hand assistance

with percussion instruments, or close placement of pt.'s own stuffed animals/toys).
   d. Draw pt.'s attention to visual stimuli by orienting pt. to his/her surroundings through verbal statements and improvised song lyrics.
6. If pt.'s participation will be active:
   a. Provide choices of musical engagement (e.g., singing, playing instruments, songwriting, moving to music).
   b. Initiate pt.'s preferred musical stimuli while assessing pt.'s response.
   c. Increase complexity of pt.'s involvement when appropriate to support maintenance of physical and cognitive functioning (e.g., if pt. is singing with the therapist, the therapist can then encourage pt. to choose an instrument to play or offer the an opportunity for improvisational or planned songwriting).
7. Observe and validate signs of fatigue or overstimulation while providing appropriate closure for pt. (e.g., MAR, offering of recorded music for pt. use post session).
8. Schedule future sessions with pt., family, and staff when appropriate.

Measurement Tools:
1. Changes in vital signs (heart rate, rate of respiration, pulse, pain level)
2. Frequency and duration of eye contact
3. Frequency and duration of purposeful physical movement
4. Pt. verbalizations
5. Frequency of pt. initiated choices
6. Observed pt. behaviors

Possible Adaptations: The therapist must adjust the choice of stimuli to meet the developmental needs of the patient. Infants will not be able to manipulate small percussion instruments but can receive tactile stimulation through swaddling and soft touch, and vestibular stimulation through rocking. For patients who are developmentally delayed, the music therapist should incorporate a balance of developmentally appropriate and chronological age appropriate songs and materials.

Population/Age Range: Preschool–adolescent

Title: *Songwriting (structured or improvised)*

Estimated Time for Implementation: 15–45 minutes

Goals: Facilitate verbal or nonverbal communication, improve self-esteem, decrease anxiety, improve choice-making and control, alleviate depression, improve coping with illness and hospitalization

Objective(s):
1. Pt. will demonstrate active participation in songwriting to extent capable.
2. Pt. will express self verbally or nonverbally depending upon ability.
3. Pt. will demonstrate improved self-esteem as exhibited by positive self-statements or positive comments about the songwriting process or product.
4. Pt. will demonstrate choice-making during songwriting interaction.
5. Pt. will demonstrate decrease in anxious behaviors.
6. Pt. will demonstrate improvement in frequency or quality of positive affect.
7. Pt. will demonstrate awareness of one positive strategy for coping with illness and hospitalization.

Response Definition:
1. Therapist will assess pt.'s level of active participation (e.g., frequency/duration of eye contact, level of verbal engagement, level of musical engagement).
2. Therapist will note frequency of pt.'s verbal or nonverbal communication attempts.
3. Therapist will note frequency of pt.'s positive self-statements or positive comments about the songwriting process or product.
4. Therapist will note frequency of pt.'s choice-making.
5. Therapist will observe changes in frequency of pt.'s anxious behaviors before and during intervention.
6. Therapist will observe pt.'s frequency and quality of positive affect before, during, and after songwriting.
7. Therapist will note pt.'s ability to verbalize positive skills for coping with illness and hospitalization.

Materials: Accompanying instrument that allows pt. participation (e.g., strumming on guitar, Q chord, portable keyboard); novel and attractive instruments such as rainstick, thunder tube, ocean drum, chimes, triangle, shaker eggs, and drums; optional: puppets or toy props for songs (must be immediately washable or owned by the pt.)

Procedural Steps:
1. Introduce self to pt.; assess developmental level, current mood state, and level of anxiety (if not already accomplished during a different intervention).

2. Based on assessment of pt.'s developmental level, attention span, and anxiety level, either directly offer choices for songwriting participation or begin by demonstrating instruments to facilitate engagement in:
    a. spontaneous song (improvised song, usually follows naturally from pt.'s active participation in music interaction, may or may not include lyrics).
    b. fill-in-the-blank (a.k.a. Cloze Technique) songwriting (pt. offers words or short phrases to complete lyrics provided by therapist, or lyrics of a familiar song).
    c. song parody (pt. rewrites lyrics of familiar, pre-existing song).
    d. blues songwriting (original lyrics created following the blues lyrical structure of AAB).
    e. musical poems (pt. and therapist create original music to original or pre-existing poetry).
    f. original song (pt. creates original lyrics and music).
3. Depending upon pt.'s developmental level and level of active participation, MT-BC may explain the specific songwriting technique, or may shape a pt.'s verbal and nonverbal responses to form the song without explaining the technique.
4. Offer pt. suggestions for broad subject areas if creating lyrics (e.g., song about something that has happened while in the hospital, song about a favorite place, song about favorite things to do, song about an imaginary place, song about a doll or toy on pt.'s bed).
5. Once a broad subject area is chosen, identify pt.'s choices for accompaniment style (e.g., accompanying instrument, fast/slow, quality such as happy/sad/angry/tired).
6. Identify pt.'s choices for musical participation (e.g., singing, speaking, playing rhythm instruments, assisting MT-BC with accompanying instrument).
7. Pt. may choose who will initiate the music.
8. For open-ended lyric writing techniques, the MT-BC may sing or speak prompts such as "I've been in this hospital for...," "If I could be anywhere right now I'd be...," etc.
9. Continue with one of the aforementioned songwriting techniques, prompting pt. for responses and choice-making whenever possible.
10. Support and validate pt. responses (e.g., while singing, therapist echoes back significant pt. verbalizations or themes).
11. Validate pt.'s negative feelings during songwriting then gradually guide pt. to identifying solutions to conflicts or negative feelings that arise during songwriting.
12. Cue pt. to bring closure to the song by deciding how he/she wants it to end.
13. If a parental consent for audio recording has been signed and pt. desires, pt. and/or therapist may create a recorded version of the completed song for the pt. to keep.
14. After finishing song and listening to a final version, assist pt. in making connections between themes in the song and conflicts/emotions experienced that are related to hospitalization or illness, when developmentally appropriate.
15. Discuss positive coping techniques that pt. could use, as developmentally appropriate.
16. Segue into a closing ritual to help pt. transition out of activity (e.g., singing the completed song once more for family or staff members if desired, singing a favorite familiar song, MAR, and/or good-bye song).
17. Schedule future sessions with pt., family, and staff when appropriate.

Measurement Tools:
1. Frequency and quality of physical participation
2. Frequency and quality of verbal and nonverbal communication efforts
3. Frequency of positive self-statements or positive comments about song or songwriting process
4. Frequency of choice-making
5. Observable signs of anxiety
6. Pt. affect
7. Pt. verbalizations

Possible Adaptations: Preteen and adolescent patients who will be hospitalized for longer than one week may engage in longer-term songwriting projects. An example might be the creation of a personal song to affirm identity or give hope and the creation of a CD recording of this song. Any songwriting technique chosen should flow naturally from the patient's engagement in music making. Songwriting techniques with higher levels of structure (e.g., fill-in-the-blank songwriting, blues songwriting) may be more effective with patients who are reluctant to participate verbally. The music therapist will vary the amount of prompting used to elicit patient responses, and the amount of structure provided depending upon the patient's level of verbal participation.

Population/Age Range: Preschool–preteen

Title: *Music-Facilitated Dramatic Play*

Estimated Time for Implementation: 20–45 minutes

Goals: Facilitate emotional expression, decrease anxiety (related to hospitalization, separation from caregivers, illness, etc.), increase verbal and nonverbal communication, identify fears related to hospitalization or illness, improve positive coping skills, improve choice-making and control

Objective(s):
1. Pt. will demonstrate active participation in music making or dramatic play to extent capable.
2. Pt. will demonstrate independent choice-making during the interaction.
3. Pt. will use instruments, voice, or puppets to express various types of affect.
4. Pt. will identify hospital or illness-related fears through play.
5. Pt. will demonstrate awareness of one positive coping skill for managing hospital-related anxiety during the musical play interaction.
6. Pt. will communicate verbally or nonverbally using puppets or instruments.
7. Pt. will demonstrate elevated mood after engaging in dramatic play as evidenced by smiles or positive comments.

Response Definition:
1. Therapist will assess pt.'s level of active participation (e.g., frequency/duration of eye contact, level of physical engagement, level of verbal engagement).
2. Therapist will note frequency of pt.'s choice-making during procedure.
3. Therapist will observe range of affect demonstrated by pt.'s use of instruments or puppets.
4. Therapist will note any hospital or illness-related fears that pt. mentions verbally or through dramatic play.
5. Therapist will observe pt.'s ability to provide positive solutions during conflicts that arise in pt.'s play.
6. Therapist will note pt.'s ability to verbalize positive coping skills for managing anxiety.
7. Therapist will note frequency of pt.'s verbal or nonverbal communication attempts.
8. Therapist will observe behaviors indicating elevated mood during or after dramatic play (e.g., positive affect, positive comments).

Materials: Novel and attractive rhythm instruments such as thunder tube, ocean drum, rainstick, drums; accompanying instrument that allows pt. participation (e.g., strumming on guitar or Q chord); optional: puppets/dolls or toy props (must be immediately washable or owned by the pt.).

Procedural Steps:

1. Introduce self to pt.; assess developmental level, current mood state, and level of anxiety (if not already accomplished during a different intervention).
2. Describe options for music-facilitated dramatic play and determine pt. participation preferences.
    a. Pt. uses instruments to musically "illustrate" a spontaneous story.
    b. Pt. uses puppets/dolls while MT-BC or family members play accompanying instruments.
    c. Pt. sings or speaks a spontaneous story song while MT-BC provides musical accompaniment.
3. Provide opportunities for choice-making (e.g., instruments, puppets, location of story, characters in story, style of musical accompaniment).
4. Initiate music or dramatic play incorporating pt.'s preferences.
5. Speak or sing brief questions to pt. to further the dramatic action.
6. Support and validate pt. responses (e.g., while singing, therapist echoes back significant pt. verbalizations or themes).
7. Validate pt.'s negative feelings during music-facilitated dramatic play then gradually guide pt. to identifying solutions to conflicts or negative feelings that arise during play.
8. Cue pt. to bring closure to the story and action of the dramatic play by deciding how she/he wants it to end.
9. Assist pt. in making connections between conflicts in the story and conflicts/emotions experienced while in the hospital, when developmentally appropriate.
10. Discuss positive coping techniques that pt. could use (or character in the story could have used), as developmentally appropriate.
11. Segue into a closing ritual to help pt. transition out of activity (e.g., singing familiar song, MAR, good-bye song).
12. Schedule future sessions with pt., family, and staff when appropriate.

Measurement Tools:

1. Frequency and quality of physical participation
2. Frequency of choice-making
3. Pt. affect
4. Pt. verbalizations
5. Frequency and quality of verbal and nonverbal communication efforts
6. Observable signs of anxiety

Possible Adaptations: Music-facilitated dramatic play is useful for patients who are reluctant to directly express their needs and fears verbally, patients with expressive communication limitations, and patients who displace their anger on family members or medical staff or direct fears and anger inward. The amount of verbal processing of themes that emerge in the dramatic play will vary depending upon the developmental level of the patient.

Population/Age Range: Preschool–adolescent

Title: *Music Permanent Product (video/audio recording, CD creation)*

Estimated Time for Implementation: 30–60+ minutes, multiple sessions

Goals: To encourage creative expression, improve self-esteem, facilitate choice-making and control, alleviate depression, improve coping with illness and hospitalization, provide a lasting gift

Objective(s):
1. Pt. will actively participate in creation of a permanent product to extent capable.
2. Pt. will express self verbally or nonverbally depending upon ability.
3. Pt. will demonstrate improved self-esteem as exhibited by positive self-statements or positive comments about the permanent product or process.
4. Pt. will demonstrate choice-making and take control of outcome of permanent product depending upon ability.
5. Pt. will demonstrate improvement in frequency or quality of positive affect.
6. Pt. will demonstrate awareness of one positive strategy for coping with illness and hospitalization.
7. Pt. will create a permanent product for family to keep.

Response Definition:
1. Therapist will assess pt.'s level of active participation (e.g., frequency/duration of eye contact, level of verbal engagement, level of musical engagement).
2. Therapist will note frequency of pt.'s verbal or nonverbal communication attempts.
3. Therapist will note frequency of pt.'s positive self-statements or positive comments about the permanent product or process.
4. Therapist will note frequency of pt.'s choice-making.
5. Therapist will observe pt.'s frequency and quality of positive affect before, during, and after creating permanent product.
6. Therapist will note pt.'s ability to verbalize positive skills for coping with illness and hospitalization.

Materials: Video camera, tripod, blank videotape, accompanying instruments or music recordings of pt.'s choice (e.g., guitar, Q chord, portable keyboard, boombox, karaoke machine), novel and attractive instruments chosen by pt., props for video (e.g., hospital equipment such as syringes, emesis basins, posters or props made by pt., items in pt.'s room such as greeting cards, signs from friends, photographs of family and pets, artwork), staff or family members as actors, labels, laptop computer, consent forms as per requirements of facility

Procedural Steps:

(Typically this is a multiple-session project for a longer-term inpatient. For this example, it is understood that previous sessions aimed at establishing rapport through active music making or music-facilitated play have already occurred.)

1. Greet pt.; assess current mood state and level of pain or anxiety (if not already accomplished during a different intervention).
2. Based on assessment of pt.'s mood state, pain and anxiety level, offer choices for creation of plan for permanent product such as:
   a. music video (with pt. composed music or pre-recorded music).
   b. video recording of pt. musical concert.
   c. CD recording of pt. composed song, improvisation, or singing with pre-recorded music.
   d. CD creation of pre-recorded music (with label and cover artwork by pt.).
3. Offer further choice making regarding permanent product such as:
   a. selection of music (recordings, live music, songwriting).
   b. who will accompany/sing.
   c. where will video/recording/creation be made.
   d. who will be involved.
   e. what kinds of instruments or props are needed.
   f. when this can be created.
   g. what could be accomplished in this session.
   h. record actual creation (dependent upon developmental level and necessary resources).
4. Support and validate pt. responses, keeping realistic goals for creation.
5. Depending upon pt.'s selection, begin writing lyrics or song, gathering items or making props, making lists, selecting actual music or instruments, transition into plan for next session.
6. Segue into a closing ritual to help pt. transition out of activity.
7. Next session: greet pt.; assess current mood state and level of pain or anxiety, continue with choice making whenever possible:
   a. write lyrics/song or add to previous created material.
   b. practice singing or playing with selected recording or karaoke, or other accompanying instruments.
   c. continue to gather/make props.
   d. practice "run through" of the permanent product when possible.
   e. plan when to record the process (when staff or family are available if needed).
   f. record actual creation (dependent upon developmental level and necessary resources).
   g. repeat previous steps for as many sessions as needed (dependent upon developmental, pain and anxiety levels, mood states and necessary resources).
8. Videotape or record the creation for a permanent product/lasting gift.
9. After finishing creation, assist pt. in making connections between themes in the pt.'s creation and conflicts/emotions experienced that are related to hospitalization or illness, when developmentally appropriate.

10. Discuss positive coping techniques that pt. used in the process of making the video/recording/creation, and how to use these with other problem areas in the hospital, as developmentally appropriate.
11. Schedule a time when staff may view finished product, live version, or concert of the creation as per pt.'s request.
12. Present and copy finished product for family as needed.
13. Schedule future sessions with pt., family, and staff when appropriate.

Measurement Tools:
1. Frequency and quality of physical participation
2. Frequency and quality of verbal and nonverbal communication efforts
3. Frequency of positive self-statements or positive comments during or about process of creating permanent product
4. Frequency of choice-making
5. Pt. affect
6. Pt. verbalizations

Possible Adaptations: Patients who have extended hospitalizations (e.g., SCT patients) may be able to produce permanent products over multiple sessions. Even younger patients may be able to create a product in a single session depending on their level of development.

Patients of all ages may put on a concert, with an instrument they are just learning or one they played pre-admission. Patients can dress for the occasion, create a stage and posters announcing the concert, as well as design programs to hand out to staff and other patients and families. Videotaping the concert enables patients to have a lasting record of their achievement that can be shared with friends and relatives who are unable to visit them during hospitalization.

Children may also create videotapes of favorite familiar songs or songs they have written. They may dance, tell jokes, display artwork, or interview staff and family on video or voice recording. Other older patients may use a music video format in which they change the original lyrics and sing or act out a video of their choice.

More intimate situations can also be recorded (e.g., family members holding or lying down next to their child and quietly singing or talking with them). Voice recorders may be less intimidating to patients and family members, and family interactions and interviews may be recorded in this way.

Patients may also want to create a recording for themselves or for a family member for a special occasion (e.g., Father's Day, birthday). Instead of creating video recordings, a patient may decide to create a CD recording and select pre-recorded music tailored to the preferences of the family member. The patient can then design a label and cover (on computer or by hand) for the CD.

Sessions with children who are actively making music may be recorded on video. Depending on the needs and desires of the family, the MT-BC may edit these later and create a montage for a poignant keepsake. Lyrics, songs, and artwork created by patients serve as permanent products and lasting gifts, which later may trigger positive memories of the hospitalization experience.

APPENDICES

Appendix A

MUSIC THERAPY AND MEDICINE

*"I certainly think that every institution should have its music therapy
and its music therapists."*

— Oliver Sacks, MD, Neurologist

What Is Music Therapy?

Music therapy is the clinical and evidence-based use of music interventions to accomplish individualized goals within a therapeutic relationship by a credentialed professional who has completed an approved music therapy program. It is an established health service similar to occupational therapy and physical therapy and consists of using music therapeutically to address physical, psychological, cognitive and/or social functioning for patients of all ages. Because music therapy is a powerful and non-invasive medium, unique outcomes are possible. In addition to its applications with hospital patients, music therapy is used successfully with persons of all ages and disabilities.

How Does Music Therapy Make a Difference for Medical Patients?

Music therapy has been shown to be an efficacious and valid treatment option for medical patients with a variety of diagnoses. Music therapy can be used to address patient needs related to respiration, chronic pain, physical rehabilitation, diabetes, headaches, cardiac conditions, surgery, and obstetrics, among others. Research results and clinical experiences attest to the viability of music therapy even in those patients resistant to other treatment approaches. Music is a form of sensory stimulation, which provokes responses due to the familiarity, predictability, and feelings of security associated with it.

What Do Music Therapists Do?

Music therapists use music activities, both instrumental and vocal, designed to facilitate changes that are non-musical in nature. Music therapy programs are based on

261

individual assessment, treatment planning, and ongoing program evaluation. Frequently functioning as members of an interdisciplinary team, music therapists implement programs with groups or individuals addressing a vast continuum of outcomes, including reduction of pain and anxiety, stress management, communication, and emotional expression.

What Can One Expect From a Music Therapist?

Music therapy utilized in a medical setting complies with the expectations and requirements inherent in the medical model of treatment. Professionally trained music therapists design and utilize individualized music experiences to assess, treat, and evaluate patients. Music therapy patient objectives are specific and relevant to medical diagnosis, course of treatment, and discharge timeline. Benefits are described in medical, and not musical, terms.

Through a planned and systematic use of music and music activities, the music therapist provides opportunities for:
- Anxiety and stress reduction
- Nonpharmacological management of pain and discomfort
- Positive changes in mood and emotional states
- Active and positive patient participation in treatment
- Decreased length of stay

In addition, music therapy may allow for:
- Emotional intimacy with families and caregivers
- Relaxation for the entire family
- Meaningful time spent together in a positive, creative way

Who Is Qualified as a Music Therapist?

Graduates of colleges or universities from more than 70 approved music therapy programs are eligible to take a national examination administered by the Certification Board for Music Therapists (CBMT), an independent, non-profit certifying agency fully accredited by the National Commission for Certifying Agencies. After successful completion of the CBMT examination, graduates are issued the credential necessary for professional practice, Music Therapist-Board Certified (MT-BC). In addition to the MT-BC credential, other recognized professional designations are Registered Music Therapists (RMT), Certified Music Therapists (CMT), and Advanced Certified Music Therapist (ACMT) listed with the National Music Therapy Registry. Any individual who does not have proper training and credentials is not qualified to provide music therapy services.

Where Do Music Therapists Work?

Music therapists offer services in medical hospitals, skilled and intermediate care facilities, rehabilitation hospitals, adult day care centers, senior centers, hospices, psychiatric treatment centers, drug and alcohol programs, schools and other facilities. In the medical setting, music therapists work with a variety of patient needs, and may work in many different hospital units, including ICU, NICU, Pre- and Post-Op, surgery, chronic pain management, cardiac care, obstetrics, emergency, pediatrics, physical rehabilitation, and outpatient programs. Some therapists are self-employed and work on the basis of independent contracts, while others are salaried hospital employees.

How Does Music Therapy Help Patients and Health Care Staff?

Dr. Walter Quan, Jr., Oncologist-Hematologist of St. Luke's Medical Center in Cleveland, Ohio, attests that:

> *"Music therapy has a wide range of applications. We see some patients whose blood pressure does come down and seems to stay down through regular use of music therapy. Another important aspect is the use in the labor and delivery room. We know that patients, who go through Lamaze training for instance, can also use music therapy to help them relax and to have pain relief in terms of labor pains."*

Music therapy is quantifiable and qualitative. Dr. Quan continues:

> *"…[I]n general as a physician you only use those things that you can measure or that have a number related to [them]… but there are a number of disciplines, and music therapy is one of them, where there is a qualitative effect which can give a lot of benefit for patients."*

Music therapists complete assessments for each patient and collect extensive data in order to write a complex patient history and develop a client-centered treatment plan. The music therapist is then able to evaluate the patient during the course of treatment. All of this contributes to the quantifiability of music therapy treatment.

Music therapy interventions are favored for the ability to meet quality of life needs. As quality of life issues and patient choice are pushed to the forefront of the national healthcare agenda, music therapy is being increasingly recognized for its unique contribution to patient quality of life.

Music therapy can help to relieve pain and reduce stress and anxiety for the patient, resulting in physiological changes, including:

- Improved respiration
- Lower blood pressure
- Improved cardiac output
- Reduced heart rate
- Relaxed muscle tension

Music therapy has been shown to have a significant effect on a patient's perceived effectiveness of treatment, self reports of pain reduction, relaxation, respiration rate, behaviorally observed and self-reported anxiety levels, and patient choice of anesthesia and amount of analgesic medication.

Why Music Therapy?

William Frohlich, President, Beth Abraham Health Services in New York, talks about music therapy as part of the total treatment modality:

"I think that the therapist plays an integral team role when you are talking about a team of physicians, a team of nurses, therapists, physical or occupational therapists and so on... included in that team needs to be a music therapist. The observations where a patient may be singing where they could not speak before or they may be walking or dancing where they could not move before – that is important for the music therapist to bring to the occupational therapist or physical therapist to become part of the total treatment modality."

Dr. Walter Quan, Jr., Hematologist-Oncologist, St. Luke's Medical Center in Cleveland, Ohio, on music therapy in the treatment of cancer:

"The mind/body relationship is particularly important in terms of looking at the immune system to treat cancer. We believe that patients who are under less stress, who are in a brighter mood, appear to do better in terms of their anti-cancer therapy. I think that music therapy and imaging and immune therapy of cancer all tie together... I think it can be helpful in conjunction with biologic therapy for cancer. A study done just relatively recently on cancer patients showed that approximately three quarters of cancer patients that had their usual pain medicines but also had the additional music therapy experienced less pain then previously... Music therapy in helping patients relax could possibly be beneficial in raising the innate immune system which could have therapeutic implications for cancer."

Susan Shurin, M.D., Chief of Pediatric-Hematology, Oncology at the Ireland Cancer Center in Cleveland, Ohio, comments on the effectiveness of music therapy in treatment of neurological impairments:

"Music therapy enables people to sometimes put words together in ways that are hard for them to do otherwise. ...[I]t often seems to be easier if [the patient] has the rhythm and cadence that comes along with music. Particularly with people with certain kinds of neurological deficits I think that [music therapy] can be very helpful. The music seems to get through to the

patient and in many ways it enables [the patient] to get through to us which [may be] very hard to do with any other modality."

Joseph Arezzo, PhD, Vice Chair, Department of Neuroscience, Albert Einstein College of Medicine, New York, talks about music therapy's role in restorative neurology:

"[T]he degree to which function can be recovered is phenomenal and we are just tapping into the extent that we can get recovery following stroke or injury or disease. We hope that music might play a particularly important role in helping [the regeneration of] those cells, in helping the individual learn to interpret the pattern and essentially to help that person learn again."

What Is AMTA?

The American Music Therapy Association (AMTA) represents over 5,000 music therapists, corporate members, and related associations worldwide. AMTA's roots date back to organizations founded in 1950 and 1971. Those two organizations merged in 1998 to ensure the progressive development of the therapeutic use of music in rehabilitation, special education, and medical and community settings. AMTA is committed to the advancement of education, training, professional standards, and research in support of the music therapy profession. The mission of the organization is to advance public knowledge of music therapy benefits and increase access to quality music therapy services. Currently, AMTA establishes criteria for the education and clinical training of music therapists. Members of AMTA adhere to a Code of Ethics and Standards of Practice in their delivery of music therapy services.

Related Resources Available from AMTA:

- *Medical Music Therapy,* edited by Jayne M. Standley
  2005. ISBN #1-884914-14-4

- *Music Therapy in Pediatric Healthcare*, edited by Sheri L. Robb
  2003. ISBN #1-884914-10-1

- *Clinical Guide to Music Therapy in Adult Physical Rehabilitation Settings*,
  written by Elizabeth H. Wong
  2004. ISBN #1-884914-11-X

- *Music Therapy with Premature Infants*, written by Jayne M. Standley
  2003. ISBN #1-884914-09-8

- *Music Therapy & Medicine*, edited by Cheryl Dileo
  1999. ISBN #1-884914-00-4

How Can You Find a Music Therapist or Get More Information?

American Music Therapy Association
8455 Colesville Road, Suite 1000
Silver Spring, MD 20910
Phone (301) 589-3300
Fax (301) 589-5175
Web: www.musictherapy.org
Email: info@musictherapy.org

Appendix B

MUSIC THERAPY IN THE TREATMENT AND MANAGEMENT OF PAIN

What is Music Therapy?

Music therapy is the clinical and evidence-based use of music interventions to accomplish individualized goals within a therapeutic relationship by a credentialed professional who has completed an approved music therapy program. Music therapy is an established health profession that uses music and the therapeutic relationship to address physical, psychological, cognitive and/or social functioning for patients of all ages and disabilities. Because music therapy is a powerful and non-invasive medium, unique outcomes are possible when interventions are directed to reduce pain, anxiety, and depression. These outcomes appear to be mediated through the individual's emotional, cognitive and interpersonal responsiveness to the music and/or the supportive music therapy relationship.

Annotated Bibliography of Research: 1992–2003

- **Reviews of Music Therapy in medical settings.**

  Standley, J. M. (2000). Music research in medical treatment. In D. Smith (Ed.), *Effectiveness of music therapy procedures: Documentation of research and clinical practice.* Silver Spring, MD: American Music Therapy Association.

  Standley, J. M. (1992). Meta analysis of research in music and medical treatment. Effect size as a basis for comparisons across multiple dependent and independent variables. In R. Spintge & R. Droh (Eds), *MusicMedicine*, St Louis, MO: MMB.

- **Music Therapy reduces pain.**

  Colwell, C. (1997). Music as distraction and relaxation to reduce chronic pain and narcotic ingestion: A case study. *Music Therapy Perspectives, 15*, 24–31.

  Edwards, J. (1998). Music therapy for children with severe burn injury. *Music Therapy Perspectives, 16*, 21–26.

  Fratianne, R. B, Presner, J. D., Houston, M. J., Super, D. M., Yowler, C. J.& Standley, J. M. (2001). The effect of music-based imagery and musical alternate engagement on the burn debridement process. *Journal of Burn Care & Rehabilitation, 22*(1), 47–53.

  Good, M., Anderson, G. C., Stanton-Hicks, M., Grass, J. A. & Makil, M. (2002). Relaxation and music reduce pain after gynecologic surgery. *Pain Management Nursing, 3*(2), 61–70.

Loewy, J. (1997). Music therapy pediatric pain management: Assessing and attending to the sounds of hurt, fear and anxiety. In J. Loewy (Ed.), *Music therapy and pediatric pain* (pp. 45–56). Jeffrey Books.

- **Music Therapy reduces physiological indicators of anxiety and reduces need for sedation and analgesia, increases completion rate, and shortens examination time during colonoscopy.**

  Smolon, D., Topp, R., & Singer, L. (2002). The effect of self-selected music during colonoscopy on anxiety, heart, rate, and blood pressure. *Applied Nursing Research, 15*(3), 126–136.

  Schiemann, U., Gross, M., Reuter, R., & Kellner, H. (2002). Improved procedure of colonoscopy under accompanying music therapy. *European Journal of Medical Research, 7*(3), 131–134.

- **Music Therapy reduces physiological indicators of pre-operative stress.**

  Miluk-Kolasa, B., Matejek, M., & Stupnicki R. (1996). The effects of music listening on changes in selected physiological parameters in adult pre-surgical patients. *Journal of Music Therapy, 33*, 208–218.

  Robb, S. L., Nichols, R. J., Rutan, R. L., & Bishop B. L. (1995). The effects of music assisted relaxation on preoperative anxiety. *Journal of Music Therapy, 32*, 2–21.

- **Music Therapy reduces cortisol in healthy adults.**

  McKinney, C. H., Antoni, M. H., Kumar, M., Tims, F. C., & McCabe, P. M. (1997). Effects of Guided Imagery and Music (GIM) therapy on mood and cortisol in healthy adults. *Health Psychology, 16*(4), 390–400.

- **Music Therapy reduces physiological and psychological indicators of distress in post–operative cardiac patients.**

  Cadigan, M. E., Caruso, N. A., Halderman, S. M., McNamara, M. E., Noyes, D. A., Spadafora, M. A., & Carrol, D. L. (2001). The effect of music on cardiac patients on bed rest. *Progress in Cardiovascular Nursing, 16*(1), 5–13.

- **Engaging in group music therapy and listening to music reduces anxiety associated with chemotherapy and radiotherapy.**

  Cai, G., Qiao, Y., Li, P., & Lu, L. (2001). Music therapy in treatment of cancer patients. *Chinese Mental Health Journal, 15*(3), 179–181.

  Harper, E. I. (2001). *Reducing treatment-related anxiety in cancer patients: Comparison of psychological interventions.* Doctoral dissertation, Southern Methodist University.

  Sabo, C. E., & Michael, S. R. (1996). The influence of personal message with music on anxiety and side effects associated with chemotherapy. *Cancer Nursing, 19*(4), 283–289.

- **Listening to music reduces nausea and emesis for patients receiving chemotherapy.**

  Standley, J. M. (1992). Clinical applications of music and chemotherapy: The effects on nausea and emesis. *Music Therapy Perspectives, 10*, 27–35.

- **Participating in Music Therapy sessions increases comfort and motivates bone marrow transplant patients during treatment.**

    Boldt, S. (1996). The effects of music therapy on motivation, psychological well-being, physical comfort, and exercise endurance of bone marrow transplant patients. *Journal of Music Therapy, 33*, 164–188.

- **Listening to music alleviates pain, fatigue, and anxiety of hospice cancer patients.**

    Longfield, V. (1995). *The effects of music therapy on pain and mood in hospice patients.* Unpublished master's thesis: Saint Louis University.

- **Music Therapy serves to decrease behavioral distress among pediatric oncology patients during needle sticks.**

    Malone, A. B. (1996). The effects of live music on the distress of pediatric patients receiving intravenous starts, venipunctures, injections, and heel sticks. *Journal of Music Therapy, 33*(1), 19–33.

- **Music provides an environment for engaging behaviors and decreasing distress behaviors for isolated pediatric oncology patients.**

    Robb, S. L. (2000). The effect of therapeutic music interventions on the behavior of hospitalized children in isolation: developing a contextual support model of music therapy. *Journal of Music Therapy, 37*(2), 118–146.

How Does Music Therapy Make a Difference?

Music therapy has been shown to be an efficacious and valid treatment option for patients experiencing pain related to a variety of diagnoses. Music therapy interventions can focus on pain management for physical rehabilitation, cardiac conditions, medical and surgical procedures, obstetrics, oncology treatment, and burn debridement, among others. Music is a form of sensory stimulation, which provokes responses due to the familiarity, predictability, and feelings of security associated with it. Research results and clinical experiences attest to the viability of music therapy even in those patients resistant to other treatment approaches.

What Do Music Therapists Do?

Music therapy utilized in the treatment and management of pain complies with the expectations and requirements inherent in the medical model of treatment. Music therapy programs are based on individual assessment and collection of extensive data for the development of complex patient histories and client-centered treatment plans. Patient objectives are specific and relevant to medical diagnosis, course of treatment, and discharge timeline.

Once goals and objectives are established, music therapists use music activities, both instrumental and vocal, designed to facilitate changes that are non-musical in nature. Through a planned and systematic use of music and music strategies, the music therapist provides opportunities for:

- Anxiety and stress reduction
- Nonpharmacological management of pain and discomfort
- Positive changes in mood and emotional states
- Active and positive patient participation in treatment
- Decreased length of stay

Functioning as members of an interdisciplinary team, music therapists also evaluate the patients during the course of treatment, implement changes that are indicated by the patient's response, and document benefits in medical, not musical, terms.

How Does Music Therapy Help Patients?

Music therapy can help to relieve pain and reduce stress and anxiety for the patient, resulting in physiological changes, including:

- Improved respiration
- Lower blood pressure
- Improved cardiac output
- Reduced heart rate
- Relaxed muscle tension

Music therapy has been shown to have a significant effect on a patient's perceived effectiveness of treatment, self-reports of pain reduction, relaxation, respiration rate, behaviorally observed and self-reported anxiety levels, and patient choice of anesthesia and amount of analgesic medication.

Music Therapy Protocol for Pain Management

"[This protocol]... is based on a cognitive behavioral model of therapy, which posits that new thoughts, feelings and body states may be conditioned to replace dysfunctional patterns. Specifically, a relaxed body and pleasant visual images may replace tension and worry when they are conditioned as a response to familiar, calming music. The conditioning process takes place when listening to this music is paired with deep relaxation through repeated practice. Over time, the music alone cues the response...

The music therapy protocol is designed to perform several functions:

1. To direct attention away from pain or anxiety, distracting the listener with comforting music.
2. To provide a musical stimulus for rhythmic breathing.
3. To offer a rhythmic structure for systematic release of body tension.
4. To cue positive visual imagery.
5. To condition a deep relaxation response.
6. To change mood.
7. To focus on positive thoughts and feelings and to celebrate life."

—Professor Suzanne Hanser, EdD, MT-BC, Berklee College of Music

Who is Qualified as a Music Therapist?

Graduates of colleges or universities from more than 70 approved music therapy programs are eligible to take a national examination administered by the Certification Board for Music Therapists (CBMT), an independent, non-profit certifying agency fully accredited by the National Commission for Certifying Agencies. After successful completion of the CBMT examination, graduates are issued the credential necessary for professional practice, Music Therapist-Board Certified (MT-BC). In addition to the MT-BC credential, other recognized professional designations are Registered Music Therapists (RMT), Certified Music Therapists (CMT), and Advanced Certified Music Therapist (ACMT) listed with the National Music Therapy Registry. Any individual who does not have proper training and credentials is not qualified to provide music therapy services.

Where Do Music Therapists Work?

Music therapists offer services in medical hospitals, skilled and intermediate care facilities, rehabilitation hospitals, adult day care centers, senior centers, hospices, psychiatric treatment centers, drug and alcohol programs, schools and other facilities. In pain management applications, music therapists can work in many different hospital units, including ICU, NICU, Pre- and Post-Op, surgery, cardiac care, obstetrics, emergency, pediatrics, physical rehabilitation, and outpatient programs. Some therapists are self-employed and work on the basis of independent contracts, while others are salaried hospital employees.

How Can You Find a Music Therapist or Get More Information?

American Music Therapy Association
8455 Colesville Road, Suite 1000
Silver Spring, MD 20910
Phone: (301) 589-3300
Fax: (301) 589-5175
Web: www.musictherapy.org
Email: info@musictherapy.org